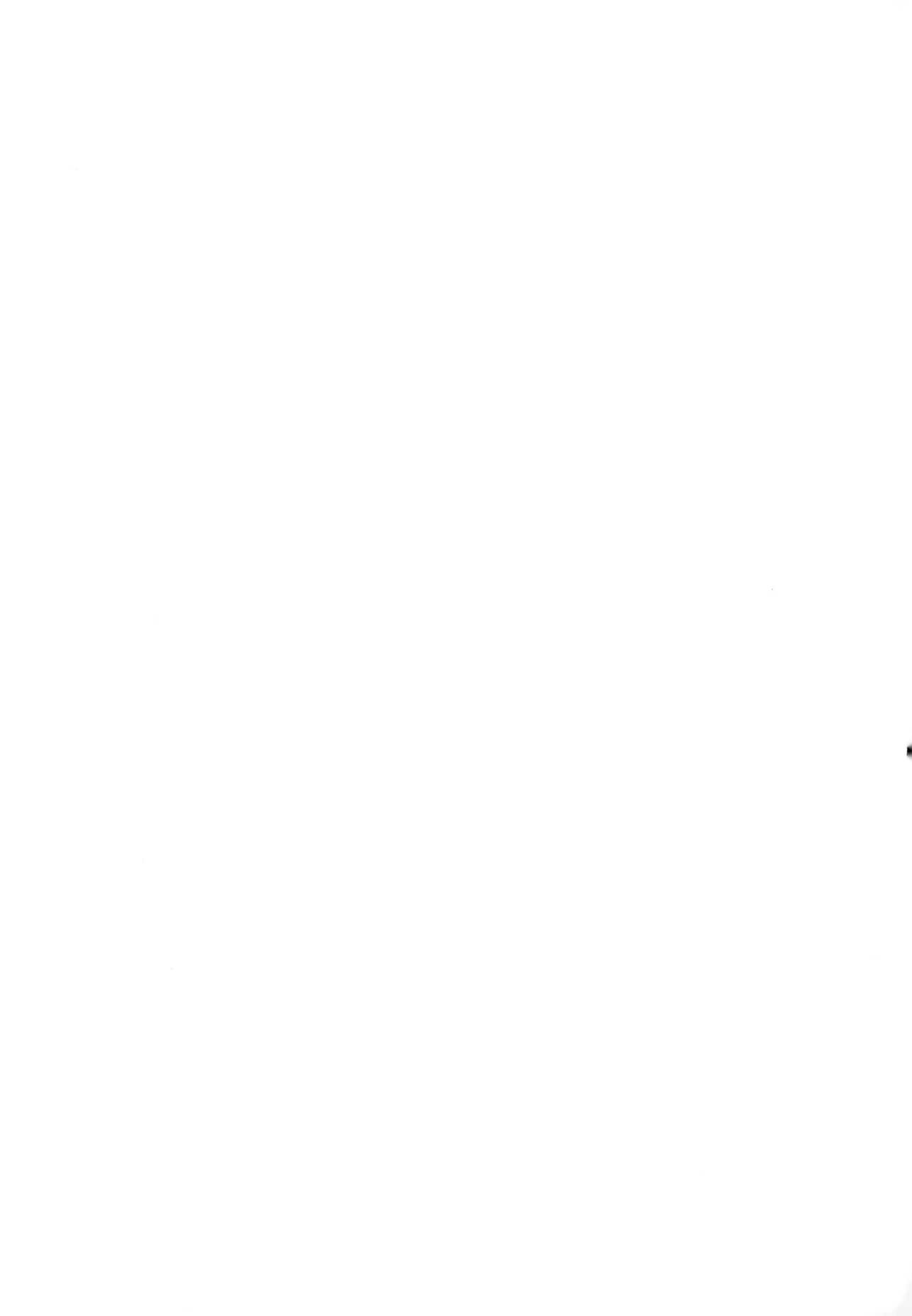

MOSES MAIMONIDES'
GLOSSARY OF DRUG NAMES

Memoirs of the
AMERICAN PHILOSOPHICAL SOCIETY
Held at Philadelphia
For Promoting Useful Knowledge
Volume 135

ISSN 0065-9738

Moses Maimonides'

GLOSSARY OF DRUG NAMES

Translated from Max Meyerhof's French Edition

Edited by

FRED ROSNER
Long Island Jewish-Hillside Medical Center

THE AMERICAN PHILOSOPHICAL SOCIETY
INDEPENDENCE SQUARE
PHILADELPHIA
1979

Published through the Imprint Series,
Monograph Publishing on Demand.
Produced and distributed by
University Microfilms International
Ann Arbor, Michigan 48106

Library of Congress Cataloging in Publication Data

Moses ben Maimon, 1135-1204.
    Moses Maimonides' Glossary of drug names.

    (Memoirs of the American Philosophical Society ;
v. 135) (Monograph publishing : Imprint series)
    Translation of Sharh asmā' al-'uqqār; translated from
the French according to the Unique Arabic Ms. #3711 of
the Aya Sofia Library, Istanbul, Turkey.
    Bibliography: p.
    1. Materia medica—Early works to 1800. 2. Materia
medica—Dictionaries—Early works to 1800. 3. Medicine,
Arabic—Dictionaries—Early works to 1800. 4. Materia
medica—Dictionaries—Arabic. 5. Materia medica—
Dictionaries—English. I. Rosner, Fred. II. Title. III. Title:
Glossary of drug names. IV. Series: American
Philosophical Society, Philadelphia. Memoirs ; v. 135.

Q11.P612 vol. 135 [RS178] 081s [615'.1'03] 79-13875
ISBN 0-87169-135-3

SARH ASMA' AL-'UQQAR

(The Explanation of the Names of Drugs)

A GLOSSARY OF MATERIA MEDICA

COMPOSED BY MOSES MAIMONIDES

Translated into English from Max Meyerhof's French Edition

according to the Unique Arabic Manuscript #3711 of the

Aya Sofia Library, Istanbul, Turkey

by

Fred Rosner, M. D.

Table of Contents

A. Preface

PREFACE

The ten authentic medical treatises of Moses Maimonides lay dormant
in manuscript form for many centuries. Over the past quarter century, Hebrew
editions of these works were published under the editorship of the late
Suessman Muntner of Jerusalem.

The past few years has seen the publication of several of these works
in English including Maimonides' treatises on Asthma (1963), Regimen of Health
(1964), Poisons (1966), Hemorrhoids (1969), Responsa (1969), Aphorisms (1970-71),
and Sexual Intercourse (1974). The present work represents one of the remain-
ing three Maimonidean treatises not yet available to the English reader. It
is an important work as described in the introductory section.

I am indebted to Mrs. Sophie Falk and Mrs. Miriam Regenworm for secre-
tarial support. I also wish to acknowledge the assistance of Mr. George W.
Corner, Editor of the American Philosophical Society, in the publication of
this book.

New York City, March 1979   Fred Rosner, M.D.

1. THE MEDICAL WRITINGS OF MOSES MAIMONIDES

Moses, son of Maimon, (Rambam in Hebrew, Abu Imran Musa Ibn Maimun in Arabic) was born in Cordova, Spain on March 30, 1135 corresponding to Passover eve of the Hebrew year 4895. His mother died in childbirth and consequently his father Dayan (judge) Maimon raised him. Persecution by the Almohades, a fanatical group from North Africa, forced the Maimon family to flee Cordova in the year 1148. Maimonides was 13 years old. The family wandered through southern Spain and northern Africa for the next ten years and finally settled in Fez, Morocco in 1158.

Little is known of Maimonides' early life and medical education. There are no sources indicating that Maimonides had any formal medical education. In his Medical Aphorisms (see below), he mentions "the elders before whom I have read"; this is the only allusion to some semi-private study of medicine. A few times he mentions the son of Ibn Zuhr from whom he heard teachings of the latter's illustrious father (the great physician Abu Marwān Ibn Zuhr) whom Maimonides held in great esteem.

Maimonides must have been an avid reader since his medical writings show a profound knowledge of ancient Greek authors in Arabic translations, and Moslem medical works. Hippocrates, Galen and Aristotle were his Greek medical inspirations and Rhazes of Persia, Al Farabi, and Ibn Zuhr, the Spanish-Arabic physician, are Moslem authors frequently quoted by Maimonides.

The Maimon family left Morocco in 1165, traveled to Palestine, landing in Acco, and from there to Egypt where they settled in Fostat (old Cairo). Maimonides turned to medicine as a livelihood only after the death of his father in 1166 and the death of his brother in a shipwreck shortly thereafter. Maimonides was left with his brother's wife and children to support and, after a year's illness following his father's death, entered into the practice of medicine. In 1174, at age 39, he was appointed Court Physician to Visier Alfadhal, Regent of Egypt during the absence of the Sultan, Saladin the Great, who was fighting in the Crusades in Palestine. It was at this time that Richard the Lion-Hearted, also fighting in the Crusades, is reported to have invited Maimonides to become his personal physician, an offer which Maimonides declined. His reputation as a physician grew in Egypt and neighboring countries and his fame as theologian and philosopher became worldwide.

In 1193, Saladin died and his eldest son, Al Afdal Nur ad Din Ali, a playboy, succeeded him. As a result, Maimonides' medical duties became even heavier as described in the famous letter he wrote to his friend, disciple and translator, French Rabbi Samuel Ibn Tibbon, in the year 1199:

> "....I live in Fostat and the Sultan resides in Cairo;
> these two places are two Sabbath limits (marked off areas
> around a town within which it is permitted to move on the
> Sabbath; approximately one and one-half miles) distant
> from each other. My duties to the Sultan are very heavy.
> I am obliged to visit him every day, early in the morning,
> and when he or any of his children or concubines are
> indisposed, I cannot leave Cairo but must stay during most
> of the day in the palace. It also frequently happens

that one or two of the officers fall sick and I must attend
to their healing. Hence, as a rule, every day, early in
the morning, I go to Cairo and, even if nothing ususual happens
there, I do not return to Fostat until the afternoon. Then I
am famished but I find the antechambers filled with people,
both Jews and Gentiles, nobles and common people, Judges and
policemen, friends and enemies, -- a mixed multitude who await
the time of my return.

I dismount from my animal, wash my hands, go forth to my
patients, and entreat them to bear with me while I partake
of some light refreshment, the only meal I eat in twenty-
four hours. Then I go to attend to my patients and write
prescriptions and directions for their ailments. Patients
go in and out until nightfall, and sometimes, even as the
Torah is my faith, until two hours and more into the night.
I converse with them and prescribe for them even while lying
down from sheer fatigue. When night falls, I am so exhausted,
that I can hardly speak.

In consequence of this, no Israelite can converse with me
or befriend me (on religious or community matters) except
on the Sabbath. On that day, the whole congregation, or at
least, the majority,comes to me after the morning service,
when I instruct them as to their proceedings during the
whole week. We study together a little until noon, when
they depart. Some of them return and read with me after
the afternoon service until evening prayer. In this manner,

I spend the days. I have here related to you only a part

of what you would see if you were to visit me ..."

Maimonides was also the spiritual leader of the Jewish community of

Egypt. At age 33, in the year 1168, shortly after settling in Fostat

(old Cairo), he completed his first major work, the Commentary on the

Mishnah. In 1178, ten years later, his magnum opus, the Mishneh Torah

was finished. This monumental work is a 14-book compilation of all

Biblical and Talmudic law and remains a classic to this day. In 1190,

Maimonides' great philosophical masterpiece, the Guide for the Perplexed,

was completed.

Maimonides died on December 13, 1204 (Tebeth 20, 4965 in the Hebrew

calendar), and was buried in Tiberias. Legend relates that Maimonides'

body was placed upon a donkey and the animal set loose. The donkey

wandered and wandered and finally stopped in Tiberias. That is the site

where the great Maimonides (Rambam) was buried.

Maimonides was a prolific writer. We have already mentioned his

famous trilogy, the Commentary on the Mishnah, the Mishneh Torah and the

Guide for the Perplexed. Each of these works alone would have indelibly

recorded Maimonides' name for posterity. However, in addition to these,

he also wrote a Book on Logic (Ma'amar Hahigayon), a Book of Commandments

(Sefer Hamitzvoth), an Epistle to Yemen (Iggereth Hashmad), a Treatise on

Resurrection (Ma'amar Techiyath Hamethim), commentaries on several tractates

of the Talmud, and over 600 Responsa. Several additional works including

the so-called Prayer of Maimonides (1) are attributed to him but are, in

fact, spurious, the prayer having been written in 1783 (1-2).

Over and above all the books we have just enumerated, Maimonides
also wrote ten medical works (3). The following is a brief examination
and analysis of these medical writings. The first is called Extracts
from Galen. Galen's medical writings consist of over 100 books and required two volumes just to catalogue and index them all. Maimonides,
therefore, extracted what he considered the most important of Galen's
pronouncements and compiled them verbatim in a small work which was in-
tended primarily for the use of students of Greek medicine. This work,
as all of Maimonides' medical books, was originally written in Arabic.
No complete Arabic manuscript exists today but several Hebrew manuscript translations are available. This work has never been published
in any language,but brief excerpts therefrom in both English and
Hebrew appeared recently in a Hebrew periodical (4). A work on the
Extracts is being prepared by J. A. Leibowitz & E. Liebes.

The second of Maimonides' medical writings is the Commentary on
the Aphorisms of Hippocrates. The famous aphorisms of Hippocrates were
translated from the Greek into Arabic by Hunain Ibn Ishak in the ninth
century. Maimonides wrote his commentary on this translation. Two incomplete Arabic manuscripts exist. A good medieval translation into
Hebrew was made by Moses ben Samuel Ibn Tibbon. In this work, Maimonides
occasionally criticizes both Hippocrates and Galen where either of these
Greeks differ from his own views. For example, in chapter five, Hippocrates
is quoted as having said, "a boy is born from the right ovary, a girl
from the left", to which Maimonides remarks "A man should be either
prophet or genius to know this". The introduction to this work was
edited in the original Arabic with two Hebrew and one German translations
by Steinschneider in 1894 (5). The entire work was published by Hasida

in 1935 (6) and again in a definitive edition by Muntner in 1961 (7).
Recently, Bar Sela and Hoff have published Maimonides' interpretation
of the first aphorism of Hippocrates (8). This is the famous aphorism
which has been called the motto or credo of the art of medicine: "Life
is short, and the art long, the occasion fleeting, experience fallacious
and judgement difficult. The physician must not only be prepared to do
what is right himself, but must also make the patient, the attendant
and the externals cooperate."

The third of Maimonides' medical works is the Medical Aphorisms of
Moses (Pirke Moshe) and is the most voluminous of all. This book is
comprised of 1500 aphorisms based mainly on Greek medical writers.
There are 25 chapters each dealing with a different area of medicine including
anatomy, physiology, pathology, symptomatology and diagnosis, etiology of
disease and therapeutics, fevers, blood-letting or phlebotomy, laxatives
and emetics, surgery, gynecology, hygiene, exercise, bathing, diet, drugs
and medical curiosities. A complete Arabic original manuscript exists in
the Gotha library in East Germany. A Hebrew translation was made in the
thirteenth century and published in Lemberg, Poland in 1834 and again in
Vilna in 1888 (9). The definitive Hebrew edition is that of Muntner dated
1959 (10). Maimonides' Aphorisms (11) were also translated into Latin in
the thirteenth century and appeared as an incunabulum in Bologne in 1489
and again in Venice in 1497, followed by several printed Latin editions (12).
Only small fragments of this work have ever appeared in a Western language
(13-16). A complete English version by Rosner and Muntner was recently
published in two volumes (17-18) and reprinted (19).

A few excerpts from this most important work will give the reader
the flavor of Maimonidean medical thinking. Maimonides speaks of

cerebrovascular disease: "one can prognosticate regarding a stroke, called apoplexy. If the attack is severe, then he will certainly die but if it is minor, then cure is possible, though difficult....the worst situation that can occur following a stroke is the complete irreversible suppression of respiration..."

Maimonides seems to be describing diabetes when he states: "Individuals in whom sweet white (humor) occurs are very somnolent (?hyperglycemia). To those who have an excess of sour white (humor), hunger occurs, then they will become extremely thirsty. When this white liquid will be neutralized, then the thirst will disappear." Maimonides explains that diabetes mellitus was seldom seen in "cold" Europe whereas it was frequently encountered in "warm" Africa. He also reports this disease to be associated with the imbibition of suave water of the Nile. (Maimonides lived in Fostat or old Cairo.) There follows the English translation of this most important aphorism No. 69 from the eighth chapter: "Moses says: I, too, have not seen it in the West (Spain, where Maimonides was born and/or Morocco where he fled from the persecution of the Almohades) nor did any one of my teachers under whom I studied mention that they had seen it (diabetes). However, here in Egypt, in the course of approximately ten years, I have seen more than twenty people who suffered from this illness. This brings one to the conclusion that this illness occurs mostly in warm countries. Perhaps the waters of the Nile, because of their suaveness, may play a role in this."

A very accurate description of obstructive emphysema is provided during a lengthy discussion of respiratory disease "...reason (for respiratory embarrassment) is narrowing of the organs of respiration, then the breast will be seen to greatly expand. This expansion will produce rapid and cut off (respirations) ..."

Clubbing of the fingers associated with pulmonary disease, already described by Hippocrates, is beautifully depicted: "With an illness affecting the lungs called 'nasal', namely phthisis, there develops rounding of the nail as a rainbow." The signs and symptoms of pneumonia are remarkably accurately described: "The basic symptoms which occur in pneumonia and which are never lacking are as follows: acute fever, sticking (pleuritic) pain in the side, short rapid breaths, serrated pulse and cough, mostly (associated) with sputum..." Hepatitis is just as beautifully described: "The signs of liver inflammation are eight in number as follows: high fever, thirst, complete anorexia, a tongue which is initially red and then turns black, biliary vomitus, initially yellow egg yolk in color which later turns dark green, pain on the right side which ascends up to the clavicle...Occasionally a mild cough may occur and a sensation of heaviness which is first felt on the right side and then spreads widely..."

So much for the Medical Aphorisms of Moses.

The fourth of Maimonides' medical writings is his Treatise on Hemorrhoids. This work was written for a nobleman, as Maimonides describes in the introduction, probably a member of the Sultan's family. There are seven chapters dealing with normal digestion, foods harmful to patients with hemorrhoids, beneficial foods, general and local therapeutic measures such as sitz baths, oils and fumigations. Maimonides disapproves of bloodletting or surgery for hemorrhoids except in very severe cases. Maimonides' whole approach to the problem seems to bespeak a modern medical trend. The Treatise on Hemorrhoids was first published by Kroner in 1911 in Arabic, Hebrew and German (20). A good general description of the work in English appeared in 1927 by Bragman (21). The definitive Hebrew edition is that of Muntner dated 1965 (22), and an English translation of the entire work was published by Rosner and Muntner (23).

In the introduction to this work, Maimonides describes the reason
for writing it:

"There was a youth, (descended) from knowledgeable, intelli-
gent and comprehending forebears, from a prominent and renowned
family, distinguished and charitable and of great means, in whom
the affliction of hemorrhoids occurred at the mouth of the rectum,
that interested me in his problem and placed the task (of healing
them) upon me. These irritated him on some occasions and he treated
them in the customary therapeutic manner until the pain subsided
and the prolapsed rectum (literally: excesses that protruded) became reduced and returned to the interior of the body so that his
(bodily) functions returned to normal. Because this (illness) re-
curred many times, he considered having them extirpated in order to
uproot this malady from its source so that it not return again. I
informed him of the danger inherent in this, in that it is not clear
if these hemorrhoids (literally: additions) are of the variety which
should be excised or not, since there are people in whom they have
once been (surgically) extirpated and in whom other hemorrhoids develop.
This is because the causes which gave rise to the original ones re-
mained and, therefore, new ones develop."

Here Maimonides provides an insight into the etiology of disease in
general in that he regards operative excision of hemorrhoids with skepti-
cism, because surgery does not remove the underlying causes which produced the hemorrhoids in the first place.

The fifth work is Maimonides' Treatise on Sexual Intercourse written
for the nephew of Saladin, the Sultan al Muzaffar Umar Ibn Nur Ad-Din.

The Sultan indulged heavily in sexual activities and asked Maimonides, his physician, to aid him in increasing his sexual potential. The work consists mainly of recipes of foods and drugs which are either aphrodisiac or antiaphrodisiac in their actions. Maimonides advised moderation in sexual intercourse and describes the physiology of sexual temperaments. There are two versions to this book, a short authentic and a longer spurious version. Both were first edited and published by Kroner in 1906 in Hebrew and German (24). Ten years later, Kroner published the true short version from the original Arabic manuscript in Granada (25). An Italian edition appeared in 1906 (26),and English (27) and Spanish (28) translations were published in 1961. The definitive Hebrew edition of both authentic (29) and spurious (30) versions of Maimonides' book on sex is that of Muntner dated 1965. A new English translation of the true work by Rosner has recently been published (31).

The sixth medical book of Moses Maimonides is his <u>Discourse on Asthma</u>. The patient for whom this book is written suffers from violent headaches which prevent him from wearing a turban. The patient's symptoms begin with a common cold,especially in the rainy season, forcing him to gasp for air until phlegm is expelled. The patient asks whether a change of climate might be beneficial. Maimonides, in 13 chapters, explains the rules of diet and climate in general and those rules specifically suited for asthmatics. He outlines the recipes of food and drugs and describes the various climates of the middle east. He states that the dry Egyptian climate is efficacious for sufferers from this disease and warns against the use of very power- ful remedies. Several Arabic, Hebrew and Latin manuscripts exist (32). The first critical edition of this work appeared in Hebrew in 1940, edited by Muntner (33). Additional manuscripts became available after World War II and a corrected, improved and revised, second Hebrew edition appeared in 1963 (34). Only 300 copies of this edition were printed and thus a third edition was published by Muntner in 1965 (35). An English version of Maimonides' book on asthma was published in 1963 (36) and a French translation in 1965 (37).

The last chapter of this work deals with concise admonitions and aphorisms which Maimonides considered "useful to any man desirous of preserving his health and administering to the sick". The chapter begins as follows: "The first thing to consider...is the provision of fresh air, clean water and a healthy diet." Fresh air is described in some detail: "...City air is stagnant, turbid and thick, the natural result of its big buildings, narrow streets, the refuse of its inhabitants...one should at least choose for a residence a wide-open site...living quarters are best located on an upper floor...and ample sunshine... Toilets should be located as far as possible from living rooms. The air should be kept dry at all times by sweet scents, fumigation and drying agents. The concern for clean air is the foremost rule in preserving the health of one's body and soul." Let our air pollution control programmers take cognizance of Maimonides' prophetic statements nearly 800 years ago.

The seventh medical work of Maimonides is his Treatise on Poisons and Their Antidotes. This book is one of the most interesting and popular works because it is very scientific and modern in its approach. It was used as a textbook of toxicology throughout the middle ages. The book was written at the request of Maimonides' noble protector, the Grand Visier and Supreme Judge Al Fadhil, who in 1199, asked Maimonides to write a treatise on poisons for the layman by which to be guided before the arrival of a physician. In the introduction, Maimonides praises

Al Fadhil and his feats in war and peace. He mentions Al Fadhil's orders
to import from distand lands ingredients lacking in Egypt but necessary
for the preparation of two antidotes against poisonings, the Great Theriac
and the Electuary of Mithridates.

The first section of the book deals with snake bites, dog bites,
scorpion, bee, wasp and spider stings. The first chapter concerns the
conduct of the victim in general. Thus Maimonides states as follows:

"When someone is bitten, immediate care should be taken to tie the
spot above the wound as fast as possible to prevent the poison from
spreading throughout the body; in the meantime, another person should
make cuts with a black lancet directly above the wound, suck vigor-
ously with his mouth and spit out. Before doing that, it is ad-
visable to disinfect the mouth with olive oil, or with spirit in
oil...Care should be taken that the sucking person has no wound in
his mouth, or rotten teeth...should there be no man available to do
the sucking, cupping-glasses should be applied, with or without fire;
the heated ones have a much better effect because they combine the
advantages of sucking and cauterizing at the same time...Then apply
the great theriac...Apply to the wound some medicine which should
draw the poison out of the body."

In his book on poisons, Maimonides also describes the long incubation
period for rabies (up to 40 days). Numerous Arabic, Hebrew and Latin
manuscripts are extant (38). A German translation was published in 1873
by Steinschneider (39). A French translation appeared in 1865 by
Rabinowicz and was reprinted in 1935 (40). An English translation of
Steinschneider's German version is that of Bragman in 1924 (42) and
Muntner's English version was published in 1966 (43).

The eighth book is the <u>Regimen of Health</u> (<u>Regimen Sanitatis</u>).
Maimonides wrote it in 1198 during the first year of the reign of Sultan
Al Malik Al Afdal, eldest son of Saladin the Great. The Sultan was a
frivolous and pleasure-seeking man of 30, subject to fits of melancholy or
depression due to his excessive indulgences in wine and women, and his
warlike adventures against his own relatives and in the Crusades. He com-
plained to his physician of constipation, dejection, bad thoughts and in-
digestion. Maimonides answered his royal patient in four chapters. The
first chapter is a brief abstract on diet taken mostly from Hippocrates and
Galen. The second chapter deals with advice on hygiene, diet and drugs in
the absence of a physician. The third extremely important chapter contains
Maimonides' concept of "a healthy mind in a healthy body", perhaps the first
description of psychosomatic medicine. He indicates that the physical well
being of a person is dependent on his mental well being and vice versa.
The final chapter summarizes his prescriptions relating to climate, domicile,
occupation, bathing, sex, wine drinking, diet and respiratory infections.

The whole treatise on the <u>Regimen of Health</u> is short and concise but
to the point. This is the reason for its great success and popularity
throughout the years. It is extant in numerous manuscripts. A Hebrew translation from the original Arabic was made by Moses ben Samuel Ibn Tibbon in
1244 and this version was reprinted several times in the nineteenth century
(Prague 1838, Jerusalem 1885, Warsaw 1886). Two Latin translations were
made in the thirteenth century. Several 15th Century incunabulae and 16th
Century editions of these Latin versions exist. A French translation by
Carcousse appeared in 1887 in Algiers (44). The Arabic text with German
and Hebrew translations was published by Kroner in 1925 (45), although he

had already published the all-important chapter 3 dealing with psychosomatic medicine 11 years earlier in 1914 (46). An English translation of
chapter 3 by Bragman appeared in 1932 (47). The definitive Hebrew edition
is that of Muntner dated 1957 (48). Two English translations of the entire
work were published: in 1958 by Gordon (49) and 1964 by Bar Sela, Hoff and
Faris (50). Another German translation by Muntner appeared in 1966 (51).
These numerous editions in many languages attest to the importance and
popularity of Maimonides' Regimen of Health.

The ninth medical writing of Maimonides is the Discourse on the
Explanation of Fits. This work has been called Maimonides' swan song as
it probably is the last of his medical works, having been written in the year
1200, four years before his death. It was also written for the Sultan Al
Malik Al Afdal and is sometimes considered to represent chapter five of the
Regimen of Health. The Sultan persisted in his over-indulgences and wrote
to Maimonides, who was himself ill, asking advice about his health. Maimonides
confirms most of the prescriptions of the Sultan's other physicians regarding wine, laxatives, bathing, exercise and the like, and near the end, gives
a very detailed hour by hour regimen for the daily life of the Sultan. The
original Arabic was edited and published with Hebrew and German translations
by Kroner in 1928 (52). English editions by Bar Sela, Hoff and Faris

in 1964 (50) and Rosner and Muntner in 1969 (23), another German
version by Muntner in 1966 (51), and another Hebrew edition by Muntner in
1969 (53) are available. The most recent edition is that by Leibowitz &
Marcus entitled "On the Causes of Symptoms" (54), in which the text is
presented in four languages (Arabic, Hebrew, Latin and English) and is accompanied by a running commentary, explanatory essays and a comprehensive
catalogue of drugs.

The final authentic medical book of Maimonides is the <u>Glossary of Drug Names.</u> This work was discovered quite recently by Max Meyerhof, an ophthalmologist in Egypt, in the Aya Sofia library in Istanbul, Turkey as Arabic manuscript No. 3711. Dr. Meyerhof edited the original Arabic and provided a French translation with a detailed commentary which he published in 1940 in Cairo (55). A Hebrew edition by Muntner appeared in 1969 (53). The work is essentially a pharmacopoeia and consists of 405 short paragraphs containing names of drugs in Arabic, Greek, Syrian, Persian, Berber and Spanish. This is the book which is translated here into English from the French edition of Max Meyerhof.

In summary, Maimonides' medical writings are varied, comprising extracts from Greek medicine, a series of monographs on health in general and several diseases in particular, and a recently discovered pharmacopoeia demonstrating Maimonides' extensive knowledge of Arabic medical literature and his familiarity with several languages. Some people feel that Maimonides' medical writings are not as original as his theological and philosophical writings. However, his medical works demonstrate the same lucidity, conciseness and formidable powers of systematization and organization so characteristic of all his writings. The <u>Book on Poisons</u>, the <u>Regimen of Health</u>, and the <u>Medical Aphorisms of Maimonides</u> became classics in their fields in medieval times.

I would like to conclude by citing a paragraph from my first paper on Maimonides (56):

"Maimonides died on December 13, 1204 (Tebet 20, 4965, in the Jewish calendar) and was buried in Tiberias, Palestine, at his own request. The Christian, Moslem and Jewish worlds mourned him. His literary ability was incredible and his knowledge encyclopedic.

He mastered nearly everything known in the fields of theology,
mathematics, law, philosophy, astronomy, ethics, and, of course,
medicine. As a physician, he treated disease by the scientific
method, not by guesswork, superstition, or rule of thumb. His
attitude towards the practice of medicine came from his deep religious background, which made the preservation of health and life
a divine commandment. His inspiration lives on through the years
and his position as one of the medical giants of history is indelibly recorded. He was physician to sultans and princes, and
as Sir William Osler said, "He was Prince of Physicians". The
heritage of his great medical writings is being more and more
appreciated. To the Jewish people he symbolized the highest
spiritual and intellectual achievement of man on this earth; as
so aptly stated, From Moses to Moses there never arose a man like
Moses, and none has since." (57)

REFERENCES:

1. Rosner, F.: The Physician's Prayer Attributed to Maimonides. Bull. Hist. Med. 41: 440-454, 1967

2. Leibowitz, J.O.: The Physician's Prayer Ascribed to Maimonides. Dapim Refuiyim 13: 77-81, 1954 (Hebr. with English summary)

3. Rosner, F.: Maimonides, the Physician: A Bibliography. Bull. Hist. Med. 43: 221-235, 1969

4. Barzel, V.: The Art of Cure: A Non-Published Medical Book by Maimonides. Harofe Haivri 2: 82-83 (Hebr.) and 177-165 (Eng.) 1955

5. Steinschneider, M.: Die Vorrede des Maimonides zu seinem Commentar uber die Aphorismen des Hippokrates. Ztschr. d. deutsch. Morgenland. Gesellsch. 48: 213-234, 1894

6. Hasida (Bocian), M.Z.: Perush lepirke Abukrat shel Ha-Rambam. Hassegullah (Jerusalem) 1934-5, nos. 1-30 (Stencil) (Hebr.).

7. Muntner, S.: Mosheh ben Maimon. Commentary on the Aphorisms of Hippocrates. Perush lepirkei Abukrat. Jerusalem: Mossad Harav Kook, 1961. XIV + 166 pp. (Hebr.)

8. Bar Sela, A. and Hoff, H.E.: Maimonides' interpretation of the first aphorism of Hippocrates. Bull. Hist. Med. 37: 347-354, 1968

9. Magid, Z. Ed. Medical Aphorisms of Maimonides (Pirke Moshe). Vilna: L. Matz, 1888, 112 pp (1st ed. Lemberg 1834) (Hebr.)

10. Muntner, S.: Moshe ben Maimon (Medical) Aphorisms of Moses in Twenty-five Treatises (Pirke Moshe Birefuah). Jerusalem: Mossad Harav Kook, 1959, XXXII + 470 pp. (Hebr.: Eng. summary). Reviewed by Levey, M.: J. Hist. Med. and Allied Sc. 17: 208-210, 1962

11. Leibowitz, J.O.: Maimonides' Aphorisms, Koroth 1: 213-219 (Hebr.) I-III (Engl. Summary) 1955

12. Leibowitz, J.O.: The Latin Translations of Maimonides' Aphorisms. Koroth 6: 273-281 (Hebr.), XCIII-XCIV (Engl. summary) 1973

13. Steinberg, W. and Muntner, S.: Maimonides' Views on Gynecology and Obstetrics. Am. J. Obst. Gynec. 91: 443-448, 1965

14. Rosner, F. and Muntner, S.: Moses Maimonides' Aphorisms Regarding Analysis of Urine. Ann. Int. Med. 71: 217-220, 1969

15. Rosner, F. and Muntner, S.: The Surgical Aphorisms of Moses Maimonides. Amer. J. Surg. 119: 718-725, 1970

16. Rosner, F.: Moses Maimonides & Diseases of the Chest. Chest 60: 68-72, 1971

17. Rosner, F. & Muntner, S.: Studies in Judaica. The Medical Aphorisms of Moses Maimonides. New York. Yeshiva Univ. Press. 1970 Vol. 1, pp 267. Reviewed by H. Gordon in Mayo Clin. Proc. 46: 698-699, 1971; and anonymous reviews in JAMA 216: 890, 1971 and Ann. Int. Med. 74: 1026, 1971

18. Rosner, F. & Muntner, S.: Studies in Judaica. The Medical Aphorisms of Moses Maimonides, New York. Yeshiva Univ. Press 1971 Vol. 2 pp 244

19. Rosner, F. & Muntner, S.: Studies in Judaica. The Medical Aphorisms of Moses Maimonides, Vol I and Vol. II, New York, Bloch Publishing Co., for Yeshiva Univ. Press 1973, pp 264 and 244

20. Kroner, H.: Die Haemorrhoiden in der Medicin des XII und XIII. Jahrhunderts. Janus 16: 441-456, 644-718, 1911

21. Bragman, L.J.: Maimonides' Treatise on Hemorrhoids. New York State Med. J. 27: 598-601, 1927

22. Muntner, S.: Moshe ben Maimon. On Hemorrhoids (Birefuoth Hatechorim) Jerusalem: Mossad Harav Kook, 1965. 32 pp (Hebr.)

23. Rosner, F. and Muntner, S.: The Medical Writings of Moses Maimonides. Treatise on Hemorrhoids and Maimonides' Answers to Queries. Philadelphia: Lippincott, 1969, XV and 79 pp.

24. Kroner, H.: Ein Betrag zur Geschichte der Medizin des XII Jahrhunderts an der Hand Zweier medizinischer Abhandlungen des Maimonides auf Grund von 6 unedierten Hanschriften. Oberdorf-Bopfingen: Itzowski, 1906, 116 (Ger.) 28 (Hebr.) pp.

25. Kroner, H.: Eine medizinische Maimonides Handschrift aus Granada. Ein Beitrag zur Stilistik des Maimonides und Charakteristik der Hebraischen Ueberzetzungsliteratur. Janus 21: 203-247, 1916. Reviewed by Seidel, E.: Mitt. z. Gesch, d. med. u. d. Naturwissensch. 17: 49-54, 1918

26. DeMartini, U.: Maimonides. Segreto dei segreti. Rome: Instituto di storia della Medicina dell'Universita de Roma. 1960. 84 pp.

27. Gorlin, M.: Maimonides "On Sexual Intercourse". (Fi'l-Jima). Brooklyn, N.Y.: Rambash Publ., 1961. 128 pp. Reviewed by Dienstag, J.I. in Tradition 4: 318-319, 1962, rejoinder by Gorlin, M., ibid 5: 322-324, 1963

28. Chelminski, E.: Notas introductorias al "Guia sobre el contacto sexual" de Maimonides. An de ars medici-Mexico 5(4): 240-248, 1961

29. Muntner, S.: Moshe ben Maimon on the Increase of Physical Vigour (M'amar al chizuk koach hagavra). Jerusalem: Mossad Harav Kook, 1965, pp 35-65 (Hebr.)

30. Muntner, S.: Pseudo-Maimonides on Sexual Life. In Sexual Life, Collection of medieval treatises (Ma'amar al razei hachajim haminiyim). Jerusalem: Geniza, 1965, 108 pp (Hebr.)

31. Rosner, F.: Sex Ethics in the Writings of Moses Maimonides. New York
Bloch Publishing Co., 1974, and 129 pp.

32. Rosner, F.: Maimonides' Treatise on Asthma. Med. Times 94: 1227-1230, 1966

33. Muntner, S.: Moshe ben Maimon (Maimonides) Sefer Hakatzereth (The Book
on Asthma). Jerusalem: Rubin Mass. 1940, XV + 168 pp (Hebr.)

34. Muntner, S.: Rabbi Moses ben Maimon. Sefer hakatzereth or Sefer hamisadim
(The Book on Asthma). Jerusalem: Geniza, 1963, 56 pp (Hebr.) Reviewed
by Dienstag, J.: Jewish Soc. Stud. 28: 38-39, 1966

35. Muntner, S.: Moshe ben Maimon on Asthma (Sefer Hakatzereth). Jerusalem:
Mossad Harav Kook, 1965, pp 67-119 (Hebr.)

36. Muntner, S.: The Medical Writings of Moses Maimonides. Treatise on Asthma.
Philadelphia: Lippincott, 1963, XXIV + 115 pp. Reviewed by Dienstag, J.:
Jewish Soc. Stud. 28: 38-39, 1966

37. Muntner, S. and Simon, I.: Le Traité de L'asthme de Maimonide (1135-1304)
traduit pour la premiere fois en francais d'apres le texte hébreu. Rev.
d'hist. méd. héb. 16: 171-186, 1963; 17: 5-13, 83-97, 127-139, 187-196,
1964; 18: 5-15, 1965

38. Rosner, F.: Moses Maimonides' Treatise on Poisons. J.A.M.A. 205:
94-916, 1968

39. Steinschneider, M.: Gifte und ihre Heilung. Virchows Arch. F. Path. Anat.
57: 62-120, 1873

40. Rabbinowicz, I.M.: Traité des poisons. Paris: Lipschutz, 1935 70 pp.
(1st ed. 1865)

41. Bragman, L.J.: Maimonides' Treatise on Poisons. Med. J. and Rec. 124:
103-107, 1926

42. Muntner, S.: Moshe ben Maimon (Maimonides), Samei hamaveth veharafuoth
kenegdam (Poisons and their antidoties, or "The Treatise to the Honored One").
Jerusalem: Rubin Mass, 1942 XX + 233 pp. (Hebr.)

43. Muntner, S.: The Medical Writings of Moses Maimonides, Vol. 2: Treatise
on Poisons and Their Antidotes. Philadelphia: Lippincott, 1966, XXXVII +
77 pp. Reviewed by DiCyan, E.: Arch. Int. Med. 119: 431-432, 1967

44. Carcousse, M.: Hygiene israelite, principes de sante physique et morale
de l'arabe par Arab Mouchi ben Mimoun. Algiers 1887, 51 pp.

45. Kroner, H.: Fi tadbir as sihhat. Gesundheitsanleitung des Maimonides
fur den Sultan al-Malik al-Afdhal. Janus 27: 101-116, 286-330, 1923;
28: 61-74, 143-152, 199-217, 408-419, 455-472, 1924; 29: 235-258, 1925

46. Kroner, H.: Die Seelenhygiene des Maimonides. Auszug aus dem 3. Kapital des diatetischen Sendschreibens des Maimonides an den Sultan al Malik Alafdahl (ca. 1198). Frankfurt A.M.: J. Kauffmann, 1914, 18 (Germ), 8 (Hebr. and Arab.) pp

47. Bragman, L.J.: Maimonides on Physical Hygiene. Ann. Med. Hist. 7: 140-143, 1925

48. Muntner, S.: Moshe ben Maimon. Hanhagath habriuth. Regimen sanitatis. Letters on the hygiene of the body and of the soul. Jerusalem: Mossad Harav Kook, 1956, XVIII + 254 pp. (Hebr.) Reviewed by Levey, M.: J. Hist. Med. and Allied Sc. 17: 208-210, 1962

49. Gordon, H.L.: Moses ben Maimon, The Preservation of Youth. Essays on Health (Fi Tadbir As-Sihha). New York; Philos. Lib. 1958 92 pp.

50. Bar Sela, A., Hoff, H.E. and Faris, E.: Moses Maimonides' Two Treatises on the Regimen of Health. Philadelphia: Am. Philos. Soc. (Trans. n.s. vol. 54, pt. 4), 1964, 50 pp

51. Muntner, S.: Regimen Sanitatis oder Dietetik fur die Seele und den Korper mit Anhang der medizinischen Responsen und Ethik des Maimonides. Basel: S. Karger, 1966, 208 pp.

52. Kroner, H.: Der medizinische Schwanengesang des Maimonides. Janus 32: 12-116, 1928

53. Muntner, S.: Moshe ben Maimon. Biyur Shaymoth Harefuoth (Lexicography of Drugs, and Medical Responses) Jerusalem 1969 Mossad Harav Kook. 164 pp

54. Leibowitz, J.O. & Marcus, S. On the Causes of Symptoms. Berkeley. Univ. of Calif. Press 1974

55. Meyerhof, J.: Un glossaire de matière médicale, composé par Maimonide (Sarh Asma al'Uqqa). Mém. Inst. Egypte, Vol. 41 LXXXVI + 256 pp. Reviewed by Sarton, G.: Isis 33: 527-529, 1941

56. Rosner, F.: Moses Maimonides (1135-1204). Ann. Int. Med. 62: 373-375, 1065

57. Leibowitz, J.O.: Maimonides on Medical Practice. Bull. Hist. Med. 31: 309-317, 1957

2. TRANSLATOR'S INTRODUCTION

According to Meyerhof, the Glossary of Drug Names by Maimonides was
known only to Ibn. Abi Usaybi'a and is mentioned by him in his Sources of
Information on the Classes of Physicians. Meyerhof believed it to be an
apocryphal book up to the time when in 1932 he was informed by Dr. Helmut
Ritter, in Istanbul, that this book exists in Arabic manuscript No. 3711 in
the Aya Sofia Library. In this book Maimonides reveals an unknown side of
his vast learning, namely, that of a philologist and linguist. The manuscript itself is very remarkable because it was written by the famous Arab
pharmacologist and botanist, Diya' ad-Din 'Abdallah, better known as Ibn
al-Baytar, the author of the greatest Arabic treatise on the simples. That
the copy of Maimonides' treatise on drug names was made by Ibn-Baytar himself is certified on the cover of the Istanbul manuscript by his pupil,
Ibn as-Suwaydi, a distinguished physician of the thirteenth century, and by
Khalil ibn Aybak as-Safadi, a well-known scholar and historian of the four-
teenth century, who were both among the owners of this precious and unique
manuscript. It is impossible to decide at exactly which period of his
medical career Maimonides would have been likely to compose such a treatise.
According to Meyerhof, it appears certain that he wrote it in Cairo, because
he frequently refers to names of plants and drugs which were, and still are
in use in Egypt. He probably composed it for the use of his Muslim friends
and pupils in Egypt and Palestine. Meyerhof, moreover, supposes that Ibn
al-Baytar copied the treatise soon after his arrival in Egypt and not from
the author's copy, because he not only made many mistakes in copying, but
also left uncorrected many mistakes of previous copyists.

The Arabic text begins with the following words: "My aim in this epitome is the explanation of the names of simple drugs which exist in our times and which are known to us and which are used in the art of medicine, and which we encounter in the medical books." Maimonides adds that he will omit the remedies that have only one well-known name and those that are too rare; he will also try to avoid repetitions and all circumstantial descriptions, in order to shorten the glossary as much as possible. He quotes as his forerunners in this work only Spanish physicians: Ibn Gulgul, Ibn Ganah, Ibn Wafid, Ibn Samagun, and Ahmad al-Ghafiqi. He then says that he intends to add popular names from "the Westland" (Morocco). There follow 405 short paragraphs containing, in alphabetical order, about 2000 names of drugs, mostly of vegetable and more rarely of mineral or animal nature. Maimonides generally gives first an Arabic name, which, however, is very often of Greek, Syriac, or Persian origin; after that, several other Arabic and Syriac names, and then names in Greek, Persian, Berber, and Spanish. These latter names, as usual among the Spanish Arabs, are given under the title of "names in the foreign language of Andalusia". They are often mutilated by the copyists, but Meyerhof was able to restore most of them with the help of Simonet's invaluable glossary. For the restoration of mutilated Berber names, the later published glossary of Moroccan Materia Medica, by Renaud and Colin, proved very useful. Meyerhof claims that it is strange that Maimonides did not mention a single Hebrew name of a plant or drug, although such names occur rather frequently in his theological writings and have carefully been collected by Löw in his great Flora of the Jews. Further, states Meyerhof, this is even more remarkable since Maimonides' older Muslim contemporary, the famous geographer, Al-Idrisi, in his hitherto unpublished "Book on Simples" (MS, Fatih Library, No. 3610, Istanbul) cites many Hebrew drug names, which he probably

copied from the works of Jewish scholars in Sicily. The absence of
Hebrew names according to Meyerhof, very likely, proves that Maimonides
composed his book mainly for the use of non-Jewish friends and pupils.

Close examination of the text again reveals Maimonides' vast knowledge of Arab medical literature, from which he took the approximately
2000 names that occur in this small but very important abstract. He utilized the drug books of his predecessors in Spain and Morocco, but very
often supplemented their knowledge by information which he had obtained
from the common people in Morocco. He must also have inspected the stocks
of drugs kept by medical men there, as he often quotes what he had seen of
root and dried flowers in their stores. He continually repeats "in our
land, al-Maghrib", thus showing that he felt at home in the West, the land
of his study during his youth, although he sometimes adds: "In Egypt or
Syria, they call this plant ....".

3. PREVIOUS EDITIONS

There are only two published versions of Maimonides' <u>Glossary of</u>
<u>Drug Names.</u> One is that of Max Meyerhof which appeared in Cairo in 1940
under the title <u>Sarh Asma' Al Uqqar</u>, in the original Arabic and accompanied
by a translation and commentary in French. Meyerhof's original intention was
to publish the work in 1935, year of the eighth centenary of Maimonides'
birth. However, textual difficulties were such that Meyerhof was forced to
consult numerous works in foreign libraries. He was further interrupted by
his professional obligations as a physician. It thus took him six years to
complete his Arabic and French edition. During the intervening years,
Meyerhof published several brief articles concerning this work. (Meyerhof,
M. Sur un Ouvrage Inconnu de Maïmonide, <u>Mélanges Maspéro</u>, Vol. 3, Cairo, 1935;
Meyerhof, M. Sur un Glossaire de Matière Medicale Composé par Maïmonide.
<u>Bull. Inst. d'Egypte</u>, Vol. 17, pp 223-235, Cairo, 1935).

The only other version of Maimonides' <u>Glossary of Drug Names</u> is the
Hebrew edition of Suessman Muntner published in 1959 by Mossad Harav Kook in
Jerusalem under the title <u>Beyur Shaymoth Harefuoth</u>. Muntner had previously
commented upon Meyerhof's work in an article in <u>Harefuah</u> (Vol. 20 #9-10, p. 77).
The present English translation is based entirely on Meyerhof's edition.

4. <u>THE UNIQUE MANUSCRIPT</u> (Meyerhof, loc. cit, pp LVII-LXI, abridged)

The only known codex containing Maimonides' <u>Glossary of Drug Names</u> is
manuscript #3711 of the Aya Sofia Library in Istanbul, Turkey. Its dimen-
sions are 25 by 17 centimeters. The manuscript itself occupies pages 64b to
102a of the codex. In the margin of the first page (64b) is an Arabic note
indicating that the manuscript belonged to the library of the Ottoman Sultan,
Mahmūd (perhaps Mahmūd the first, who reigned from 1730 to 1754).

The manuscript was written in its entirety by Ibn al-Baytar and comprises
38 folios with 17 lines on each page. The writing is Maghribian, very legible,
nearly calligraphed, and richly punctuated and vocalized. The first essay
is entitled <u>Missive of Hunain Ibn Ishaq the Physician, on Weights & Measures</u>.
It comprises pages 64a to 68a. It is followed by <u>The Book of Qusta ibn Luqā
of Ba'labakk on Weights & Measures</u>. This essay is much longer than the previous one and comprises pages 68a to 74b of the manuscript. Pages 71a and b,
in the margins have several corrections in a handwriting different from that
of Ibn al Baytar who himself made not a single correction in the entire
manuscript.

Then follows the <u>Kitab Sarh al- 'Uqqār ta'lif as-Saih ar-Ra'is Abu
'Imran Mūsā ibn 'Abdallāh al-Isrā'ili al-Magribi</u> (The Book on the Explanation of Medicinal Drugs, composed by the master and leader Abū 'Imran Mūsā,
son of 'Abdallāh, the Israelite, the Maghribian). This treatise occupies
twenty-seven and one-half folios, from pages 74b to 102a. After a two-and-
a-half page introduction, there follow, in the order of the semitic alphabet,
short articles or paragraphs arranged in chapters, that form the content of
the <u>Glossary of Drugs.</u> Meyerhof, and after him Muntner, in their French and
Hebrew editions respectively, numbered the 405 articles which contain approximately 1800 drug names.

In the original Arabic manuscript, the articles or paragraphs follow each other without punctuation. However, the titles are written in red ink with letters slightly larger than those of the text. The addition of diacritical points and of vocalization is considerable, contributing greatly to the identification of many drug names. It is remarkable that the author, Maimonides (or perhaps the copyist Ibn al-Baytar) mostly uses the vulgar forms of the name in usage in Maghrib or in Egypt, in placing vowels differently from the classic vocalization, and at an end of many names, instead of the nunnation there is a sukun. The signs of tasdid and damma, placed by Ibn al-Baytar, resemble each other and are easily confused. Sometimes he placed negligible vocalizing signs such that one can err, as in the first name utrugg. On the other hand, the sixth name ustuhudus is perfectly vocalized.

One might suppose that a manuscript copied shortly after the death of the author, Maimonides, by a specialist of universal reputation such as Ibn al-Baytar, would be a perfect copy. But quite the contrary is in fact the case. The number of words which lack diacritical points and vocalization, where the copyist only gives the sometimes doubtful writing of the name, is large. One must also add a considerable number of instances where Ibn al-Baytar overlooked rather obvious errors, or where he himself committed absurdities. For example, in article #123, instead of harasat al-baqar ("pearl of cattle"), which was the well-known name of concretions of beef biliary calculi in medieval Egypt, Ibn al-Baytar wrote gazarat al-baqar ("carrot of cattle") which makes no sense at all. He never tried to correct obvious errors in the text of Maimonides and even less so the numerous errors of the copyist which crept into the text. On Folio 38a, he forgot to insert in red ink the titles of eight articles and that of chapter Ha. The same

is true of article 304 where the title fawaniya is omitted by the copyist Ibn al-Baytar.

Even worse, on Folio 92a, he forgot to write the title of article #252
nailufar, and attached this article to the previous one. He then placed the
names nailufar and nisrin as titles of the following articles, thus causing
a great confusion, and he also omitted the title of the article which should
have followed, i.e. nargis, and attached it to the previous article. Ibn
al-Baytar did not even mention the confusion of articles 251 to 252 which he
produced, and did nothing to rectify it. In addition, at the bottom of
folio 96a, he gave to article 315 the title fil instead of filzahra, and to
article 316 which explains the previous name, he gave the defective title
fahzahrag. Furthermore, the number of names either altered or completely
mutilated is great.

All the above is noted by Max Meyerhof in the introduction to his
Arabic edition and French translation. Meyerhof was thus forced to spend
many months in reestablishing the original form, and not always was he
successful. He was immensely aided by Renaud and Colin from Rabat, particularly for certain Berber and old Castilian names.

Meyerhof suggests that the incorrectness of the text might be due to the
fact that Ibn al-Baytar either copied the manuscript in great haste, or
during the period when he was young and inexperienced such as shortly after
his arrival in Egypt in 1220, approximately 20 years after the death of the
author, Moses Maimonides.

5. CONTENT OF THE GLOSSARY OF DRUG NAMES
    (Meyerhof, loc. cit. pp LXII-LXVII, abridged)

The Book on the Explanation of Drug Names is an alphabetical glossary
of synonyms of medicinal drugs, as Maimonides, the author, himself expounds in his brief introduction. He defines his goal in declaring that
he did not intend to describe simple remedies nor to discuss their use -
but to explain some but not all of their names, that is to describe their
synonyms. For this reason, he excluded from his list well-known drugs and,
of course, those with only one name. As examples of the latter one might
mention camphor (kafur), ambergris ('anbar), musk (misk), violet (banafsag),
fig (tin) and cantharides (dararih) which are often described among the
simple remedies in Maimonides' medical and theological works, but which are
lacking in his glossary of synonyms of drugs.

The book represents a type of work that was in vogue particularly in
Maghrib, the west of the Musulman world. In fact, Maimonides himself mentions five extant works by Spanish authors from which he was inspired:
four are Musulman and one Jewish. The latter is the Talhis of the celebrated Abu' 1-Walid (Yonah) ibn Ganah. The four others are the Book of
Simple Drugs of Ibn Wafid, the Explanation of Drugs by Ibn Gulful, the
Collection of Simple Drugs by Ibn Gulgul, the Collection of Simple Drugs
of Ahmad al-Gafiqi and the Book of Simple Drugs of Ibn Samagun. It is sur-
prising that Maimonides did not know the important treatise of drugs by
his coreligionist Ibn Biklaris.

In general, Maimonides' work shows occidental inspiration. This is
graphically illustrated in the concluding words of his introduction: "I
have added thereto all that is reputed among the inhabitants of Maghrib....
I give preference to the interpretation which seems to me the one most

accepted by us in Maghrib". This phrase "by us in Maghrib" is repeated again and again throughout the glossary. Maimonides frequently adds "the inhabitants of Egypt call it...". It is, therefore, certain that he wrote his glossary in Egypt, as all his other medical writings.

By contrast, Maimonides' scientific thinking, has its origin in the west, in Spain and in Morocco, where he spent his years of study. Maimonides is known for his philosophic, theologic and other medical works. A book of medical lexicography such as the Glossary of Drug Names reveals a totally unknown or ignored aspect of the scientific activity and ability of Maimonides. Many works of this type appeared after Maimonides in both the Eastern and Western Musulman worlds. As in these other works of drug synonyms, the 405 articles of Maimonides' Glossary of Drug Names are of unequal length, sometimes comprising only a few words; other times articles occupy up to 15 lines or nearly an entire manuscript page. Maimonides, in general, gives the best known name of a drug as the title for an article and then follows it with synonyms in Arabic, ancient Greek, Syriac, Persian, Berber and Spanish. The latter language is designated by the words fi'agamiyyat al-Andalus ("in the foreign tongue of Andalusia"). It is the Andalusian dialect of old Castillian derived directly from the Latin. Works of medical writers of Musulman Spain have greatly contributed to the knowledge of this language of which only rare documents exist (see R. Dozy and W. H. Engelmann Glossary of Spanish and Portuguese Words Derived from the Arabic 2nd edit. Leyden and Paris 1969).

As he states in his preface, Maimonides also added many terms in popular usage ('anima), particularly in Maghrib but also in Egypt. As a consequence of this, he often vocalizes these terms according to the popular pronounciation, deviating from the classic vocalization of the great Arabic dictionaries.

His manner of vocalizing the popular Egyptian dialect corresponds to the pronunciation heard to this day in the bazaars of Cairo. For the Moroccan dialect, one observes much analogy with the modern terms as refined by Renaud and Colin in their edition of _Tuhfa_. Such terms are derived sometimes from the Greek or Latin and othertimes from Spanish.

In some articles, Maimonides furnishes useful explanations of different drugs that have the same name, or of different species of the same drug. His remakrs are in part novel and unedited and complete the dictionaries of technical terms in use by the Arabs. The names of drugs in Arabic writings are, in general, given in Arabic and in Greek, Syriac and Arabicised Persian. Spanish-Arabic authors also add the names in Berber and ancient Castillian. Maimonides copied the latter names from his predecessors, and quite accurately. The alterations of names are attributable to the copyists. For Arabic, his native tongue, and for Syriac (neo-Aramaic), a language closely resembling Hebrew, he had no difficulty at all, and his transcriptions are, for the most part, correct.

By contrast, Greek and Persian were not familiar to Maimonides, and he occasionally confused the two languages, or wrote their Arabic forms incorrectly. Thus he wrote _nabtafilun_ instead of _bantafilun_ (pentaphyllon) and inserted this paragraph in Chapter _nun_. In this error, he follows several Arabic authors who made the same mistake because of their lack of knowledge of the Greek language. (For example, Ibn Sina, Canon I, 378).

One is struck by the fact that Maimonides, in his _Glossary_, did not mention a single name in Hebrew. This is even more astonishing in view of the fact that Maimonides was perfectly familiar with the names of simple remedies in the Hebrew language. Immanuel Löw, in his fundamental work _Die Flora der Juden_ (Vienna, 1934, vol. IV, p. 75), discussing the subject of simple vegetables, notes that the Bible contains 117 names of plants, whereas the _Mishnah_

contains 320. Löw also found many of these names in the <u>Mishneh Torah</u>,
Maimonides' monumental codification of all Biblical and Talmudic law and
the only work of Maimonides written in Hebrew. Many of these names are
also explained in Maimonides' own <u>Luminary</u> (<u>As-Sirag</u>) or Arabic commentary
on the <u>Mishnah</u>. Maimonides thus knew perfectly well the names of plants and
drugs in Hebrew. In spite of this, he failed to use a single synonym in
Hebrew, probably because he wrote his <u>Glossary</u> primarily for the use of his
non-Jewish pupils. His other medical writings also do not contain Hebrew
terms, probably for the same reason.

It seems certain, according to Meyerhof, that even to Jewish physicians
of Maghrib and Egypt, Arabic medical terms were better known as the Hebrew
names. The physician-druggist Kohen al-'Attar, who lived a half century
after Maimonides, introduced some rare Hebrew names in his synonyms of
drugs. By contrast, the great Musulsam scholar al-Idrisi who died in 1166,
in his famous <u>Collection of Drugs</u>, included everywhere among the numerous
synonyms he mentions, Hebrew names transcribed in Arabic characters. He
did this because of his relations with Jewish physicians with whom he came
in contact at the court of the Kings of Palermo. There thus exists the
curious fact that Hebrew synonyms of drugs are lacking in the work of the
greatest Jewish Sage, yet they are found in part in the work of one of the
greatest Musulman scholars of the same century. As to the Arabic synonyms,
Maimonides, in his <u>Glossary</u>, gives the same names that one finds in his other
medical writings.

6. BIBLIOGRAPHY
(Meyerhof, loc. cit. pp LXXI-LXXVI)

'ABD AL-LATĬF, Relation de l'Egypte par Abd-Allatif médecin arabe de Bagdad...
by Sylvestre de Sacy. Paris 1810

'ABD AR-RAZZĀQ, Kachef er-Roumoŭz (Revelation of Enigmas) of Abd er-Rezzaq
ed-Djezairy...Translated and annotated by L. Leclerc. Paris 1874

ACHUNDOW, Die pharmakologischen Grundsaetz (Liber fundamentorum pharmacologiae)
des Abu Mansur Muwaffaq bin Ali Harawi...translated by Abdul Chalig Achundow
from Baku, is Histor. Studien aus dem Pharmakolog. Institut der Kaiserl.
Universitaet Dorpat...vol. III. Halle 1893

'ALI IBN AL-'ABBĀS, Kamil as-Sinā'a at-tibbiyya (Arabic text), by 'Ali ibn
al-'Ăbbās al-Magūsĭ. Cairo, Būlāq 1294

ANASTASE, Nubkhab ad-Dakhair fi Ahwal al-Djawahir, or Choix des trésors enfouis
dans la connaissance des pierres précieuses,by Ibn al-Akfani. Transcription, with lexicographic, scientific and literary notes by P. Anastase-
Marie de St.-Élie. Cairo 1939

ASMA'Ĭ, Kitāb an-Nabāt wa's-Sagar (Arabic text), by "Abd al-Malik al-Asma'Ĭ,
ed. A. Haffner, Beirut 1908

BAILLON, Traité de botanique médicale phanérogamique by H. Baillon, Paris 1883

BEDEVIAN, Illustrated Polyglottic Dictionary of Plant Names. Cairo 1936

BERENDES, Des Pedanios Dioskurides aus Anazarbos Arzneimittellehre in fuenf
Buechern. Translated by J. Berendes. Stuttgart 1902

BERGGREN, Guide français-arabe vulgaire des voyageurs et des Francs en Syrie
et en Egypte. Arabic Druggist (p. 881-884). Upsalla 1844

BERUNI, Kitāb as-Saĭdana (Book of Drugs), by Abu'r-Raihan al-Beruni, unedited
manuscrit of the Bibliotheque Orhan Gazi in Brousse (Anatolia).

BOTICA, (Botica La oficina de farmacia o repertorio universal, etc.)
Segun el plan de la utlima edicion de Dorvault... by D. José de Pontes
Y Rosales, etc. Madrid 1872-1878

BOULOUMOY, Flore du Liban et de la Syrie, by L. Bouloumoy. Paris 1930, 2 vol.
one being an atlas of 508 plates.

BROCKELMANN (Lex.) Lexicon syriacum authored by Carolo Brockelmann, 2nd edition,
Halis Saxonum 1928

BROCKELMANN, G.A.L., Geschichte der arabischer Literatur. 2 vol. Weimar-Berlin
1898-1902. Supplement, Berlin 1936-39

CHAU-JU-KUA, His Work on Chinese and Arab Trade in the Twelfth and Thirteenth
Centuries, entitled Chu-fan-chi. Translated from the Chinese and Annotated by Fr. Hirth and W. W. Rockhill, St. Petersburg 1911

CHOPRA, Indigenous Drugs of India, their Medical and Economical Aspects, by
Chopra. Calcutta 1933

CLUSIUS, Caroli Clusii Atrebat. Rariorum aliquot stirpium per Hispanias ob-
servatarum Historia...Antwerp, 1576

DAMIRI, Ad-Damiri's Hayāt al-Hayawān (A Zoological Lexicon). Translated from
the Arabic by A.S.G. Jayacar. London and Bombay 1906-1908, 2 vol.
(the second incomplete).

DAWUD, Tadkirat Ūlī al-Albāb by Dāwūd al-Antākī. First edition of the Arabic
text in three volumes. Cairo 1281 of Hegira.

DIOSCORIDES, Pedanii Dioscuridis Anazarbei De Materia medica libri quinque,
ed. Max Wellmann. Berolini 1907-1914, 3 vol.

DOZY, Supplément aux dictionnaires arabes by R. Dozy. Leyden 1881, 2 vol.

DRAGENDORFF, Die Heilpflanzen der verschiedenen Voelker und Zeiten by George
Dragendorff. Stuttgart 1898

DUCROS, *Essai sur le droguier populaire arabe de l'inspectorat du Caire*, by
     M.A.H. Ducros, Mém. prés. a l'Inst. de'Egypte...Vol. XV. Cairo 1930

DYMOCK, Pharmacographis Indica. *A History of the Principal Drugs of Vegetable*
     Origin Met with in British India, by William Dymock, C.J.H. Warden and
     David Hooper. London, Bombay and Calcutta, 1890-1893, 3 vol.

ENCYCLOPÉDIE DE L'ISLAM, Leyden and London 1913-1936, 4 vol.

FIGARI, *Studii scientifici sull'Egitto e sue adiacenze*...by Antonio Figari
     Bey. Lucca 1864-1865, 2 vol.

FIHRIST (Ibn an-Nadim) *Kitab al-Fihrist*. Mit Anmerkungen herausgegeben von
     Gustav Flügel. Leipzig 1871-1872

FORSKAL (Flora), *Flora Aegyptiaco-Arabica*...detexit, illustravit Petrus
     Forskal...ed. Carsten Niebuhr. Hauniae 1775

FORSKAL (Mat. Med.), *Materia Medica Kahirina*, in *Descriptiones animalium*, etc.
     observ. Petrus Forskal...ed Carsten Niebuhr. Hauniae 1775

FRAENKEL, *Die Aramaeischen Fremdwoerter im Arabischen*, by Sigmund Fraenkel,
     Leider 1886

FREYTAG, *Lexicon arabico-latinum*...Georgii Wilhelmi Freytagii. Halis Saxonum
     1830-1837, 4 vol.

GALEN, *Claudii Galeni opera amnia*, ed. W. Kuehn. Leipzig 1821-1833, 20 vol.

GHAFIQI, *The abridged Version of "The Book of Simple Drugs" of Ahmad ibn*
     Muhammad al-Ghafiqi...ed. by M. Meyerhof and G. P. Sobhy. Cairo 1932-1938

GHAFIQI (ms.) Illustrated manuscript of the first part of the *Livre des*
     Simples of 'Ahmad al-Ghafiqi, conserved as n° 7508 in the Osler library,
     McGill University. Montreal (Canada)

HEHN, *Cultivated Plants and Domestic Animals in their Migration from Asia to*
     Europe, by Victor Hehn, ed. by J. St. Stallybrass. Longdon 1891

HERRERA, Libro de Agricultura, by Gabriel Alonso de Herrera. Medina del Campo 1569

HEYD, Histoire du commerce du Levant au moyen âge, French edition, Stuttgart
1878 (two reimpressions), 2 vol.

HONIGBERGER, Thirty-five Years in the East, etc. by John Martin Honigberger
London 1852, 2 vol.

HOOPER AND FIELD, Useful Plants and Drugs of Iran and Iraq by David Hooper
and Henry Field, in Field Museum of Natural History, Botanical Series,
vol. IX n° 3. Chicago 1937

IBN ABI USAIBI'a, 'Uyūn al-Anbā fī Tabaqāt al-Atibbā ("Sources of information
on the classes of physicians") by Ibn Abi Usaibi'a, ed. Aug. Mueller,
Arabic text. Cairo 1882

IBN AL-BEITHAR, Traité des Simples par Ibn al-Beithar. Translation of Dr.
Lucien Leclerc, in Notices et Extraits des Manuscrits de la Bibliothèque
Nationale. Paris 1877-1883, 3 vol.

IBN AL-BEITHAR (text) Kitāb al-Gāmi' li-Mufradat al Adwiya wa'l Agdiya, by
Diyā' ad-Din...ibn al-Baītār. Cairo-Būlāq 1291, 4 vol.

IBN 'AWWAM, Le livre de l'agriculture d'Ibn-al-Awam (Kitab al-Felahah), translated from the Arabic by J.J. Clément-Mullet. Paris 1864-1867, 3 vol.

IBN SĪNĀ, Kitāb al-Qanun fi't-Tibb, by Abu 'Alī al-Husain ibn Sīnā. Cairo,
Bulaq 1294, 3 vol.

IDRISI, Kitāb al-Gāmi' li-Sifāt Astāt an-Nabāt, etc. ("Collection of descriptions of the diversities of plants, etc."). Manuscrit (vol. 1 only) n° 3610
of the Fatih library in Istanbul (author: Sheriff Muhammad al-Idrisi;
died in 1166)

IBN AL-QIFTI'S Ta'rīh al-Hukamā'...edited by Julius Lippert. Leipzig 1903

ISSA, Dictionnaire des noms des plantes en latin, français, anglais et arabe,
by D'Ahmed Issa Bey, Cairo 1930

KEIMER, Die Gartenpflanzen im alten Aegyten, by Ludwig Keimer. Hamburg 1924

KOHEN, Minhāg ad-Dukkān wa-Dustūr li'1-A'yān, by Ab '1-Munā ibn Abī Nasr al-
    Isrā'īlī, called Kohēn al-'Attār. Cairo-Būlāq. 1287 of Hegira

LAGUNA, Pedacio Dioscorides Anazarbeo, acerca de la Materia medicinal. Trans-
    lated from the Greek into vulgar Castilian by the Doctor Andres de Laguna.
    Salamanca 1570

LANE, An Arabic-English Lexicon... by Edward William Lane, London 1863-1893,
    8 vol. (incomplete)

LANGKAVEL, Botanik der spaeteren Griechen. Berlin 1886

LAOUST, Mots et choses berbères, etc. by E. Laoust. Paris 1920

LAUFER, Sino-Iranica...by Berthold Lauter, in Field Museum of Natural History,
    Anthropol. Series, vol. XV, p. 185-630. Chicago 1919

LECLERC, Histoire de la médecine arabe, by Lucien Leclerc. Paris 1876, 2 vol.

LISAN, Lisān al-'Arab, by Gamāl ad-Dīn ibn Manzūr. Cairo-Būlāq 1300-1304
    of Hegira

LOEW, Die Flora der Juden, by Immanuel Löw (Veroeffentlichungen der Alexander
    Kohut Memorial Foundation, vol. II-IV et VI). Vienna 1924-1934

LUERSSEN, Medicinisch-pharmaceutische Botanik, etc...by Chr. Luerssen, 2 vol.
    Leipzig 1879-1882

MALOUF, An Arabic Zoological Dictionary (in Arabic) by Amin Malouf (Amin al-
    Ma'luf), Cairo 1932

MANHAG, Al-Manhag al-Munīr fī Asmā'al-'Aqāqir. Anonymous manuscript n° H 187
    of the private library of M. Meyerhof.

MECHITHAR, Mechithar des Meisterarztes aus der 'Trost bei Fiebern...aus dem
    Mittelarmenischen uebersetzt...by Ernst Seidel. Leipzig 1908

MEYER, Geschichte der Botanik by Ernst Meyer. Koenigsberg 1854-1857, 4 vol.

MEYERHOF, (Chichm), Histoire du Chichm, remède ophtalmique des Egyptiens, in Janus (Leyden 1914), p. 265-273

MEYERHOF, (Bazar), Der Bazar der Drogen und Wohlegerüche in Kairo, in Archiv fuer Wirtschafstforchung im Orient (Weimar 1918), fasc. 1-4

MUNHASSAS, Kitāb al-Muhassas...by 'Alī ibn Ismā'īl...ibn Sīda, 17 vol. Cairo, Būlāq 1316-1321 of Hegira

MUSCHLER, A Manual Flora of Egypt, by Reno Muschler, 2 vol. Berlin 1912

NAGM AD-DĪN, Le Livre de l'art du traitement de Najm ad-Dyn Mahmond...text, translation, glossaries...by D. P. Guigues. Beirut 1903

NIHAYA, Nihāyat al-Arab fī Funūn al-Arab by Sihāb ad-Dīn Ahmad ibn 'Abd al-Wahhāb an-Nurairī, Cairo 1342/1934-1356/1937. (12 volumes have appeared to date)

PLINY, C. Plinii Secundi naturalis historiae libri XXXVII, numerous good editions indicated by Sarton, I, 249

POST, Flora of Syria, Palestine and Sinai...by Georges Post. Second edition... by J. E. Dinsmore. Beirut 1932-1933, 2 vol.

QĀMŪS, Al-Qāmūs al-Muhīt, by Abū Tāhir Magd ad-Din Muhammad ibn Ya'qūb al-Firūzābādī, 3rd edition. Cairo, Būlāq 1301-1302 of Hegira, 4 vol.

RAMIS, Bestimmungstabellen zur Flora von Aegypten, by D'Aly Ibrahim Ramis. Jena 1929

RAZI, Kitāb Manāfi' al-Agdiya wa Daf' Madārrha, by Abū Bakr Muhammad ibn Zakariyyā' ar-Rāzī, Cairo 1305 of Hegira

RENAUD-COLIN, see Tuhfa.

SCHLIMMER, Terminologie medico-pharmaceutique et anthropologique francaise-persane..., by Joh. L. Schlimmer, Teheran 1874

SCHWEINFURTH, Arabische Pflanzennamen aus Aegyten, Algerien und Jemen, by G. Schwinfurth. Berlin 1912

- 1 -

SERAPION, Les noms arabes dans Serapion "Liber de simplici medicine". Essai
de restitution et d'identification...by D'Pierre Guigues. Paris 1905

SICKENBERGER, Die einfachen Arzneistoffe der Araber im 13. Jahrhundert by
E. Sickenberger, in Pharmaceutische Post (Vienna 1891-1895, n⁰ 1-1001
of Ibn al-Beithar-Leclerc, incomplete)

SIMONET, Glosario de voces ibericas y latinas usadas entre los Mozárabes...
by Fr. J. Simonet. Madrid 1889

STEINGASS, A Comprehensive Persian-English Dictionary...by F. Steingass.
London 1892

STEINSCHNEIDER, (Heilm.), Heilmittelnamen der Araber, by Moritz Steinschneider.
Reprint from the Wiener Zeitschrift Fuer die Kunde des Morgenlandes,
vol. XI-XIII. Frankfurt 1900

STEINSCHNEIDER (Hebr.), Die hebraeischen Uebersetzungen des Mittelalters und
die Juden als Dolmetscher...by Moritz Steinschneider. Berlin 1893

SUWALDI, Kitāb as-Simāt fi Asmā' an-Nabāt ("Book of stigmata on the names of
plants"), by Ibrahim ibn Ahmas ibn Tarhān ibn as-Suwaidi. Autographic
manuscript (?). Arabic n⁰ 3004 of the Bibliothèque Nationale in Paris.

TAG, Tāg al-'Arūs min Gawāhir al-Qāmūs..., by Muhammad Murtada az-Zabīdi.
Cairo, Būlāq 1306-1310 of Hegira, 20 vol.

THEOPHRASTUS, Theophrastus' Enquiry into Plants...with an English Translation
by Sir Arthur Hort, (The Loeb Classical Library). London 1916, 2 vol.

TRABUT, Répertoire des noms indigènes des plantes...dans le Nord de l'Afrique,
by Dr. L. Trabut. Algier 1935

TSCHIRCH, Handbuch der Pharmakognosie, by A. Tschirch. Leipzig 1909-1923, 3 vol.

TUHFA, Tuhfat al-ahbab, glossaire de la matière médicale marocaine. Text
published for the first time with translation, critical notes and index,
by H.P.J. Renaud and Georges Colin. (Publ. de l'Inst. des Hautes Etudes
marocaines, vol. XXIV). Paris 1934

VULLERS, Joànnis Augusti, <u>Lexicon persico-latinum etymologicum</u>...Bonnae
    1855-1867, 2 vol. and supplement

WATT, <u>The Commercial Products of India, Being an Abridgement of "The Dictionary</u>
    <u>of the Economic Products of India"</u>, by Sir George Watt. London 1908

WIEDERMANN (Beitr.), <u>Eilhard Wiedemann's Beitraege zur Geschichte der Natur-</u>
    <u>wissenschaften</u>, vol. I-LXXIX. Erlangen 1904-1928

YĀQŪT, <u>Jacut's geopgraphisches Woerterbuch</u>...herausgegehen von Ferdinand
    Wuestenfeld. Leipzig 1866-1870, 6 vol.

YULE-BURNELL, <u>Hobson-Jobson. A Glossary of Colloquial Anglo-Indian Words</u>, etc.
    by Henry Yule and A. C. Burnell. New Edition. London 1903

ZENKER, <u>Dictionnaire turc-arabe-persan,</u> by Jules Théodore Zenker. Leipzig
    1866-1876, 2 vol.

I regret that two important works concerning Indian and Assyrian
materia medica were not at my disposition. They are:

  K.-R. KIRTIKAR and B.-D. BASU, <u>Indian Medicinal Plants</u>, second edition, 1936.
    Calculla 4 vol.

  R. CAMPBELL THOMPSON, <u>The Assyrian Herbal; a Monograph on the Assyrian</u>
    <u>Vegetable Drugs</u>. London 1934

TRANSLATION INTO ENGLISH OF MAX MEYERHOF'S RENDERING
OF THE TEXT TOGETHER WITH HIS COMMENTARIES

(pp 3-204 of the 1940 Meyerhof edition)

MAIMONIDES' INTRODUCTION

(fol. 74ᵛ)   In the name of God, the Merciful and Compassionate!
God is my support and my reward!

THE BOOK ON THE EXPLANATION OF DRUGS

COMPOSED BY

THE MASTER AND LEADER ABŪ 'IMRĀN MŪSĀ IBN 'ABDALLĀH,

THE ISRAELITE, THE MAGHRIBIAN

He said: my aim in this epitome is the explanation of the names of
simple drugs which exist in our times, and which are known to us, and which
are used in the art of medicine, and which we encounter in the medical books.
Of these well-known simple remedies, I will only mention those to which are
ascribed more than one designation, be it because of the difference in
languages, or be it because of various names in the same language. For a
single remedy may carry several names by the representatives of the same
language, (fol. 75ʳ) as a consequence of a coincidence in naming, or a
difference in the origin of the terminology by the inhabitants of various
regions. I will not mention any of the known and reputable remedies, concerning which physicians are in agreement, in that they only give a single
widely accepted name, Arabic or foreign. Because the goal of this epitome
is neither the definition of the different kinds of remedies by means of their
description, nor a discussion of their usefulness, but rather uniquely

the explanation of some of their names by their synonyms. Similarly,
I will not mention a known and established remedy, as (for example) the fig,
the grape and other similar fruits just because their Greek names are mentioned in the books which have been transmitted to us, for their writers

have mentioned and explained them, except in the case where these Greek
names are endowed with a large quantity of synonyms for the remedy in
question. I will also silently omit any remedy which carries a name that
is little used, or unknown, and which does not have a great utility in
medicine.

I will classify the enumerated remedies in alphabetical order, but
I will avoid repetitions. If, for example, a remedy has two names, the
first of which begins with an alif and the second with a bā', and if these
two names are mentioned in chapter (or letter) alif, I will not again mention the second in chapter (or letter) bā'. All this is done with the
goal of abbreviating and rendering (the material) into the most easily
remembered form because, in spite of the effort which would be necessitated
by research into a specific name, it will serve as a powerful aid to
(fol. 75ᵛ) one's memory to remember the numerous names of the remedy
in question. My goal is to reduce the volume of this epitome, in order
to facilitate the task of those who wish to remember it, and to increase
thereby its utility. The first term by which I introduce the series of
names of a remedy is the one which is most common but least known among
professionals, because the foreign name of many remedies is more known
and familiar to physicians than its Arabic name.

For the explanation of these names I base myself upon the book of Ibn
Gulgul regarding the interpretations of the drug, upon the book of Abu'l-
Walid ibn Ganāh, upon the collection composed in Spanish by a more recent
writer named al-Ghafiqi, and upon the writings of Ibn Wāfid and Ibn Samagūn.
I have added thereto all that is reputed among the inhabitants of Maghrib
without being contested by the medical authorities. When the commentators
are not in accord about a certain point, I give preference to the interpretation which seems to me the one most generally accepted in Maghrib. I

then mention it as such as the most reputed. And in cases of divergence of views, I cite the preponderant opinion.

May God guide us in the path of truth.

CHAPTER ALIF

1) UTRUGG   Citron, cedrate (lemon), Citrus medica L.

MAIMONIDES: It is the "medicinal apple".

MEYERHOF: [Theophrastus IV, 2; Dioscorides I, 115; Serapion 46;

         Ghafiqi 11; Ibn al-Beithar 16; Tuhfa 21; ʿAbd ar-Razzāq 6;

         Issa 51, 19; Loew III, 278 ff.]

This designation tuffāh mā'ī is the translation from the Greek.
Suwaidi (fol. 279a) writes more correctly tuffāh māhī and explains that
the adjective is not derived from mā' meaning "water", but from Māh
meaning Media. The name utrugg derives from the Persian turung
(Vullers 1, 439) and from the Sanskrit mātulunga (Laufer 301). The
cedrate (Citrus medica RISSO var. cederata) appears to have been the
first species which, coming from the Indies, reached the Mediterranean
countries around the third century before the Christian era. Its name
passed into Hebrew (etrōg meaning Citrus medica L. lageniformis ROEM.),
and its fruit still plays a role at the Jewish festival of Tabernacles.
The assertion of Loret (Le cédratier dans l'antiquité, Paris 1891), according to which this tree was known in Egypt around 1500 BCE, is considered erroneous (Loew, loc. cit.).

ʿAbd al-Latif, celebrated physician of Baghdad and younger contemporary of Maimonides, in his Description de l'Egypte (p. 31) mentions a half dozen citrons of different species that he saw in Egypt,
among them a compounded lemon which was the product of a lemon tree
grafted upon a citron tree (according to the Jewish physician Ibn
Gumaiʾ, another contemporary of Maimonides). See the scholarly commentaries of Sylvestre of Sacy (Abd al-Latif p. 115-117) and of Clément-
Mullet (Étude sur les noms arabes de diverses familles de végétaux;

Journal Asiatique, 6th series Vol. 15, p. 17-41. The author enumerates
approximately fifty Arabic names of aurantiaceae).

2) ARZ   Cedar, pine

MAIMONIDES: This is the "male pine" (sanawbar dakar), and it is non-edible.
It is the one from which one extracts the tar. The cyprus
(sarw) is a type of pine (arz).

MEYERHOF: [Theophrastus III, 4-13; Dioscorides I, 69-77; Serapion 470;
Tuhfa 298, 352, 381, 458; Issa 43, 14; 139, 15; Loew III, 14 ff.]

The explanation of the name arz is not yet certain. This name designates a type of cedar, as well as a type of pine. The name "male pine" is
the translation of arrhēn peukē of Theophrastus (I, 9,3) and of Dioscorides,
and refers on the one hand to the Aleppo pine (Pinus halepensis MILL) and
on the other hand to the Pinus Laricio POIR. The Arab name "female pine",
translated from the Greek peukē theleia, designates the parasol pine
(Pinus Pinea L.) whose fruit has edible seeds. See below item 317 (sanawbar).
The origin of the Arabic name is the Aramaic arza (Brockelmann, Lex. 47b).

3) IFSINTĪN   Absinth (wormwood)

MAIMONIDES: In medical writings, it is frequently called kašūt rūmi.
It is that which is known in Spanish under the name yerba
batra. One also calls it ušainīsa.

MEYERHOF: [Theophrastus VII, 9, 5; Dioscorides III, 23; Ghafiqi 27;
Ibn al-Beithar 113; Tuhfa 1; ʿAbd ar-Razzāq 5 and 454; Loew
I, 379 ff; Issa 22, 1.]

Afsantin, afsintīn or, more rarely, ifsintīn, is the Arabic transcription of the Greek apsinthion, passed through the Aramaic. The name kašut

rūmī (Greek dodder) is described by Issa. The Spanish names yerba batra
(a modern Spanish name for absinth is hierba santa) and ajenjo (one should
read aršamīsa or ašenšu instead of ušaínīsa. In Ghafiqi Ms. fol. 18 one
reads ūšainsī), are also found in Simonet (18 and 613). An ancient Arabic
name of this Artemesia absinthium L. is damsīsa. The plant does not grow in
modern Egypt, where the name dasīsa serves to designate the bastard absinth
(Ambrosia maritima L.) (Schweinfurth 58, and Issa 12, 15). See below at
number 186 (kašūt).

4) ANZARŪT   Sarcocol

   MAIMONIDES: It is also called ʿanzarūt; it is a Persian ocular (kuhl)
            remedy. Its Greek name is sarkokolle.
   MEYERHOF: [Dioscorides III, 85; Serapion 38; Ghafiqi 37; Ibn al-Beithar
            171 and 1599; Tuhfa 35; ʿAbd ar-Razzāq 19; Issa 26, 14.]

   It is a resinous gum derived from a Persian umbelliferous plant which
one thought everywhere to be Penaea mucronata L; Dymock (I, 178) has demonstrated that it is derived from the Astragalus sarcocolla DYM.

   The name kuhl fārisī ("dried Persian collyrium") was in use in Egypt
(according to Ibn al-Beithar 171). The Greeks employed it as a cicatrizant,
as the name sarkokolla indicates. The Arabs utilized it as a strong purgative, and as an ocular remedy. The name of this drug is derived from the
Persian anzarūt or angarūt (Vullers I, 126). One finds this resin at the
druggists at the bazaars of Cairo (Ducros II).

5) ISFANG AL-BAHR   Marine Spronge

   MAIMONIDES: This is the "foam of the sea" (ragwat al-bahr), and it is
            also called the "cream of the sea" (zabad al-bahr). It is the
            "cloud" (gaïm), and one also calls it gamām (same meaning).

It is that which the people of Maghrib know under the name
naššāfa ("which dries"), and one also calls it "wool of the sea"
(sūfat al-bahr).

MEYERHOF: [Theophrastus IV, 6; Dioscorides V, 120; Serapion 41; Ghafiqi 105;
Ibn al-Beithar 75; ʿAbd ar-Razzāq 36.]

The Arabic name isfang or isfung, today in Egypt isfing, is derived from
the Greek spongia or spongos. It is the common sponge (Euspongia officinalis L.)
which served both in surgery in the form of a tampon, and, calcined, as a
remedy for external and internal usage. Regarding the nature of the sponge,
Theophrastus and other scholars of antiquity, as well as certain Arab writers -
for example Idrisi and Abu'1-ʿAbbās an-Nabāti - took it for a plant, whereas Aristotle and the majority of Arab authors recognized its animal nature.
Simonet (p. 187) wished to derive the Arabic name isfang from the Latin
spongia, but the latter is already found in   Ibn Sina.

6) USTŪHŪDŪS   Lavender Stoechas

MAIMONIDES: The Stoechas, which physicians employ in Maghrib and in
Egypt, is the same plant which the people of Maghrib call
al-halhāl. It is waša'i'aš-šaih, and one also calls it
aršanīsa; it is sunbul al-ahāniya. I have learned from
eminent scholars, who display scientic zeal in the study of
plants, that it is not the same Stoechas mentioned by Galen,
but something which possesses the same (medicinal) qualities.
As to the true Stoechas, it has larger leaves than the aforementioned, and thicker inflorescences (waša'iʿ). It grows
in the vicinity of Toledo.

MEYERHOF: [Dioscorides III, 26; Ghafiqi 28; Ibn al-Beithar 62; Tuhfa
13; ʿAbd ar-Razzāq 8; Issa 106, 5; Loew II, 73 ff; Ducros 6.]

One is dealing with the Labiate <u>Lavandula Stoechas</u> L. (Arabic Stoechas).
The Arabic name <u>ustūhūdūs</u> is the transcription of the Greek genitive
<u>stoïkhados</u>. The name <u>lavandula</u>,in turn,is derived from the Syriac <u>lebonta</u>,
whereas the Hebrew name of this plant is <u>ēzibyōn</u>. Issa cites Arabic names
unknown to Maimonides, and the latter (cites) several names which are not
encountered in any other location. <u>Sunbul</u> signifies "spike",and <u>wašīʿa</u>
"bobbin, spindle" or, in botany, an inflorescence in the form of a terminal
spike. That of the Stoechas, having a beautiful light blue color, carries
the name <u>wašaʾiʿ aš-šaīh</u> (spindle of the old man). Concerning the name
<u>aršanīsa</u>, it might be a corruption of <u>artemisia</u> (in modern Castilian
<u>artemisa</u>; Ibn Biklaris in Dozy I, 18 also gives the form <u>aršamīsa</u> for the
lavender Stoechas. See also number 3),and was inscribed in this paragraph
by error. The medical usage of this drug is primarily for diseases of
nerves. One finds dried flowers thereof in the bazaars of Cairo (Ducros).

7) IKLĪL AL-MALIK   Melilot (sweet clover)

<u>MAIMONIDES</u>: This is the "tree of love" (<u>šagarat al-hubb</u>); its Berberic
name is <u>tīrāzan</u>,and this is the <u>dāršāh</u>. It is called
<u>coronilla</u> in Spanish,and consists of two species: one (fol.
76ᵛ) has pods resembling tails of scorpions,and is known
by the name "scorpioid melilot" (<u>iklīl al-malik al-muʿaqrab</u>).
I have learned that the roots imported from Syria,and utilized
as theriac (antidote) against the bite of venomous animals,
and known by the name of "serpent root" (<u>ʿirq al-hayya</u>),are
the roots of this species of melilot.

<u>MEYERHOF</u>: [Theophrastus VII 15, 3; Dioscorides III, 40; Serapion 21;
Ghafiqi 30; Ibn al-Beithar 128; <u>Tuhfa</u> 4; ʿAbd ar-Razzāq 2;
Issa 116, 20; Loew II, 465.]

The Melilotus officinales L. was in usage as an emollient since the Greek epoch, until our time. Its Arabic name signifies "royal crown", and it is derived from the Syriac and Hebrew kĕlīl malkā. I have come across the Berberic name, under the term tizara, in (the writings of) the oculist Muhammad al Ghafiqi. (Meyerhof, M. Le Guide d'oculistique de Mohammad ibn Qassoum ibn Aslam al-Ghafiqi of the 12th Cent. Barcelona 1933, p. 178.) The Persian name dār-šāh is not found in the dictionaries, but one does find šāh-afsar (Vullers II, 393). The arabicized Spanish name (frequently corrupted fur-fulia or qornulia) coronilla real (modern Castilian would be corona de rey) is the translation from the Arabic (Simonet 135-136). One cultivated the melilot in Spain (Ibn ʿAwwām II, 309 ff).

The "scorpioid melilot" may be one of the following papilionaceous plants: Coronilla scorpioïdes KOCH, Scorpiurus, or Ornithopus, all of which have pods resembling tails of scorpions, and were employed against the sting of this animal (Dragendorff 324). The "serpent root" mentioned by Maimonides is, according to Issa (1224), that of the verticil myriophyllum (family Haloragidaceae).

8) IDHIR   Schoenus

MAIMONIDES: It is well known to us in Maghrib under the name "straw
            of Mecca" (tibn Makka), and its flower (spike) is the gawz ginā.
MEYERHOF: [Theophrastus IX, 7; Dioscorides I, 17; Serapion 9; Ghafiqi 2;
          Ibn al-Beithar 29; Tuhfa 34; ʿAbd ar-Razzāq 9; Issa 16, 16;
          Ducros I; Loew I, 694 ff.]

This drug is one of the graminaceae, Andropogon Schoenanthus L. or Andropogon Laniger Desf. (odorous rush, straw of Mecca, etc.), whose root is astringent. It is still sold in the bazaars of Cairo (Ducros). Ğawz ǧīnā

is a corruption of the Persian name of the plant gōr giāh (grass of the
evening primrose) (Vullers II, 1044).

9) ATL   Tamarisk with gallnuts

   MAIMONIDES: This tree is well known by this name in Egypt. It is the"green-
            ish one" (an-naddār), and the simsār, although one also says
            that the simsār is the wood of box trees (hasab al-baqs).The
            oriental tamarisk (atl) is one species of tamarisk (tarfā);
            its kernels (habb al-atl) are those that the people of Egypt
            call"the savory" (al-adba).

   MEYERHOF: [Theophrastus V 4, 8 myrikè; Dioscorides I, 89 akakallis;
            Serapion 43; Ghafiqi 6; Ibn al-Beithar 17; Tuhfa 23;'Abd ar-Razzāq
            21; Issa 177, 2; Loew III, 398 ff; Ducros 56.]

      Atl is the Arabic name of a tree of North Africa and Arabia (called)
   Tamarix articulate Vahl. (Tamarix orientalis Forsk), It is an ancient
   Semitic name, in Assyrian aslu, Egyptian'sr copte oci (see Keimer Die
   Gartenpflanzen, etc., vol. 1, p. 56, #109 ff and p. 155), Hebrew eshel.
   The tree does not produce any fruits, and its "kernels" or "fruits" are
   nothing but gallnuts provoked by the sting of a cynips. One sells the
   gallnuts of the tamarisk (tamr el-atl) in the bazaars of Cairo (Ducros 56).
   They are reddish pieces, rich in tannin, employed as an astringent and
   depurative remedy, and also as a coriaceous substance. Maimonides here
   fails to mention two names frequently employed to describe these gall-
   nuts: the Persian kasmāzak (see below number 200) and the Berber takkawt
   (Tuhfa 23). The name tarfā designates the tamarisk in general,and in particular Tamarisk gallica and Tamarisk nilotica BGE.   (Schweinfurth 45).
   Simsār is the Persian name of a young sprout of the boxtree (Vullers II,463).

10) ĀS   Myrtle

    MAIMONIDES: Its most widely known name by the people of Maghrib is

                ar-ra'ihān and by the people of Egypt al-marsīn.

    MEYERHOF: [Theophrastús I, 10-14 etc., (myrrhine); Dioscorides I, 122,

              (myrsine); Serapion 13; Ghafiqi 9; Ibn al-Beithar 69;

              Tuhfa II, 272; 'Abd ar-Razzāq II; Issa 122,19; Loew II,

              257-274, (very important!); Ducros 4.]

    Ās is derived from the Semitic name of the Myrtus communis L.,
in Assyrian āsu, in Aramaic āsā. The Hebrew name hadas is found, among
others, in the Hebrew works of Maimonides (Loew II, 258). Ra'ihān in
Arabic means "odoriferous" and in general designates the basil (plants).
Marsīn is obviously the Arabic transcription of the Greek name myrsine.

11) UŠNA   Flowery lichen, etc.

    MAIMONIDES: This is the "gray hair of old age" (šaibat al-'agūz) and
one also says   simply aš-šaiba.

    MEYERHOF: [Theophrastus III 8, 6 (phaskos); Dioscorides I, 21 (bryon);

              Serapion 48; Ghafiqi 3; Ibn al-Beithar 85; Tuhfa 59;

              'Abd ar-razzaq 10 and 979; Issa 186, 13; Loew 23 ff.]

    The Arabic name ušna comes from the Ayriac šantā and today de-
signates all sorts of mosses and lichens sprouting on the bark of trees.
In Egypt, one sells at least eight types at the bazaars; one uses it as
a substitute for yeast in the making of bread (J. Müller. Revue Mycologique,
Dec. 1881 and G. Schweinfurth, Archiv. f. Wirtschaftsforsch. im Orient
1-2, 1918). They are primarily Ochrolechia, Lecanora esculenta and
Usnea florida HOFFM.)

12) AQĀQIYĀ   Acacia juice (gum arabic)

MAIMONIDES: This is the juice of the acacia pod (qarad); this pod
            is the fruit of the gum tree (sant), which is well known
            in Egypt. I will speak thereof under the letter sīn.

MEYERHOF: [Theophrastus I, 2 (akantha); Dioscorides I, 101 (akakia);
          Serapion 6; Ibn al-Beithar 1735 and 1758; Issa 22; Loew
          II, 377-391; Ducros 143]

   Akakia in Dioscorides designates the tree; to the Arabs it is the
juice of its fruits. It is employed as an astringent remedy in medicine,
as well as by the tanners and curriers of Cairo (Ducros 29 and 143).
The tree in question is the mimosa of Egypt (Acacia arabica Willd. var.
nilotica Del) which will be discussed in number 278.

13) IĠĠAS   Plum

MAIMONIDES: Its most familiar name to us in Maghrib is al-burqūq;
            the inhabitants of Spain also call it ʿuyun al-baqar
            ("eyes of beef"). It is aš-šāhalük, and it is also
            termed aš-šahalūǧ.

MEYERHOF: [Theophrastus I, 10-13 etc. (kokkymelon); Dioscorides I,
          12; Serapion 32 and 274; Ghafiqi 10; Ibn al-Beithar 21;
          Tuhfa 45; ʿAbd ar-Razzāq 26; Issa 149, 1: Loew II, 163-169.]

   The fruit of Prunus domestica L. was called barqūq in Maghrib
(from the Greek praï-or brekokkia which Dioscorides I, 115 designates
as the apricot) (from the Latin praecox. See Langkavel p. 5). Today,
everywhere, it is the Arabic name for the plum. The names šāh-lūk and
šāh-lūg are Persian, and refer to a sort of large white plum (Dozy I,
178 and Kohen p. 136). Regarding the cultivation of the plum tree in
Spain, see Ibn ʿAwwam I, 319-321.

14) ANGURA   Roman nettle and others

MAIMONIDES: It is habb an-nisā (kernels of women); one calls it

al-qurrais and in Maghrib al-hurraiq; in Spanish (fol.

77) anifis. It is the nabāt an-nār (the "plant of

fire"); there are two species, one white and one black.

MEYERHOF: [Theophrastus VII, 7,2 (akalyphé); Dioscorides IV, 93 (akaléphé);

Serapion 272; Ghafiqi 74; Ibn al-Beithar 165; Tuhfa 10;

ʿAbd ar-Razzāq 26; Issa 186, 6; Loew III, 479-481.]

Angura designates different species of nettle,(including) the

small nettle (Urtica urens L.), and above all the Roman nettle (Urtica

pilulifera.L.); their seeds are still sold to this day in the bazaars

of Cairo as diuretics and emollients (Ducros 17). Qurrais and hurraiq

designate "that which burns". Anifis is probably a corruption of

akaléphé, or perhaps of orticax (Simonet 410). The Spanish name today

is ortiga. Ghafiqi (ms. fol. 40a) has artalīqā.

15) AZFĀR AT-TĪB   Ungues Odorati (Fragrant nails;
                                        Byzantine cockroaches)

MAIMONIDES: This is al-fāʾih ("the fragrant one")

MEYERHOF: [Dioscorides II, 8 (onyx); Serapion 44; Ghafiqi 111;

Ibn al-Beithar 104; ʿAbd ar-Razzāq 52; Ducros 152.]

This drug is constituted by (using) the opercula of gastropods

(Murex inflatus, Strombus lentiginosus, Pleurotoma Babyloniae etc.),

which vaguely remind one of nails or claws. When fresh, these opercula

emit an odor of spikenard. One still sells them in the bazaars of

Cairo (Ducros) as laxatives, and for fumigation.

16) ANAGALIS   Pimpernel

    MAIMONIDES: It is the 'uśbat al-'alaq (the "blood sucking herb"), and
               one also calls it ādān al-fār ("ears of a mouse"). There
               are two species, one is the one which is called cardenella
               in Spain, and which has blue blossoms. The other has red
               blossoms, and is the one which one calls naśanitāla.

    MEYERHOF: [Dioscorides II, 178; Ghafiqi 18; Ibn al-Beithar 197; Tuhfa
               3,8; 'Abd ar-Razzāq 58; Issa 14, 12; Loew III, 77.]

    This plant is the primulacea Anagallis, of which one species has
blue blossoms, the Anagallis caerulea ALL.(field pimpernel), and
another (species) has red blossoms, the Anagallis arvensis L. (red
pimpernel). The name ādān al-fār, which also designates the myosotis
(forget-me-not; mouse ear), was amply discussed by Renaud and Colin
(Tuhfa 3). I   add that, according to Loew, this translation from
the Greek anagallis derives from Hunain b. Ishāq, who added the adjective nabatī ("nabatean"). The Spanish names are mentioned by
Simonet (102). Naśanitāla is the Arabic corruption of the ancient
Hispanic la xintella.

17) AMĪRBĀRĪS   Barberry

    MAIMONIDES: One also calls it barbārīs. It is atwān and as-sawsal;
               its Persian name is az-zaraśk; one also says zaratk.

    MEYERHOF: [Serapion 17; Ghafiqi 15; Ibn al-Beithar 146; Tuhfa 18;
               'Abd ar-Razzāq 54; Issa 30,18; Loew I, 287 ff; Ducros 164.]

    The plant in question, Berberis vulgaris L, is not mentioned in
the Greek works of botany. The reading amīrbāris is a frequent
corruption of ambarbāris, a name whose origin has not been elucidated

(? from the Syriac). Zirišk is the Persian name of the kernels (fruits) of the plant; it is found in medical books of the Syrian vernacular. Atwān seems to be an error of the copyist for atwār or atrār (Issa), and Sawsal is only known as the name of another plant, Anarrhinum orientale BTH. (Issa 15,5). Maimonides does not make mention of the Berberic name of the drug, argis, a name which is well known in Morocco. The root of Berberis is still for sale in the bazaars of Cairo under the name ʿūd ar-rīh ("odoriferous wood"), and the fruits are sold as astringents under the name tamr al-amīrbārīs (Ducros 57 and 164).

18) ANĞUDĀN   Leaves of asafoetida

MAIMONIDES: This name is applicable to the leaves of the plant whose
              resin is called al-hiltīt (asafoetida).

MEYERHOF: [Theophrastus VI, 3 etc; Dioscorides III, 80; Serapion 30
             and 37; Ghafiqi 34; Ibn al-Beithar 158; Tuhfa 14;
             ʿAbd ar-Razzāq 55; Issa 82, 8; Dymock II, 147 ff; Ducros
             89; Loew III 452-455.]

The plant in question is the umbelliferous Ferula asafoetida L. (Ferula Scorodosma BENTH, and HOOK), and others, the silphion of the Greeks. As to the latter, the Arabs had different names for the parts of the plant which were used as drugs. We will find it again below in number 31. In Egypt and in Syria, the resin is called abū kabīr. Asafoetida, the fetid gum resin employed against hysteria and nervous afflictions, carries the name hiltīt. The name anğudān is the Arabic form of the Persian anğudān or anguyān. I think that this name is related to the Sanskrit hingu (Chopra 171).

19) ANĪSŪN   Anise

MAIMONIDES: This is the seed of the "Roman fennel" (rāziyāniǧ rumī);
            it is the same as that which the people of Maghrib know
            under the name "sweet grain" (ḥabba ḥulwa), and it is the
            "sweet cumin" (al-kammūn al-ḥulw).

MEYERHOF: [Theophrastus I, 12,1; Dioscorides III, 56; Serapion 35;
          Ghafiqi 32; Ibn al-Beithar 159; Tuhfa 33; 'Abd ar-Razzāq
          23; Issa 140, 5; Ducros 12; Loew III, 468.]

The Greek name ánison is probably derived from the ancient Egyptian;
the plant Pimpinella anisum L. appears to have originated from Egypt
and from Cyprus. The seeds are sold in Cairo under the name of yansūn
(Ducros). The cultivation of the two types of anise in Musulman Spain
was described by Ibn 'Awwam (II, 249 ff). In certain Indian dialects
(Bombay), the name of the drug today is still erva-dos, from the
Portuguese herva doce (Dymock II, 131).

20) UQHUWĀN   Matricaria (feverfew) and varieties

MAIMONIDES: This is what is called in Arabic al-qurrās, and in Spanish
            poplinaira; one also calls it manzanilla and ǧašūniš
            (guijones).

            This herb resembles the camomile (bābūnaǧ), and there are
            several species, colored white and yellow. The name of
            the white one in Greek is amárakon, and that of the yellow
            one amáranton.

MEYERHOF: [Theophrastus VII, 7,2; Dioscorides III, 138; Serapion 7;
          Ghafiqi 48; Ibn al-Beithar 121; Tuhfa 25; 'Abd ar-Razzāq
          53,58,187; Issa 48,6; Ducros 9; Loew I, 375-378.]

This has to do with the compound (plant) Chrysanthemum Parthenium
Pers., and of several related species, corresponding to the parthénion
of the Greeks. The Spanish name manzanilla most likely designates the
camomile (Anthemis, see number 39), whereas the name of the matricaria
is magarzo or magarzuela (Simonet 325 and 343). The other Spanish
name poplinaira and guijones have been explained by Simonet (257 and
456). The name Uqhuwān is derived from the Persian Ākahwān(Vullers I, 113).
The tops of the Chrysanthemum Parthenium Pers. are sold by Egyptian
druggists as sudorifics under the name Uqhuwān bābūnig and karkās
(Ducros). The cultivation of the camomile in desert lands, cultivation which requires very little irrigation, was in use in Spain, and
is found described in Ibn Awwam (II,309 ff.).

21) ĀSĀRŪN   Asarum

MAIMONIDES: In Spanish it is ušra (asaro) and one also calls barbāla
            (bobrella).

MEYERHOF: [Dioscorides I, 10; Ghafiqi I; Ibn al-Beithar 61; Tuhfa 36;
            Abd ar-Razzāq 18; Issa 23,15; Loew I,223; Ducros 5.]

This has to do with the rhizome of the aristolochochia Asarum
Europaeum L. (asarum) which is imported into Islamic lands from the
Extreme Orient, India   and from Persia. One still sells it in the
bazaars of Cairo under the name nārdin barrī ("wild nard"). Regarding
the Spanish names cited by Maimonides, one should read asaro and (asara)
bacara (Laguna 18, Simonet, 24). It was a well known emetic prior to
the introduction of the root of ipecac. For the Spanish names, see
Simonet 24 and 32. Barbālla is an error of the copyist, because this
Arabicized Castilian name (bobrella) designates long aristolochia

(Simonet 49). In the text of Ghafiqi (ms. fol. 60a) one finds the writing būyāla.

22) ABHUL   Savin (juniper) and varieties

MAIMONIDES: This is al-'ir'ar and barātwā; there exists (fol. 77ᵛ) one species whose name is "tree of God" (šaǧarat Allāh); and the deodar (ad-dabīdār) is also one of its species.

MEYERHOF: [Dioscorides I, 76; Serapion 2; Ghafiqi 5; Ibn al-Beithar 7; Tuhfa 26; 'Abd ar-Razzāq 16; Issa 102,17; Loew III, 355 ff.]

Abhul is, in general, the Arabic name of the savin juniper (Juniperus Sabina L.);'ar'ar - this is how Arabic dictionaries vocalize it - is that of the common juniper (Juniperus communis L.). The savin is also called the male 'ar'ar. The name barātwā is an Arabic transcription of the Syriac barutā which is derived from the Greek bráthy. Šaǧarat Allāh,"tree of God", is the translation of the Sanskrit name devadāru, which designates the deodar cedar of India (Cedrus Deodara LOUD). In Egypt and in Syria, where the common juniper doesn't exist, one gives the name habb al-'ar'ar to the fruit or to the berry of the cade Juniper (Juniperus oxycedrus L.) which is sold in the bazaars as a diuretic (Ducros 73).

23) AFAÏTIMŪN   Dodder

MAIMONIDES: The most familiar name in Spain is as-su'aïtira (the "little thyme").

MEYERHOF: [Dioscorides IV, 177; Serapion 168; Ghafiqi 80; Ibn al-Beithar 112; Tuhfa 32;'Abd ar-Razzāq 7; Issa 63, 6: Loew I, 453-461.]

This is a well known parasitic plant (Cuscuta Epithymum L.) which

causes devastation in artificial meadows‚by implanting and sustaining
itself upon lucerns, clovers, etc. with the help of its suckers.   The
Arabs have erroneously considered as a special type the dodder which
attacks plants fit for fodder, and have distinguished it from the one
which infests thyme, origan and other similar plants.   See below kušut
at number 186.   The Arabicized Greek name epithymon is usually written
af ītimūn.

24)   UŠNĀN AL-QASSĀRĪN   Fuller's glasswort

MAIMONIDES: This is al-gāsūl‚and in Arabic one calls it al-hamd and
               al-hurd; in Spanish šawka yarbāta; and in Berber tagaīgaīt.
               It is by this last name in particular that it is known in
               Morocco.   Its name in ancient Greek is adárkes.   The burned
               ashes of this plant constitute al-qaly (alkali); I will
               speak thereof in chapter qāf. The vegetable glasswort‚with
               which one washes one's hands‚is well known.

MEYERHOF: [Dioscorides V, 119; Serapion 515; Ghafiqi 76; Ibn al-Beithar
             87; Tuhfa 38; ʿAbd ar-Razzāq 25 and 734; Issa 161, 6; Loew
             I, 645 ff.]

    See the statement of Loew concerning soapy plants in the Orient,
and A. Steiger and J.J.Hess, Soda, in Vox Romanica II (Zurich and Leipzig
1937), pp. 53-76. Gāsūl and hamd are generic names designating vegetables
employed as a substitute for soap, particularly by the desert Bedouins.
Ušnān (al-qassārīn, "fuller's") is the name of Salsola kali L; gāsūl
specifies the Salicornia fruiticosa L.(in modern Egypt, Schweinfurth 61).
Šawka(in Arabic) means "spine, spinous plant"‚and yerbata is a Spanish
corruption, perhaps of herba barbata (Simonet 32 and 616). The Catalonian

name of Salsola Kali is barella espinosa, whereas other halophyte plants
are called gazul or aguazul in Andalusian. The Berberic name should be
pronounced tagirist (Renaud, Tuhfa 225). The identification of the Greek
term adárkês with usnān is erroneous, since Dioscorides designates as
adárkês a crust which forms on the plants by the evaporation of salt waters.
Regarding the subject of qaly, see below at number 345.

25) AFARBIYŪN   Euphorbia (Spurge) Resin

MAIMONIDES: One also calls it furbiyūn. Its Berberic name by which it
            is well known in Maghrib is tākūt. The people in Egypt call
            it lubāna maġribiyya ("Maghribian incense").

MEYERHOF: [Dioscorides III, 82; Serapion 399; Ibn al-Beithar 1673; Tuhfa
          249 and 323; ᶜAbd ar-Razzāq 885; Issa 80, 12; Loew I, 602-607;
          Ducros 173.]

The Arabic name is derived from the Greek euphórbion and designates
the spurges with resin (Euphorbia resinifera Berg.) and other plants which
grow at the southern border of Mount Atlas in Morocco. The precise
Berberic name is not tākūt, as Maimonides and Ibn al-Beithar write it,
but tikiut (Renaud and Colin, according to Tuhfa). Today one sells this
yellow and black resin in the bazaars of Cairo under the name of farbiyūn
or liban maġrabī (Maghribian incense). Very irritating, it is not employed except for external usage as a vesicant (Ducros).

26) ASĀBI ᶜAL-ᶜADĀRĀ   "Fingers of virgins" (a black grape)

MAIMONIDES: This is a black grape with oblong grains which resembles
            painted fingers; it grows in the (valley) Sierra (Sarā).

MEYERHOF: [ʿAbd ar-Razzāq 33; Ibn al-Beithar 93; Issa 190, 6.]

This name is lacking in the majority of treatises on simple drugs, but was known to Kohen (122 last line) and to Freytag (I, 478). Ibn al'Awwam (I, 607) mentions these "fingers of virgins" among the Spanish grapes as a black grape with oblong grains, and describes its cultivation. One introduces the grains of the grape into tubes of seeds, in order to give them an elongated form. In addition, I found in Dozy (I, 816), according to the Muhīt al-Muhīt, that the black grapes were called asābi ʿalʿabd ("fingers of slaves"), and the red ones asābi ʿal-ʿadārā or asābi ʿal-ʿarūs ("fingers of a young married woman"), because they resemble fingers colored with henna on the occasion of Arabic festivals. The Orientalist J. G.Wetzstein, who lived for a long time in the Near East, states in the introduction of a botanical work (K. Koch, Die Bäume and Sträucher des alten Griechenlands - 2nd edit. Berlin 1884 p. XIII): "In Damascus, the dessert of a meal throughout the entire year consists of fresh fruits....in August grapes, particularly the transparent 'fingers of virgins' grapes of delicious tables grown in the gardens of the city." Ibn al-Beithar gives the synonym ʿinab baqari ("grape of beef"), Issa (calls it) ahdāq al-baqar ("sloes of beef"). As to the name sarā, I have translated it Sierra, thinking of the Sierra of Morena, or the Sierra of Cordova, mountains well known to the Arabic Spanish scholars. Nevertheless, this orthography is little used; in general one writes šarā or šārra (Encyclopédie de l'Islam, I, 350; and Simonet 514). Al-Idrisi (Edrisi. Description de l'Afrique et de l'Espagne. ed. Dozy and De Goeje. Leyden 1866 p. 71 of the French text) states that the grape ʿadārā was, in his epoch (12th century), a product of Sūs Aqsā in the south of Morocco.

27) ITMID   Stibium (sulfide of antimony)

MAIMONIDES: There exist mines thereof in Maghrib and in the Orient.

The one which is found in Maghrib is called Ruhl az-zurqa

("dry dark collyrium") by the Maghribians, and the one which

is found in the Orient is called Ruhl isbahānī ("dry colly-

rium from Ispahan").

MEYERHOF: [Dioscorides V, 84; Galen XII, 236; Serapion 17; Ghafiqi

106; Ibn al-Beithar 18; ʽAbd ar-Razzāq 20; Ducros 197.]

The substance in question is Stibium (native antimony); its princi-

pal minerals are stibium (sulfide of antimony) and palmated galena

(antimony sulfide of lead). The Greek names stibi (Dioscorides) and

stimmi (Galen) and the ancient Latin stibium, as well as the Arabic

itmid or atmud, and its medieval Latin corruption antimonium are, in the

final analysis, derived from ancient Egyptian s.d.m.y. (copte CTHM stim).

One has found this black painted collyrium in many tombs of ancient

Egypt, and one still sells it in our times in the bazaars of Cairo under

the name kohl hagar, kohl iswid, kohl galā, etc. (Ducros). The mines of

galena of Tortosa in Spain (from al-Maqqari, according to Levi-Provencal.

L'Espagne Musulmane au Xe siècle, Paris 1932, p. 177) were esteemed, and

probably furnished the Maghribian kohl. But the best kohl came from the

mines of Kirmān (Southern Persia). P. Guigues (Serapion 17) speaks of its

preparation and of the sophistication of kohl in Syria.

28) USRUNG   Minium (red lead)

MAIMONIDES: This is al-basaliqūn and one also calls it sāliqūn. Its

most widely known name in Maghrib is az-zarqūn; it is

"burnt lead" (rasās muhraq).

MEYERHOF: [Dioscorides V 88b; Galen XII, 235; Serapion 5 and 42;

Ghafiqi 110; Ibn al-Beithar 74; Tuhfa 54; ʿAbd ar-Razzāq 853.]

Minium is a mixture of the oxide and peroxide of lead, and has a red color. The names isranğ, isrinğ, sirinğ, sāliqūn, sarīqūn, etc. are Persian (Vullers I, 97), but are derived from the Greek syrikón. (Nevertheless, Dozy and de Goeje derive this name from the Persian āzarqun or "color of flame". See Edrisi's Description de l'Afrique et de l'Espagne, Leyden 1866 p. 312 ff.). Azarcon is still today the Spanish name of minium. The Greek name (Dioscorides) was sándyx. One produced the minium by burning ceruse, of which we will be concerned below in number 29. See also number 32.

29) ISFĪDĀĞ   Ceruse (white lead)

MAIMONIDES: It is also called isbidāğ ar-rasās; it is al-bāruq ("the

glittering"), and its name among the people (fol. 78ʿ) is

al-bayād ("the white").

MEYERHOF: [Dioscorides V 88a; Galen XII, 243; Serapion 14; Ghafiqi 109;

Ibn al-Beithar 73; Tuhfa 37; ʿAbd ar-Razzāq 22.]

This drug is the white of ceruse, basic carbonate of lead. The Arabic name derives from the Persian sapid ab ("white water or lotion") also written isfidāb, safīd āb, sapidāğ, safīdāğ, etc. (Vullers I, 98 and 216). It is interesting to mention that the popular name of ceruse noted by Maimonides has survived until our days in Spain in the form albayalde (in Portuguese alvaiade).

30) INFĪHA   Rennet

MAIMONIDES: This is al-'aqid ("rennet"), and its name among the people

of Maghrib is al-yanaq.

MEYERHOF: [Dioscorides II, 75; Galen XII, 274; Serapion 36; Ghafiqi 112; Ibn al-Beithar 172 and 2322; Tuhfa 44; ʿAbd ar-Razzāq 24.]

One is dealing with stomach rennet of young ruminants, called pitya by the Greeks. The name yanaq is also encountered in Ibn al-Beithar (2322) who designates it as an Andalusian term. (Ghafiqi, ms. fol. 56a also vocalizes al-yanaq, but he doesn't touch the subject of the origin of this name.) Nevertheless, it is difficult to find its origin, the modern Spanish name being cuajo.

31) USTURGĀZ   Root of asafetida

MAIMONIDES: It is said that this is the root of the levage (al-kāšim), and it is also said that this is the root of the asafetida (al-hiltīt).

MEYERHOF: [Theophrastus III, 1-2; Dioscorides III, 80; Ghafiqi 36; Ibn al-Beithar 84; Issa 82,8; Loew III, 455.]

This last designation is more exact. The term usturgāz derives from the Persian šuturgāz ("camel pasture"), and is applicable to many plants. It is often confused with ušturhār ("camel thorn") which designates certain thistles and spinous plants. Ušturgāz is perhaps the equivalent of "other magydaris" mentioned by Dioscorides at the end of his paper. See above number 18.

32) UBBĀR   Lead

MAIMONIDES: This is ar-rasās, al-usrub, al anuk and al-qalaʿi.

MEYERHOF: [Dioscorides I, 98 and V, 81; Serapion 185 and 412; Ibn al-Beithar 13 and 1042; Tuhfa 39, ʿAbd ar-Razzāq 29 and 30.]

In dictionaries this word is vocalized abbār or ābār. This word designates "black lead" or burnt or calcinated lead (lead sulfide),

which is mentioned by the majority of Arabic medical authors by the name
rasās muhraq or usrub. The word rasās sometimes means tin; qala'i always
means that. This latter term is derived from the name Qala', a town on
the western coast of the peninsula of Malacca, from which the Musulman
merchants imported tin into the lands of the Occident. See above paragraph 28 (usrung̈).

33) ANDRĀSIYŪN   Peucedanum (porc fennel)

MAIMONIDES: It is also called g̈ahanīk; it is the one which is known to us
under the name yarba tūra (yerva tora).

MEYERHOF: [Theophrastus IX, 14-20; Dioscorides III, 78; Serapion 240;
Ghafiqi 33; Ibn al-Beithar 176 and 2310; Tuhfa 211; Issa
137, 5; Loew III, 465.]

This plant is the "porc fennel", peukédanon of the Greeks, the
Ombelliferous Peucedanum officinale L. The Arabicized name andrasion
is undoubtedly derived from the Greek, but one has not yet identified its
origin. The name g̈ahanīk seems to be Persian (giyāh-i-namnak? Steingass
p. 1108). Its spelling reminds one of the name g̈ablahank (Ghafiqi 212)
which, however, refers to the sesamoid (Reseda alba L.).

The Spanish name is found in Tuhfa under the more correct form
yarbātun which is derived from the Latin herbatum (Simonet 617). Laguna
(323) gives the Castilian and Catalonian forms, yervatun and herbatur
(respectively), whereas the modern Castilian name is ervato (Botica 831).
The herbaceous part of the plant was used as an anti-hysteric.

34) ĪRASĀ   Blue iris

MAIMONIDES: One also calls it Īras. Physicians specifically designate
by this name the azure lily (as-sawsan al-asumāng̈unī).

MEYERHOF: [Theophrastus I, 7 and VI, 8; Dioscorides I, 1; Serapion 487; Ibn al-Beithar 216; Tuhfa 28; ʿAbd ar-Razzāq 31; Issa 100,12; Loew II, 1-4; Ducros 108.]

It is the Iris florentina L. The vocalization īrasā and īras is little used in Arabic as transcription from the Greek iris. The term asumānǧūnī is derived from the Persian asumān-gūn, "blue sky". The name īrisā is borrowed from Aramaic. In the Jewish-Aramaic dialect of Palestine, one said īrūsa (from the Greek genitive ireos). The rhisome of the iris is sold in the bazaars of Cairo under the name gidr el-banafsig ("root of violet") and ʿiro et-tīb ("fragrant root") or gurmet el-banafsig. It is used as a detergent and emmenagogue (Ducros). See below article 272.

35) UFIYŪN   Opium

MAIMONIDES: This is a remedy with very celebrated virtues, and known by this name. Certain types of people call it al-marqad(instead of al-murqid, "the soporific"). It is the dried milky juice of the black poppy; it resembles robs (concentrated juices of fruits).

MEYERHOF: [Theophrastus I, 12,2; Dioscorides IV, 64; Serapion 502; Ibn al-Beithar 116 and 2120; Tuhfa 40; ʿAbd ar-Razzāq 12; Issa 134,7; Loew II, 364-370; Ducros 8.]

The orthograph ufiyūn instead of afiyūn is unusual, but it corresponds better to the Greek ópion whose transcription produced the Arabic word.

The Palestinian Talmud mentions opium under the name opion. The cultivation of poppy (Papaver somniferum L.), as well as the production of opium, has since a long time been prohibited in Egypt where it bloomed,

particularly in the desert of Thebe, until the beginning of the nineteenth century. Opium was introduced and sold secretly, particularly in
the form of aromatic electuaries known by the name manzul,but less and
less, as a result of police surveillance. Kohen (p. 128, line 12) states
that,in his epoch (13th century),the best opium was prepared in Abu Tig
in Upper Egypt.

36) UMĀLĪ   Eleomel (oil of honey)

MAIMONIDES: This is something which flows from the trunk of a tree in
           Palmyra, much thicker than honey. It is what one calls
           duhn al-ʿasal ("oil of honey, eleomel").

MEYERHOF: [Dioscorides I, 31; Ibn al-Beithar 137; ʿAbd ar-Razzāq 57.]

   The Arabic name is alaūmālī, exact transcription from the Greek
elaíomeli, given by Ibn al-Beithar. Maimonides seems to have taken the
first syllable al for the Arabic clause and suppressed it. Dioscorides
states that eloeomel is an oily excretion which flows from the trunks
of olive trees near the oasis of Palmyra in Syria. Arabic physicians do
not seem to have given an exact description of this substance,but simply
copied the clause from Dioscorides. According to Bathandier (Bulletin
Commercial, March 1901), in 1900 near Mansoura (al-Mansura, Lower Egypt),
there were many olive trees which, during the summer, secreted an oily
substance called by the natives ʿasal zaitun ("honey of olive tree");
that was a pathologic excretion caused by insects and containing 52%
mannite (sugar of manna). Kohen (p. 139, line 30) gives the additional
name ʿasal Dāwūd ("honey of David") to eleomel. See the paper by Hooper
and Field on the "honey of the willow" (p. 168).

37) ADNĀB AL-HAÏL("horse's tails")   Salsify (goat's beard)

MAIMONIDES: This plant is also called "goat's beard" (lihyat al-taïs);
it is not the cynomorium (al-tarātīt), but it seems to be
a type of aviculary (quddāb), much smaller than the latter.

MEYERHOF: [Theophrastus VII, 7,1; Dioscorides III, 43; Serapion 151;
Ibn al-Beithar 2014; Tuhfa 199 and 428; 'Abd ar-Razzāq 407;
Issa 182, 4.]

There is in this name an element of confusion. To all the Arabic
writers the singular danab al-haïl ("horse's tail") designates the horsetail (Equisetum), the Arabic name being the translation of the Greek
(hippouris) and Latin names. The synonym lihyat at-taïs is nevertheless
in usage for the salsifys of the meadow (Eragopogon pratensis L.), whose
Greek name was also translated into Arabic ("goat's beard"). The comparison with the aviculary (Polygonum aviculare.L:) proves that Maimonides
was considering the salsify of the meadow, although the latter is a compound (plant), whereas the aviculary appertains to the family of Polygonacea.
That which is sold today in the bazaars of Cairo under the name lihyat
et-taïs is neither one nor the other, but the herb of the meadow sweet
(Spiraea Ulmaria L.), a rosaceous plant that one uses as a vulnerary and
sudorific tonic (Ducros 205).

CHAPTER BĀ'

38) BISBĀSA   Mace

    MAIMONIDES: This is ad-darkīsā, and according to some manuscripts,
               darkīsī; it is al-ğārkun and it is said that it is at-
               tālisfir.

    MEYERHOF: [Serapion 83 and 489; Ibn al-Beithar 281 and 464, 846 and
               1443; ʿAbd ar-Razzāq 131; Issa 122, 6; Loew II, 60-62;
               Ducros 37.]

Mace is the false aril or arillode of the nut of the nutmeg tree
(Myristica fragrans Houtt.) The name bisbāsa or bisbās in Spain designated (in the past) and today in Morocco designates the fennel. (Tuhfa
358 and Dozy I). In Cairo, it always had the name mace (Ducros 37).
Dār-kisā is its Persian name passed into Syriac, and from there into
Arabic pharmacology, whereas ğārkūn is the Arabicized form of the Persian
čārgūn ("four colors?") (Vullers I, 498 and 786). Tālisfar was considered a Greek word (telésphoron) which was passed into Persian, and
which designated the peel of the root of an Indian tree ("olive tree"),
which was employed against intestinal hemorrhages and dysentery (Vullers
II, 529). It was identified by Hunain, translator of the Materia Medica
of Dioscorides, as makir (Dioscorides I, 82) and the latter by other
Arabic writers as mace, an opinion contested by Al-Ghafiqi and others
(confusion between macis and macer).It is Dymock (III, 373 ff) who has
proven that the name tālisfar is derived from the Sanskrit word tālīsa-
pattra and designates the branches of the common yew (Taxus baccata L.),
known as a venemous drug of India. However, Chopra (p. 560) states
that in India, under the name tālis-patra, druggists sell

the leaves and the shoots of many other plants, as for example, the
Abies webbiana Lindi. See also number 212.

39) BĀBŪNAǦ   Camomile and varieties

MAIMONIDES: One also says bābūnak and bābūnaq. This is the "flower
            (apple) of the earth" (fuqqāh al-ard) and the "sweet basil
            of beef" (habaq al-baqar). Its Spanish name is mašanālla
            (manzanilla) and its Greek name khamaímelon (fol. 78ᵛ)and
            also khamaímêlís. It has both yellow flowers and white
            flowers.

MEYERHOF: [Theophrastus VII 8, 3; Dioscorides III, 137; Serapion 144;
            Ghafiqi 151; Ibn al-Beithar 220; Tuhfa 86, ʿAbd ar-Razzāq
            53 and 123; Issa 18, 5; Loew I, 375-378.]

It is above all the Roman camomile (Anthemis nobilis L.). The name bābūna
(from which the others are derived) is Persian. Fuqqāh al-ard is probably
an error of the copyist for tuffāh al-ard ("apple of the land" i.e.
potato), translation of the Greek khamaímélon. Ibn al-Beithar gives the
Spanish name maqārǧa; this is magarza, Castilian name of Matricaria, as
we have seen in number 20. Anthemis nobilis does not grow in Egypt.
The herb is imported and sold in the bazaars by the name babūnig or ših
babūnig (Meyerhof 269). It is often confused with the feverfew (Ducros 6).
Various species of camomile were cultivated in Spain as medical plants
(Ibn ʿAwwam II, 309 ff).

40) BĀDRANǦŪYA   Melissa (balm)

MAIMONIDES: One also says bādranbūya. It is a type of fragrant plant which we call "lemony basilisk" (habaq turungī) because its aroma

is like that of the lemon. In Egypt one calls it at-turungān

("lemony"), and its Persian name is marmāhūr.

MEYERHOF: [Theophrastus VI, 1,4; Dioscorides III, 104; Serapion 64; Ghafiqi

145; Ibn al-Beithar 221; Tuhfa 72; ʿAbd ar-Razzāq 123; Issa 117,

4; Loew II, 75.]

This plant is the labiate Melissa officinalis L., known to the Greeks

by the names melissophyleon and melittaïna. Its synonyms in Arabic are

very numerous (see Ibn al-Beithar, Ghafiqi and Issa). Maimonides only gives

the names of Persian origin: bādrang-būya signifies "odor of lemon", turungān

"lemony". Marmāhūr is not the Persian name of the melissa, but that of another

labiate, probably the "Egyptian origan" (Origanum maru L.). The latter erron-

eously carries its French name, because it doesn't exist in Egypt. In Spain,

many species of melissa were known and even cultivated. They were used to

attract the bees to their hives (Ibn ʿAwwam II, 273-275). One of the French

names of melissa is "piment des ruches" (pimento of hives). The Arabicized

Persian names of the melissa have survived in the Spanish vernacular:

bedarangi, albedarrumbe and torongil (Botica 747).

41) BĀQILLĀ   Bean

MAIMONIDES: This is al-ǧirǧir and its most well-known name in the cities

is al-ful.

MEYERHOF: [Theophrastus III and VIII; Dioscorides II, 105; Serapion 202;

Ghafiqi 127; Ibn al-Beithar 224; Tuhfa 76; ʿAbd ar-Razzāq 155;

Issa 189,1; Loew II, 501-503.]

The marsh bean (Vicia faba L.), kyamos Hellēnikós of the Greeks, was

cultivated in Egypt since the earliest times; it has been found at prehistoric

sites. One of its Egyptian names p.r, Coptic <u>fel</u>, <u>feli</u> (see L. Keimer.
<u>Sur Quelques Petits Fruits en Faience Emaillée datant du Moyen Empire</u>,
<u>in Bull. de l'Inst. Franc. d'Arch. Orientale du Caire</u>, Vol. 28, 1929,
pp. 86 ff) was transferred into Aramaic <u>fula</u> and into Arabic. The bean
is today called <u>fūl</u> in all of North Africa, in Syria and in Palestine.
The other name <u>bāqilā</u> or <u>bāqillā</u> seems to be of Aramaic origin (Fraenkel
139), but this term is not at all encountered in the Syrian literature.
Ibn 'Awwam (II, 81-89) discusses at length the cultivation of the bean
in Spain.

42) <u>BULLŪT</u>   Oak acorn

<u>MAIMONIDES</u>: This is what the people of Egypt know by the name <u>tamrat al-</u>
<u>fū'ād</u> ("heart fruit, heart shaped"); its tree is <u>as-sindiyān</u>,
and it is <u>al-qandawār</u>.

<u>MEYERHOF</u>: [Theophrastus III, 3-8 and others; Dioscorides I, 106;
Serapion 326; Ghafiqi 121; Ibn al-Beithar 339; <u>Tuhfa</u> 87 and
370; 'Abd ar-Razzāq 169; Issa 152, 9; Loew I, 621-630;
Ducros 42.]

The vocalization <u>bullūt</u> is found only in Maimonides; everywhere else it
is written <u>ballūt</u>. This name designates the oak and its fruit the acorn;
it is derived from the Aramaic <u>ballūtā</u>. The Hebrew Biblical name of the
acorn is <u>allōn</u>, related to the Assyrian <u>allūnu</u>. In Egypt, the name <u>tamrat</u>
<u>al-fu'ād</u> was still employed in the 16th century by Dāwūd (I, 163), but
is no longer in usage today. In the bazaars one sells the acorns of
<u>Quercus pedunculata</u> EHRENB, under the name of <u>ballūt</u> (Ducros). <u>Sindiyān</u>
is a Persian name which designates different species of oak, particularly

the holm-oak (green oak, Quercus Ilex. L.). The name qandawār, which is
lacking in the other (botanic) dictionaries, is mentioned by Dozy (II,411),
according to Ibn Biklāris, as a synonym for ballūt. The form of this name
is Persian. See below ğaft al-ballūt (aril of the acorn) in number 83.
The Arabic name has been preserved in the modern Spanish vernacular: bellota,
meaning acorn.

43) BUNDUQ   Hazelnut (Corylus Avellana L.)

MAIMONIDES: This is al-ğillawz.

MEYERHOF: [Theophrastus I, 12 and III, 3; Dioscorides I, 125; Serapion

            16; Ghafiqi 198; Ibn al-Beithar 357 and 502; Tuhfa 64;

            'Abd ar-Razzāq 200; Issa 58, 13; Loew I, 616-620.]

   The name bunduq is derived from the Greek (Pontikón karyón, "Pontus nut").
As to the name ğillawz, it is derived from the Persian galūz or ğalūz, corrupt form
of čil-ğuza("forty nut"), which designates the pine or the sapin and its
fruit (Vullers I, 587). From these result the confusions discussed by
Renaud and Colin (Tuhfa p. 64).

44) BĀDĀWARD   Thistle (acanthus)

MAIMONIDES: It is not aš-šukā'ī (wild artichoke, Onopordon Acanthium L.)
             as certain people have considered it; (rather) it is the
             "white thorn" (aš-šawka al-baïdā'), and an-nuqd, and the "wild
             carthamus" (al-'asfur al-barri), and al-marğūn, and one calls
             it in Arabic 'uss(?).

MEYERHOF: [Theophrastus IV, 4,6 (ákorna); Dioscorides III, 12 (akantha

            leukế); Serapion 65; Ghafiqi 143; Ibn al-Beithar 222; Tuhfa

            66; 'Abd ar-Razzāq 163 and 969; Issa 139,17.]

The name of this plant is the Arabic form of the Persian bād-āward
("brought by the wind", probably because the spherical capitulum of this
thistle is rolled by the wind across the plains), and corresponds to the
ákantha leuké ("white thorn") of Dioscorides. Above all, it designates
the common thistle or acanthus (Picnomon Acarna Coss.), but also certain
Carduacea (types of echinops or globe thistle) and other compounded plants
(Carthamus, Picridium). Thus is explained the name of the "wild carthamus"
which is vocalized in our text ʿasfur instead of ʿusfur. Nuqd is the Arabic
name of numerous species of compounded plants (Asteriscus, Carthamus,
Odontospermum, Picridium etc., see Issa, Arabic index p. 21). The other
names have not yet been determined. The name bādāward was transformed
in French into bedegar or bedeguard, a term which designates the gall
produced upon the eglantine (sweetbrier) by the sting of a hymenopteros,
Cynips Rosae.

45) BASAD   Coral

MAIMONIDES: This is the coral (al-marǧān), the same plant. Its Greek
           name is korállion. People are of different opinions re-
           garding the designations al-basad and al-marǧān. Some say
           that the plant itself is al-marǧān, and that al-basad de-
           signates its thin branches; others say that al-basad de-
           signates its roots which spread out in the earth. This
           plant grows at the bottom of the sea.

MEYERHOF: [Dioscorides V, 121; Serapion 56; Ghafiqi 182; Ibn al-Beithar
          282; Tuhfa 73; ʿAbd ar-Razzāq 134; Ducros 215.]

Dioscorides did not clearly express himself regarding the nature of
coral. Pliny and the Arabs took it for a plant which petrifies when one

extracts it from the sea. Until 1677, one of the questions posed at the doctoral examination in pharmacy in Paris was: "is coral a plant?" (Dorveaux. Une thèse de pharmacie, Paris 1901). It was not until 1711, thanks to the researches of naturalist Count Marsigli, that the animal nature of coral (Corallium rubrum Lam.) was definitively established.

The name basad is one of the Arabic forms of the Persian term bussad, bissad or bistām (Vullers I, 239-241). Marğān (vulgar murgan) is Arabic, but is probably derived from (the Greek) margaritēs ("pearl"), according to Dozy II, 578. Concerning the types of coral sold at the bazaars of Cairo, see Ducros numbers 104 and 215.

46) BARDĪ   Papyrus

MAIMONIDES: This is al-hāqī.

MEYERHOF: [Theophrastus IV, 8; Dioscorides I, 86; Serapion 88;
          Ghafiqi 161; Ibn al-Beithar 257; Tuhfa 84; ʿAbd ar-Razzāq
          160; Issa 66, 11; Loew I, 563-575.]

The Cyperus Papyrus L. was one of the characteristic plants of Egypt. Its ancient Egyptian name twf and Coptic šoouf passed into Hebrew sūf. The origin of the Arabic name bardī has not been clarified. The name hāqī and the name hafā' (Issa) appear to me to be mutilations of halfā (Loew I, 567). Today the name birdī in Egypt (where the papyrus no longer exists) designates an aquatic plant, the reedmace Typha augustata B. and C., from which one manufactures mats. Such is also the case, according to Renaud-Colin (Tuhfa), in North Africa.

47) BARANĞMAŠK   Type of basil or mint (Calaminintha
                                                        officinalis?)
MAIMONIDES: One also says falanğamašk and baranğamašk. It is
            al-qaltamān and asābiʿ al-fatayāt (the "fingers of young

maidens"); it is the well known "clove basil" (habaq qaranfulī).

MEYERHOF: [Dioscorides III, 43 (?); Serapion 74; Ibn al-Beithar 1676; Tuhfa 327; 'Abd ar-Razzāq 317 and 714; Issa 127, 1; Loew II, 78ff.]

Ibn al-Beithar or his predecessors identified this drug with the âkinos of Dioscorides, within which one wished to recover Thymus or Calamintha Acinos or the villous basil Ocimum pilosum WILLD. The Arabic name is derived from the Persian, and is explained by Vullers (I, 110) as afrang-mušk ("Frankish musk") or as palang mišk (I, 371) "leopard musk", because of the motley appearance and aromatic odor of the plant. This latter explanation alone was adopted by Laufer (586). Dymock (III, 90) declares that in India palang mišk or birang mišk are the fruits of an unidentified labiate imported from Persia. Schlimmer (367) states that in Persia the name fereng mišk is applicable to the leaves of the labiate Melissa Calamintha L. (Calamintha officinalis Monch.)whose fruit is employed in India as an aphrodisiac (Dragendorff 678). Habaq (plural ahbāq) is the generic name of certain odoriferous labiates (basil, thyme, mint, etc.) and qaranful (qaranful is the popular pronounciation) meaning "clove" designates the aroma of the plant. Qaltamān is undoubtedly an Arabicised form of the Greek kalaminthê. (Dioscorides III 35).

48) BĀDARŪǦ   Large basil

MAIMONIDES: One calls it in Arabic ar-raihān * (fol. 79ʳ); it is al-hawk and al-humāhim and al-habaq an-nabatī (Nabatean basil).

* there is a blank space here in the manuscript, but it is certain that the word raihan or raihan makakī was there

Its Greek name is bāsīlīq (basilikón); this plant is the

basil with the large leaves well known to everybody. It

is known to us (i.e. in Maghrib) under the name of "chamberlain's

cap", tartūr al-hāǧib.

MEYERHOF: [Theophrastus I, 6-7, etc.; Dioscorides II, 141; Serapion 73;

Ghafiqi 144; Ibn al-Beithar 223 and 892; Tuhfa 72 and 179;

'Abd ar-Razzāq 125; Issa 126, 4; Ducros 112; Loew II, 78-83.]

This is the large species of basil (Ocimum Basilicum L.), the well-

known aromatic labiate. The name bādrūǧ or bādrōz is Persian. The

Arabic synonyms given by Maimonides are found in the majority of authors;

for the others see Issa. The name hawk, which comes from the Aramaic

hawkā and passed into Hebrew, is, according to Loew (II, 79), the origin

of the Arabic habaq (see the preceding article). Tartūr is the Arabic

designation of a long and pointed bonnet which was worn by certain func-

tionaries; it reminds one, by the popular name mentioned by Maimonides,

of the form of the flowers of the basil. The arabic name al-habaq is pre-

served in Spanish as albahaca, which designates the large basil.

49) BAHĀR   Buphthalmon (oxeye)

MAIMONIDES: This is al'-arār in Arabic, and it is known to the people

of Maghrib by the name "rose of donkeys" (ward al-hamīr)

and in Spanish raisuttaqa; this is 'ain ahlāh.

MEYERHOF: [Dioscorides III, 139; Serapion 79; Ghafiqi 152; Ibn al- Beithar

365; 'Abd ar-Razzāq 135; Issa 17, 18; Loew I, 370; Ducros 46.]

The name bahār may be Persian ("Springtime") or may be derived from the

Arabic root b.h.r. "sparkling (by its beauty"). The bouphthalmon of the

Greeks and the bahār of the Arabs designated a yellow compound (plant) such as <u>Anthemis arvensis</u> L., <u>Chrysanthemum coronarium</u> L., <u>Anacyclus valentinus</u> L., etc. The cultivation of white buphthalmon in Musulman Spain is described by Ibn ʿAwwām (II 264-265). In modern Spain, the name of the wild camomile is still <u>albihar</u>. In the bazaars of Cairo, one sells by the name <u>bahār</u> the yellow capitula of <u>Anthemis tinctoria</u> L. (Ducros). I cannot explain the Spanish name <u>raisuttaqa</u>,which is corrupted (? <u>raiz rustica</u>); the modern name is <u>manzanilla loca</u>. The nameʿ<u>ain ahlāh</u> is the corruption of a Syriac term that we encounter in Ibn al-Beithar (22) in its correct form ʿ<u>ain aglā</u> which means "open eye". According toʿAbd ar-Razzāq, the name <u>bahār</u> is in usage in Maghrib at the present time for the cultivated narcissa.

50) <u>BAHMAN</u>   Behen root

MAIMONIDES: That which is utilized of this plant is only its root; it
            is for this reason that this name designates this root in
            particular. There are two types, one red and one white.
            The name of white behen in Spanish is <u>yerba šāna</u>. As re-
            gards the red (behen), it does not grow in the Maghrib but
            in the land of <u>al-ʿIrāq</u> (Mesopotamia).

MEYERHOF: [Ghafiqi 639; Serapion 283; Ibn al-Beithar 367; <u>Tuhfa</u> 71;
           ʿAbd ar-Razzāq 132; Issa 45, 13 and 174, 10; Ducros 47.]

    Ghafiqi has already remarked that a discussion arose among Arab
writers concerning this plant. He himself describes three different
types whose roots were used as <u>bahman</u>. This latter name is Persian and
designates the month of January,during which this root is unearthed
and eaten (Dymock II, 303). The white behen is still sometimes sold in
the bazaars of Cairo. It is, according to Ducros, the root of the composite <u>Centaurea Behen</u> L. The nature of red behen has not been established.

- 39 -

The majority of modern writers are in favor of the plumbaginaceous
Statice Limonium L., but this opinion is contested by Loew (III,68).
The Spanish name yerba sana designates a type of mint (Simonet 616).
See the discussion of this question by Meyerhof-Sobhy (Ghafiqi) and
Renaud-Colin (Tuhfa).

51) BAWRAQ   mineral soda, impure natron

MAIMONIDES: It is a type of natron (natrūn), one of the salts that
            form in Egypt. Armenian soda (bawraq armīnī) is the
            cream of the soda; it is superior to the other.

MEYERHOF: [Dioscorides V, 113; Serapion 61; Ghafiqi 188; Ibn al-
           Beithar 381; Tuhfa 92; ʿAbd ar-Razzāq 137; Ducros 232.]

   The name bawraq is derived from the Persian bawra or bura and designates both the borate of soda as well as the crude natron which de-
posits itself on the shores of the lakes of Wādi Natrūn in Egypt. One
also finds it in the province of Behera (lower Egypt) and in el-Kāb
(upper Egypt). (See A. Lucas, The Occurrence of Natron in Ancient
Egypt, in Journal of Egyptian Archaelogy Vol. 18: 62-66, 1932.) This
natron, impure carbonate of soda, was designated by the ancient Egyptians
by the word n.t.r.y. See Erman's Wörterbuch, p. 90 (Hebrew neter) from
which is derived its Greek name nitron which passed into the Arabic
language. The Arabic bawraq simultaneously designates saltpetre and
borate of soda. This term passed into Latin in the form borax (Cf.No.383).

52) BAZRQUTŪNĀ   Psyllium (fleawort)

MAIMONIDES: This is asfiyūs, and its name in Spanish is bsīl (psillio).

MEYERHOF: [Dioscorides IV, 69; Serapion 62; Ghafiqi 163; Ibn al-
           Beithar 278; Tuhfa 55, 69; ʿAbd ar-Razzāq 87 and 138;
           Issa 143, 4; Loew III, 63; Ducros 36.]

These are the seeds (bazr, bizr) of the "herb of fleas" (Plantago
psyllium L.) known to the Greeks by the name psyllion (from psylla,
flea), because its brown seeds resemble fleas or bugs. Hence the Syriac
name qtōnā ("bug") from which is derived the Arabic name. As to the
name asfiyūs, I accept the explanation of Vullers (I, 901, 99), which
means that the term asbiyūs or asfiyūs is Persian and derives from
asp-gūš ("horses' ear"). In the bazaars of Cairo one still sells
al-bargūti "bed-bug", as a soothing, refreshing and ophthalmic remedy
(Ducros). The name bizr-qutūnā is preserved in the Spanish language
in the form zargatona.

53) BAQLA YAMĀNIYYA ("vegetable of Yemen")   blite

   MAIMONIDES: Its Arabic name is as-sadah, in Spanish blitu (blito);
                 it is al-yarbūz, and one also calls it ğarmūz and kastağ.
                 One of these types is the one which is called riğl al-ğarād
                 ("grasshopper foot").

   MEYERHOF: Theophrastus VII, 1-3; Dioscorides II, 117; Serapion 49;
              Ibn al-Beithar 318; Tuhfa 67; ʿAbd ar-Razzāq 145; Issa
              11, 13; Loew I, 352-354.

   Blite is the plant Albersia Blitum Kunth; in Greek bliton. The
names sadah and kastağ are found in different forms in Issa. The term
riğl al-ğarād is applicable to several different plants; for example,
the common yew. Yarbūz and ğarmūz are derived from the Syriac zarbūzā
which is, according to Loew, a name borrowed from Persian, but it is lacking in the Persian dictionaries, and exists only in Turkish (yarpuz,
term designating a type of marjoran). Blite is very widely prevalent,
and its variety oleracea is cultivated in Europe and   India as a

substitute for spinach. Ibn ʿAwwām(II, 152) describes the manner of
sowing blite in Seville.

54) BITTĪH   Watermelon and melon

MAIMONIDES: This is a well-known plant, known by this name (bittīh)
in all Arab countries. There are round ones (fol. 79ᵛ)
and oblong ones; among the latter is the one whose name in
Greek is muluniyā (melonia). Egyptians call the melon al-
bittih al-asfar (the "yellow melon"), because they call the
watermelon (addulāʿ) al-bittih al-ahdar (the "green melon").

MEYERHOF: [Dioscorides II, 134-135; Serapion 58; Ibn al-Beithar 303,
780, 1739; Tuhfa 347; ʿAbd ar-Razzāq 171-172; Issa 50, 12ff;
Loew I, 550-553.]

The watermelon (Citrullus vulgaris SCHRAD.) was known to the ancient
Egyptians and the Hebrews as its name abtiah proves, rendered in the
Septuagint as pepón and passed into Syriac (fattihā) and Arabic (bittiha).
Regarding the different types, see Clément-Mullet (Études sur les noms
Arabes de diverses familles de végétaux, in Journal Asiatique, sixth
series, vol. 15 pp 90-122, January-February 1870), Guigues (in Serapion
58), Issa and Loew. Bittih asfar was probably a melon (Cucumis Melo,
variety Chate Naud, called in Egypt today ʿAbdillāwī). ʿAbd al-Latif (34)
explains this name as a derivative of ʿAbdallāh ibn Tāhir, governor of
Egypt in the tenth century, who probably introduced this species.
Bittih ahdar or hindi ("Indian watermelon") corresponds to dullāʿ of the
Maghribians and the Syrians. It is the round and green watermelon which
is well known in Egypt. See below number 98, and Hehn (239ff). Concerning the cultivation of the melon in Spain, see Ibn ʿAwwām II, 215-221.
Compare also below number 98 (dullāʿ).

55) __BUHŪR MARYAM__ ("Incense of Maria")   Motherwort, marigold and sowbread

__MAIMONIDES__: Modern botanists believe that this denomination applies to
the roots of the herb called __ādiryūn__, which is known in
Spain as "the gilded" (__ad-dahabiyya__) because its flowers
(blossoms) have the color of gold. It is called __ḡarḡaritiyya__
in Spain, and, if its flowers fall, there comes out something like a paw; it is this which one calls "lion's paw"
(__kaff al-asad__). The name of this plant in Greek is __kyklāminos__.
It is not the same plant as __ṡaḡarat Maryam__ ("the tree of
Maria") but the latter is a plant different from __buhūr__
__Maryam__ and its name in Greek is __kyklaminos__.

__MEYERHOF__: [Theophrastus IX, 9; Dioscorides II, 164-5 and III, 96;
Serapion 85; Ghafiqi 137; Ibn al-Beithar 247,1307,1524,
1693; __Tuhfa__ 12, 89; 'Abd ar-Razzāq 159; Issa 36, 17 and 63,
12 and 107, 5; Loew I, 288-289 and III, 77-79; Ducros 153.]

The Arabs have designated approximately ten plants by the name __buhur__
__Maryam__ ("incense, fumigation of Maria") or __ṡaḡarat Maryam__ ("tree or herb
of Maria"). __Ādaryūn__ derives from the Persian __ādar-gūn__ ("color of fire",
Vullers I, 24) and designates the marigold (__Calendula officinalis__ L. or
__Calendula arvensis__ L.). __Kaff al-asad__ ("lion's paw") is the translation of
léontopétalon of Dioscorides, and designates the berberidacea __Leontice__
__Leontopetulum__ L. Finally, the __kyklaminos__ of the Greeks is the __Cyclamen__
__europoeum__ L. See number 364. The Greek name is frequently encountered
in the distorted form __faqlaminus__. Issa (107,5) instead of __ādaryūn__, gives
__ādarbūya__ as the Persian name, and, instead of __ḡarḡaritiyya__, gives __hadibiyya__
as the Arabic name, and both of them to designate __Leontopetalum.__

56) BUZAIDĀN   Undetermined

MAIMONIDES: The majority of commentators state that it is the plant
called "fox testicles" (husā'at-ta'lab),but this is incorrect; it is a tree imported from   India.

MEYERHOF: [Ghafiqi 140-141; Serapion 90, 115, 196 and 495; Ibn al-Beithar
373; Tuhfa 80, 419; 'Abd ar-Razzāq 133, 870 and 916; Issa 129;
8-11; Loew II, 296.]

Nearly all Arabic and Persian physicians have, in effect, identified
the Persian designation būzidān with the roots of orchidaceae which are
called "testicles of the dog or fox", and in modern Egypt denominated
al-musta'gila. They have, further, assimilated it with the satyrion of
Dioscorides (III, 128), an aphrodisiac remedy whose botanical identity
could not be established. Certain authors state that this remedy grows in
Egypt from which it is exported to other countries in the Musulman Orient.
But Maimonides lived in Egypt, and certainly was very familiar with drugs
sold in the bazaars of Cairo in his epoch; furthermore,the name of the
drug is Persian, and it is not likely that an Egyptian drug was sold in
Cairo by the Persian name būzidān. In fact, we read in Avicenna (Ibn Sina I,
272) that būzidān was"a woody Indian remedy";and we find in Dymock (II,
281ff) that in the Indian bazaars, under the name būzidān,certain roots of
Trachydium etc. are sold, but above all a rhizome of the composite
Tanacetum (or Pyrethrum) umbelliferum BOISS. The plant was discovered by
the botanist Aitchison in the valleys of Afghanistan; its root is imported into Persia and oriental India where it is sold as a galactagogue
and fattening remedy for women. It is a rhizome of approximately 20 to 30
centimeters in length, resembling brown wood. I suppose it is the "Indian
wood" that Maimonides speaks of (see below number 391).

After having written this commentary, the confirmation of my opinion
came to me from the manuscript of al-Ghafiqi which states (fol. 57a:
"Abū zaidān is an Indian remedy; those who claim that it is the husā at-ta⁽
lab (Orchis Morio, etc.) are in error. Certain people (physicians) maintain
that it is the al-bahaǧ (Orchis hiricina L., satyrium)."

57) AL-BALL W'AŠ-ŠALL   Types of elder trees

MAIMONIDES: These are two types of herbs with very similar properties.
            They both have a common Arabic name al-⁽ubab. The name of
            one of these two types is aktē in Greek, and its Spanish name
            is yādqu (yezgo); it is ar-raq⁽a and ar-rabraq. The name of
            the other is khamaiaktē in Greek (fol. 80ᵗ) , and in Spanish
            sabūdna (sambuco, sauco).

MEYERHOF: [Theophrastus I, 5, 8; Dioscorides IV, 173; Serapion 278;
            Ibn al-Beithar 124; Tuhfa 208 and 427; Issa 162, 8-9;
            Loew I, 332; Ducros 120.]

The two names are often vocalized bull and ǧull. These are the
equivalents of the plants aktē and chamaiaktē which are the black elder
tree (Sambucus nigra L.) and the small elder tree or dwarf elder (Sambucus
Ebulus L.). Bull is the corruption of the Spanish ebul or ébol (Simonet 51).
Both grow in Syria but not in Egypt. Contrary to the assertion of Maimonides,
the name ⁽ubab is given to certain solanaceae, but not to caprifoliaceae to
which belong the elder trees. The two other names are not mentioned by
other authors, except raq⁽a which is encountered (but) with a totally
different meaning. In contrast, the Spanish names are still well-known
in our times (Simonet 611): yezgo is still found in Tuhfa in the form
yadquh; it designates the dwarf elder. The other name was mutilated by
the copyist: it should read sabūqu (sambuco) (Simonet 573), which designates

the black elder. It is not superfluous to remark that many Arab writers confused the name bull with bul, which is the Arabicized Indian name of the "bel Indian" fruit derived from the Indian tree Aegle Marmelos CORR. The flowers of the black elder are sold in the bazaars of Cairo by the name zahr el-bailisān ("flowers of the small balm"), as a sudorific and resolutive (Ducros).

After having completed this commentary, I found the following explanation among the synonyms in Ghafiqi (Ms. fol. 60b): "Aqti is al-hamān (the elder) which we will mention under the letter hā'; it is a well-known plant which is called šabūqa (sambuco, sauco) in Spanish. There is(also) a small species which is called yādqa (yezgo). Dioscorides gave a description of both types. I am not aware of any more ignorant commentators than those who have written in their books that akte is an Indian plant which has two species: one is as-sull and the other al-bull. It is a nonsense which they have repeated after ar-Razi who promulgated it in his book which he called Al-Kāfi ("The Sufficient"). In addition, one finds many erroneous opinions in the commentaries of ar-Rāzi, and this is one of them. For if akte is the name for al-bull and aš-šull, as ar-Rāzi maintains, it is a different akte from the one which Dioscorides so named in Greek. The ignorance of certain commentators goes so far that they affirm that akte is identical to al-bull and aš-šull, and that yezgo and sauco are called chamaiakte in Greek. This is a major error because Dioscorides called chamaiakte only the small species of the two, and that one is yezgo, whereas he calls both species (together) akte."

The names aš-šull, wa'l-bull, wa'l-full are also found in the celebrated "Perfect Book of the Medical Art" (Kitāb Kāmil as-Sinā'a at-Tibbiyya) composed in 983 C.E. by the Persian physician 'Ali Ibn al-'Abbās al Magusi

(edit. Bulaq 1291 A.H. II, 103), but it designates an Indian drug already
mentioned by Ibn Sarābiyun (9th cent.) and later by Ibn Sinā (Canon I,
271,406 and 435ff). These are thus not Spanish names, but Indian names.
Bull is the equivalent of Aegle Marmelos, full refers to Jasminum Zambac,
and šull has not yet been determined. It is probable that the Arabic-
Spanish physicians of the tenth century transferred the names bull and
šull to the species of elder which were best known in their lands. I
found the same confusion in Suwaidi (fol. 44a).

58) BANǦ   Henbane, mullen and hemlock

MAIMONIDES: There are two species: the seeds of one are white, those of
the other black. The white and small seeds are al-banǧ and
the black ones aš-šawkarān. One also calls it as-saïkarān
and in Spanish barbāška (verbasco). One further calls it
balmānda (milmandro). The name of šawkarān in Greek is
kôneion; it is maknasat al-andar ("the broom of the granary"),
aš-šawka al-yahūdiyya ("the thorn of the Jews") and aš-šawka as-sawdā'
("the black thorn").

MEYERHOF: Theophrastus IX, 15-20; Dioscorides IV, 78, IV, 68, IV, 103;
Serapion 72, 134 and 478; Ghafiqi 162 and others; Ibn al-
Beithar 356,375,1262-1263, 1350; Tuhfa 77 and 455; ʿAbd ar-
Razzāq 129,848 and 875; 76,167 and 195; Issa 48, 13; 77,19;
96,3-5; 187,12; Loew III, 354, 359ff; Ducros 19,43 and 119;
Dymock II, 628, III, 319ff.

In this chapter Maimonides confused several venemous drugs which in
part carry the same names. Banǧ is an Indian name (bhanga) passed through
the Persian bang into Arabic. It designates the Indian hemp (Cannabis

sativa var indica) and was later employed to designate other intoxicating drugs, notably the henbanes (Hyoscyamus albus, niger, muticus). Sikrān, saïkarān, šukrān, etc. derive from the semitic root s.k.r., which is very ancient and designates all sorts of intoxicating drugs. It is for this reason that one attributed these names both to the hemlock (Cicuta and Conium) as well as to the henbanes and to the mullen (Verbascum). The Arabic names miknasat al-andar (in ʿAbd ar-Razzāq musallih al-andar) and sikrān al hawt ("inebriate the fish, the whale"), as well as barbāškā, only designate the latter plant. But šawka yahūdiyya and šawka sawdāʾ are today in usage to designate a totally different plant, the rolling thistle (Eryngium campestre L.), an ombelliferous plant. As is evident, the confusion in this paragraph is considerable. In Cairo, one still sells flowers, leaves and seeds of the white henbane (bing, DUCROS). The name bing today, in the popular language of Egypt, signifies any soporific or narcotic remedy. Formed therefrom is the verb bannig yebannig, meaning to chloroform, to narcotise. It appears that the henbane was also cultivated in Spain (Ibn ʿAwwām II, 311-312). Balmānda is an error of the copyist for malmāndru; this is an ancient Castilian name (melmendro or milmandro, according to Simonet 357).

59) BAQLA HAMQĀʾ   Purslain

MAIMONIDES: This is ar-riǧla and al-farfah and al-farfiz and al-baqla al-mubāraka ("blessed legume"). The Syrians call it al-farfahīn, and the name of the wild species of this plant is péplion in Greek.

MEYERHOF: [Dioscorides IV, 168; Serapion 50; Ibn al-Beithar 313; Tuhfa 68; ʿAbd ar-Razzāq 139; Issa 147, 10; Loew III, 70-75; Ducros 24.]

For the explanation of the Arabic names, I refer the reader to the discussion by Renaud and Colin in Tuhfa. Farfiz is probably a corrupt reading for furfir ("purslain"). This vegetable (Portulaca oleracea L.) has been known in the Orient for a very long time. The names farfah and farfahin (the reading of Ibn al-Beithar farfag and farfagin is faulty) are probably derived from the Persian perpehen through the intermediary of the Syriac farfahina (Loew, Fraenkel 143). The druggists of Cairo sell the seeds of the wild purslain or the satanic purslain (Portulaca silvestris L) by the name bizr er-rigla eš-šetani. The seed is imported from India, and recommended as a vermifuge (Ducros). Regarding the cultivation of the purslain in Spain, see Ibn ʿAwwam I, 149-151. See below number 112.

60) BASAL AL-FAR   Squill

MAIMONIDES: This is al-isqil and al-ʿunsul, and it is known in Maghrib by
              the name "onion of pork" (basal al-hinzir) and its Greek name
              is skilla,* and in Berber uhkal.

MEYERHOF: [Theophrastus I, 6 and VII, 12-13; Dioscorides II, 171;
              Serapion 250; Ibn al-Beithar 1593; Tuhfa 31 and 308;
              ʿAbd ar-Razzaq 15 and 669; Issa 185, 15; Ducros 40; Loew II,
              188-194.]

The Arabic name signifies "onion of rat". The bulb of the squill, the liliacea Urginea maritima BAKER, is utilized up to the present time as a poison against rats. Isqil is the Arabic transcription of the Greek name skilla. The Aramaic name was hasuba, from which is derived hasab of the Mishnah (Loew). The origin is perhaps the Assyrian hasbu (Barth).

* in the text an error of the copyist: kata gene instead of the name skilla
  which I have inserted

For other Arabic names (bussa'il, 'unsēl, 'unsulān, basal Fir'awn) see
Loew. The Berberic name seems to have been corrupted. G. S.Colin
(Etymologies magribines, in Hespéris 1927, number 49) gives agufāl.
In Egypt one sells the bulbs of squill in the bazaars as a rat poison
and to obtain, by friction, irritation and even vesication of the skin
(Ducros). For certain superstitious ideas linked to the squill, see
Ibn 'Awwām II 373ff.

61) BASAL AZ-ZĪR   Grape hyacinth

MAIMONIDES: This is "the earth chestnut" (qastal al-ard) and al-bulbūs.
Al-qa'bīl is one of its species, and this qa'bīl is a
small species of edible onion which is imported from Syria
into Egypt.

MEYERHOF: [Theophrastus I, 6; Dioscorides II, 170; Serapion 53;
Ghafiqi 135; Ibn al-Beithar 337; 'Abd ar-Razzāq 170; Issa
121,8; Loew II, 184-187; Ducros 39.]

This drug is the bulb of the "hairy hyacinth" (Muscari comosum MILL),
well known to the Greeks by the name bolbós or bolbos edódimos ("edible
bulb"). The Arabic name is found faultily transcribed in the majority
of Arab writers; it is not basal az-zir but basal az-ziz ("hairy bulb"),
so named because of the tuft of fruitless flowers which terminates its
inflorescence. Suwaidi (article basal nabat, fol. 50a of the manuscript)
distinctly states: "One of its species is known as basal az-ziz, with
two zai' among which is a yā' with a vowel placed below it. Qastal al-ard
in general is the name of the oriental hyacinth, and qa'bīl that of the
amaryllaceae Pancratium maritimum L. ("sea narcissus"). The bulbs of
these plants are easily confused. Ducros found the bulb of the "onion

of wolf" (<u>Ornithogallum umbellatum</u> L.) in the bazaars of Cairo by
the name <u>basal az-zir</u>.

62) <u>BALĀDUR</u>   Oriental cashew nut

<u>MAIMONIDES</u>: This is <u>anaqardiyā</u>.

<u>MEYERHOF</u>: [Serapion 51; Ghafiqi 126; Ibn al-Beithar 347; ʿAbd ar-Razzāq
128; Issa 166, 122; Loew I 202-204; Ducros 41; Laufer 482ff.]

The Arabic-Persian name is the translation of the Sanskrit name
<u>bhallātaka</u> (Dymock I, 389) or <u>bhallatamu</u> (Chopra 385), in Chinese
<u>p'o-lo-te</u> (Laufer 582ff), and designates the "nut of the swamp", fruit
of the Indian tree <u>Semecarpus Anacardium</u> L. The resinous and tart juice
of this fruit is employed in   Oriental India to corrode warts and
to mark linen. The fruit is cordiform. Its name <u>anakardia</u> it not ancient Greek - it was unknown to Dioscorides - but Byzantine. The
cashew nut is found mentioned for the first time by Paul of Egina
(7th century) in his book VII, chapter II, 38 as an ingredient of the
"antidote of Theodoret". Popular Oriental belief attributed to this
fruit the property of fortifying one's memory and sharpening one's intelligence. A Jewish legend (Loew p. 203, according to Steinschneider)
attributes the superior intelligence of our Maimonides to a strong dose
of cashew nut. According to an Islamic legent, the great Arabic historian Ahmad ibn Yahyā al-Balāduri, who lived in Baghdad in the 9th
century, is supposed to have died following the absorption of too
strong a dose of the same remedy. This drug is still sold in the
bazaars of Cairo (Ducros 41).

63) <u>BARINGĀSIF</u>   Wormwood

<u>MAIMONIDES</u>: This is <u>aš-šawāsirā</u> and "the musk of geniuses" (<u>misk al-ǧinn</u>).

Its name in Greek is artemisia; it is a type of southern-
wood (qaisūm).

MEYERHOF: Dioscorides III, 113; Serapion 455; Ghafiqi 150; Ibn al-
Beithar 255; Tuhfa 456; 'Abd ar-Razzāq 162 and 940;
Issa 22, 13; Loew I, 384-385; Ducros 139.

The plant in question is wormwood (Artemisia vulgaris L., compositae),
a very common herb. The name bilingāsif or biringāsif is the Arabic
form of the Persian biringāsp (Vullers I, 227). Sawāsirā is a borrowed
name in the Syriac language suvāsrā (Loew); misk al-ğinn is an Arabic
name which is in usage both for wormwood and for Teucrium Polium L.
(Ibn al-Beithar 1352 and 2134, Tuhfa 101). Southernwood (Artemisia
Abrotanum L.) is a relative of wormwood. In the bazaars of Cairo, instead of wormwood, a related but much larger plant, the "tree wormwood"
(Artemisia arborescens L.), known by the name šeba, is sold (Ducros).

64) BAHRĀMĪǦ   (Salix balchia), here clematis

MAIMONIDES: It is zayyān in Arabic, and in Spanish yarba du-fuaqu
(yerba do fuego), and one also calls it hāl balbaška (?),
and in Greek lepidion. It is the wild jasmine (fol. 80)
(al-yāsamin al-barrī); its odor is penetrating.

MEYERHOF: Dioscorides IV, 180; Ghafiqi 154; Ibn al-Beithar 1506;
Tuhfa 206; Issa 52,3.

In this chapter Maimonides followed al-Ghafiqi who erroneously
identified bahrāmaǧ as Clematis. Bahrāmaǧ is the Persian designation of
a willow of central Asia (Salix balchia or Salix Caprea?); see the
discussion of this name by Meyerhof and Sobhy (Ghafiqi). All the other
Arabic names are in accord with Clematis augustifolia JACQ. or

Clematis flammula L. The Spanish name (Simonet 614) signifies "herb
of fire", and is also found translated into Arabic ('uşbat an-nār).
Lepidion is not the Greek name of this plant, but klématis. The other
supposed Spanish name appears to be a corruption of malva visco, and is
not therefore in its (proper) place here. See below number 390.

65) BASBĀYIG   Common polypody

MAIMONIDES: This is as-sakiraglī, which means "having many feet"
            (katir al-arğul). One also calls it adrās al-kalb
            ("teeth of a dog"). One likewise calls it 'aliğuniyā(?)
            and polypódion in Greek. In addition, one calls it šutur
            'ali and sağiriglā, and its name in Spanish is barbūdiyu
            (polipodio), and in Berber tištiwin. By this last name,
            it is well known to the people of Maghrib.

MEYERHOF: [Theophrastus IX 13,6; Dioscorides IV, 186; Serapion 82;
            Ghafiqi 170; Ibn al-Beithar 280; Tuhfa 88; 'Abd ar-Razzāq
            181; Issa 146,9; Loew I, 12.]

    This is the polypody (Polypodium vulgare L.), a fern whose rhizome
contains tannic acid and serves as a remedy against diarrheas. Nearly
all the aforementioned names are translations from the Greek polypodion,
"having many legs". Basbāyig comes from the Persian (bas meaning many; and
pāyak meaning small foot; Vullers I, 238). Sakiragli and sağirigla
are transcriptions from the Syriac sagi ragle or regla which has the
same meaning. (See the studies of Fleischer on the Supplément aux
Dictionnaires Arabes bv Dozy. part 3 in Bèrichte der phil. - hist.
Klasse der Koenigl. Saechs. Gesellschaft der Wissenschaften 1864 p. 13).

'Aliǧuniyā is perhaps a mutilation of the Latin name filicula (fern) and šutur ʿalī another corruption of the Syriac name. The Berberic name is usually encountered in the form tištiwān or ištiwān (Renaud in Hespéris, 1931, 144). As to the Spanish name, see Simonet (468): purpodia is equivalent to polipodio in modern Castil ian.

66) BUTM   Terebinth and lentisk

MAIMONIDES: It is a known tree. The wild terebinth is ad-darw (the lentisk) and it is, as one states, the mastic tree (mastakā).

MEYERHOF: [Theophrastus III-V, IX; Dioscorides I, 71; Serapion 59 and 84; Tuhfa 178, 317 and 329; ʿAbd ar-Razzāq 322; Issa 131, 14; Loew I, 191-195.]

The tree in question is the anacardiacea Pistacia Terebinthus L. which furnishes edible fruits (habba hadrāʾ, "green kernel") and a resin, which was the terebinth of the ancients (the terebinth of today is extracted from coniferous trees). Kohen (p. 125, last line) gives the Persian name binäst for the resin of the butm (the terebinth). See below number 320. The name butm is Semitic (Assyrian butnu; Hebrew botem; Aramaic botnā etc.). Darw is the Arabic name of the lentisk (Pistacia Lentiscus L.) which, in effect, furnishes the resin called mastic. See Tuhfa number 251, and below our commentary on number 156 (habba hadrāʾ). Concerning the cultivation of the terebinth in Spain, see Ibn ʿAwwām II, 368-370.

67) BADANǦ   Embelia Ribes

MAIMONIDES: It is also called biranǧ. It is an Indian remedy which has the form of a hazelnut with a pulp.

MEYERHOF: [Serapion 5; Ghafiqi 171-172; Ibn al-Beithar 259; Issa 75,5; Dymock II, 349-354.]

Badang is the Arabic name, derived from the Sanskrit vidanga, of
the seeds of the myrsinacea Embelia Ribes BURM. whose Persian name is
birang, and in Hindustani babrang (Dymock). Nevertheless, its seeds do not
have the bulk of a hazelnut but only of a grain (fruit) of pepper.
Maimonides probably confused them with another Indian drug, the nut of
the bonduc (Caesalpinia Bonducella FLEM.), which is called rata in
Arabic. The fruits of the Embelia ribes were imported into Persia and
the western part of the Islamic world via Afghanistan. It is for this
reason that in Arabic they also carry the name birang kãbili (birang
from Kaboul). It is a vermifuge whose seeds contain embelic acid. An
Anglo-Indian physician (Harris, in Lancet, July 23, 1887) recommended
them as an excellent remedy against tapeworm. One no longer finds them
in the bazaars of Cairo, but only in those of   Oriental India. To
this day, the Indian druggists in the Punjab designate the vermifuge
fruits of Myrsine africana L. by the name bebrang, (Chopra 586).

CHAPTER ǦĪM

68) ǦUMMĀR   Palm-cabbage

MAIMONIDES: One also calls it hass an-nahl ("palm lettuce"); it is the
            heart of the palm tree. By contrast, the plant known to
            the Maghribians by the name al-ǧummār is a very small spe-
            cies of palm tree.

MEYERHOF: [Dioscorides I, 109, 5; Ibn al-Beithar 512; Tuhfa 107;
          Abd ar-Razzāq 207; Loew II, 325ff; Ibn ʿAwwām I, 323.]

As Renaud and Colin expounded in Tuhfa, the term ǧummār designates
both the "heart", that is the pith (fecula amylaceae) contained within
the trunk of the date tree Phoenix dactylifera L., as well as its terminal bud whose tender leaves are eaten as the artichoke. Here we are
dealing with the latter vegetable because Maimonides gives the synonym
"palm lettuce". The other designation refers to the dwarf palm (Chamaerops
humilis L.) whose "heart" is currently eaten, and is well-known in Morocco.
In Egypt, today, the term ǧummār only designates the terminal bud of the
date tree. It is rarely eaten, being considered as a delicacy and ex-
pensive dish. See below numbers 176 (Talʿ), 204 (Kufarrā) and 206 (Kāfūr).
It should be noted that Kohen, who lived in Cairo half a century after
Maimonides, gives (middle of p. 127) ǧubn annahl ("cheese of the palm
tree") as a synonym for ǧummār. He thus speaks of the pith or the heart
of the palm tree which has a marked resemblance to white cheese.

69) ǦAWZ ǦUNDUM   Edible lichen

MAIMONIDES: One also calls it ǧawz kundum. It is "the fat of the earth"
            (šahmat al-ard), "the charcoal of the earth" (ǧamr al-ard),
            and "the earth of honey" (turbat al-ʿasal). To us (in Maghrib),
            it is called ad-dādi.

MEYERHOF: [Serapion 287; Ghafiqi 222; Ibn al-Beithar 538; Issa 86; Loew I,
25ff and II, 63.]

The identification of this drug has been in doubt for a long time.
Leclerc (Ibn al-Beithar) first considered it not as an earthy substance but
as an edible lichen, probably <u>Lecanora Sphaerothallia esculenta</u> EV.(Sickenberger
63). Adrisi (p. 81), in approximately 1150 C.E., had already given a good description thereof: "It is something which grows in deserts surrounded by barren
mountains. It grows between the rocks, is yellowish and does not exceed the
height of a claw...". In effect, this lichen forms starchy tubercles which
grow in the Persian, Kurdish and North African deserts with an extraordinary
rapidity after the rains (Schlimmer 12-14). They serve as nourishment for
nomadic peoples in times of famine. A Persian legend claims that the troups of
Alexander the Great were saved by the edible lichen during their march across
the desert of Sistan. One also identifies it with the Biblical manna. The
name <u>gawz gandum</u> is Persian and signifies "wheat kernel". For <u>dādi</u>, see below
numbers 86 and 327.

70) <u>ǦĀWARS</u>   Common millet, sorgo

MAIMONIDES: This is a type of millet of birds (<u>duhn</u>); and the "Indian millet"
(al-ǧāwars al-hindi) is <u>sorgho</u> (<u>data</u>).

MEYERHOF: [Theophrastus IV and VIII; Dioscorides II, 97; Serapion 285;
Ghafiqi 201; Ibn al-Beithar 460; <u>Tuhfa</u> 96; Abd ar-Razzāq 218;
Issa 133, 17; Loew I, 738-46.]

<u>Ǧāwars</u> is the arabicized form of the Persian <u>ǧāwers</u> which corresponds
to the Greek <u>kéngchros</u> and to the common millet (<u>Panicum miliaceum</u> L.) of
modern botanists. <u>Duhn</u> is the Arabic name of <u>sorgho</u> or small millet, nourishment of the Sudanese people. (<u>Pennisetum spicatum</u> KCKE). Finally <u>dura</u> -

* In Issa one finds all the Arabic names; however, his identification of
<u>gawz gundum</u> with <u>Garcinia Mangostana</u> is erroneous.

the vocalization <u>dara</u> is probably an error of the copyist - is the large
millet (<u>Sorphum vulgare</u> PERS.). See the discussion of these names by
Renaud and Colin (<u>Tuhfa</u>) and in Ibn ʿAwwām II, 74-77.

71) ǦAWZ BAWWĀ   Nutmeg

<u>MAIMONIDES</u>: This is ǧawz at-tīb ("the aromatic nut"), and one also calls
          it ǧarbuwwā.

<u>MEYERHOF</u>: [Serapion 286 and 295; Ghafiqi 193; Ibn al-Beithar 526;
          <u>Tuhfa</u> 98; ʿAbd ar-Razzāq 196; Issa 122, 6; Loew II, 60,62;
          Dymock III, 192-197; Ducros 68.]

    This well-known Indian spice carries other Arabic names (see Issa).
The name of the title is Persian: <u>gawz</u> means nut, and <u>buwā</u> or <u>buyā</u> means
scented aroma. The name ǧarbuwwā (ǧaz-buwwā?), which is not encountered
anywhere else, is probably a corruption of the known name. The Greeks
didn't mention this drug save during the Byzantine epoch. Occidental
Europe didn't know of it until the 18th century of the Christian era.
One sells nutmeg (<u>Myristica fragrans</u> HOUTT.) in the Egyptian bazaars under
the name <u>gōz</u> or <u>gōzet et-tib</u> ("perfumed nut"); Ducros erroneously translates "good or agreeable nut". Since the suppression of the traffic of <u>hasis</u>
and other stupefying (drugs), the lower Egyptian population makes use of
the tea plant and nutmeg as stimulants.

72) ǦAʿDA   Germander

<u>MAIMONIDES</u>: This al-ǧuʿaïda. Its name in Spanish is <u>yerba balira</u> and
          one also says <u>badlira</u>. Its Greek name is <u>polion</u>.

<u>MEYERHOF</u>: [Theophrastus I, 10, 4; Dioscorides III, 110; Ghafiqi 208;
          Ibn al-Beithar 488; <u>Tuhfa</u> 101; ʿAbd ar-Razzāq 208; Issa 179,11.]

In general one identifies the name ǧu'da or ǧa'da with a labiate,
the mountain pennyroyal (Teucrium Polium L.); ǧu'aida is a diminutive of
this name and designates, according to Ibn al-Beither 488, a wild species.
The Spanish name, according to Simonet (615), is read yerba pedilare and
derives from the Latin herba pedicularis, "lousewort", a name which is
also applicable to stavesacre (Delphinium Staphisagria L.).

73) ǦAZAR   Carrot

MAIMONIDES: One calls it (fol. 81^z) in Arabic as-subātiyya ("scarlet"),
in Roman bišnāqa (visnaga), in Persian astafilina, in
Spanish isfannāriyya, and its name is also nahšal. The name
of its wild species is bahārina(?) (or laǧārna?).

MEYERHOF: [Theophrastus IX, 15,5; Dioscorides III, 52; Serapion 289;
Ghafiqi 207; Ibn al-Beithar 481; Tuhfa 93; 'Abd ar-Razzāq 201-
212; Issa 694; Loew III, 447-449.]

It is the carrot (Daucus carota L.) whose Spanish name in our times
is zanahoria (derived from isfannariya). The name ǧazar is of Persian
origin; the Roman name visnaga in effect derives from the Latin pastinaca
and designates parsnip (Dozy I, 83; Simonet 430; Laguna 317). As to the
name astafilina, it is not Persian but of Greek origin (staphylinos);
it is still in use in Maghrib and Syria in the form istuflin. Nahšal
(here, and in number 258 in our manuscript it is orthographed nahsak) is
the Persian name of the wild carrot (see number 258) whose seeds are
called dūqū (see below number 94). The name bahārina whose reading is
uncertain because it lacks diacritical points in our
manuscript, is not found anywhere else. Its form resembles harahabina
of Mishnaic tractates (Loew), which designates eryngium (Eryngium campestre L.).

If one should read <u>lagárna</u>, one would think of a Spanish name. See number 94. Concerning the cultivation of the carrot in Spain, see Ibn ʿAwwām II, 176-179.

74) <u>ǦIRǦIR</u>   Rocket (plant)

MAIMONIDES: In Arabic one calls it <u>al-katā</u>,and its Greek name is euzómon; in Spanish <u>arūqa</u> (eruca). Its wild species is called aïhaqān in Arabic.

MEYERHOF: Theophrastus VII, 1-5; Dioscorides II, 140; Serapion 284; Ghafiqi 202; Ibn al-Beithar 473; <u>Tuhfa</u> 95; ʿAbd ar-Razzāq 210; Issa 77, 12; Loew I, 491-493.

The name <u>ǧirǧir</u> is generally identified with the rocket (<u>Eruca sativa</u> MILL.) which still carries the name <u>gargir</u> in Egypt,even to the present time. The Latin name <u>eruca</u> became <u>oruga</u> in modern Castilian (Laguna 224; Simonet 410). <u>Katāh</u> is, according to Ibn al-Beithar (1890), the Arabic name of the seeds of the rocket, whereas <u>aïhuqān</u> designates the wild rocket (<u>Brassica Erucastrum</u> L.), as is indicated by Maimonides. The cultivation of the two types of rockets in Musulman Spain has been described by Ibn ʿAwwām II, 301ff.

75) <u>ǦULLINĀR</u>   Balauste (Wild pomegranate)

MAIMONIDES: It is <u>balaustion</u> (in Greek). Its Arabic name is <u>ar-ragat</u> and <u>al-mazz;</u> it is the blossom of the wild pomegranate and its petioles (<u>aqmāʿ</u>); it does not produce fruits. As to the calyx (ǧunbud) of the pomegranate, it falls from the inflorescence of the cultivated pomegranate and resembles the wild pomegranate.

MEYERHOF: Dioscorides I, 111; Serapion 293; Ghafiqi 194, Ibn al-Beithar

494; Tuhfa 94 and 287;ʿAbd ar-Razzāq 205; Issa 151, 3; Loew

III, 95; Ducros 65.⌉

This name in Arabic is vocalized ǧullanār; it derives from the Persian
gulnār (gul-i-ānār, "rose or blossom of the pomegranate"). The name mazz
(al-Asmaʿi) is vocalized mizz by several dictionaries. See below number
243 (muzz). The blossom of the wild grenadier (Punica granatum L.) is
sold as an astringent in the bazaars of Cairo. It is still called gulnār
or nārmišk, whereas the blossom of the cultivated pomegranate carries the
name gunbad er-rummān (Ducros). The cultivation of the wild pomegranate
tree is discussed by IbnʿAwwām (I, 259ff).

76) ǦAWAŠIR   Opopanax of druggists

MAIMONIDES: It is al-barūtā.

MEYERHOF: ⌈Theophrastus IX, II; Dioscorides III, 51; Serapion 476;

Ghafiqi 206; Ibn al-Beithar 459; Tuhfa 108;ʿAbd ar-Razzāq

204; Issa 129, 1; Loew III 458-459; Ducros 62.⌉

One derives this name from the Persian gāw-šir, "cow's milk", or from
gawar šir(Vullers 947), "milk of opopanax" (gawar). The name barūtā is undoubtedly of Syrian origin; Loew gives the name bārurā after the Syriac
lexicographer Bar Bahlūl. Opopenax is the concreted resin of an umbelliferous plant Opopanax Chironium KOCH. This brownish-red gum resin
is sold in the bazaars of Cairo as an antispasmodic and laxative (Ducros).

77) ǦANTIYĀNĀ   Gentian

MAIMONIDES: It is al-kušad; its name in Spanish is bišlišku (basilisco)
             and one (also) calls it "serpent's remedy" (dawā' al-hayya).

MEYERHOF: ⌈Dioscorides III, 3; Ghafiqi 204; Ibn al-Beithar 515; Tuhfa

102;ʿAbd ar-Razzāq 232; Issa 86, 22; Loew I, 653; Ducros 66.⌉

This name is the Arabic transcription of gentiáne of the Greeks
(Gentiana lutea L. of the modern Greeks). The Spanish synonym is no longer
found in actual Spanish: Renaud-Colin (Tuhfa 102) explains it, according
to Ibn Biklāris, as derived from "royal", being that it is the legendary
king Gentius who is supposed to have discovered the properties of this plant.
Simonet (43) considers possible the derivation of this word from basilisco,
because the root of this drug was used against the bite of poisonous rep-
tiles; this is further confirmed by the last Arabic name "root of the
serpent". Moreover, we find "Basilisca; id est gentiana..." in a Latin
glossary composed in approximately 700 C.E. in Spain or in Southern
France (Edited by J.L.Heiberg, with the title Glossae medicinales. Kgl.
Danske Videns-kabernes Selskab, Hist.-phil. Meddelelser IX, 1, Kōbenhavn
1924, p. 12). And in Ghafiqi (Ms. fol 105b): "basilisqun, this is al-
basiliska, the Andalousian name for gantiyana"). Kušād or gušād is the
Persian name of gentian. In the bazaars of Cairo the root of Gentiana lutea
L. is sold as a stomachic; even today it still carries the name of "ser-
pent's remedy" (Ducros).

78) **GĪBSĪN**   Gypsum

MAIMONIDES: It is the gypsum stone (hagar al-gabs) before it is calcined (burned); it is the "plaster of bakers" (gibs al-
farrānīn). It is a brilliant and white stone. One also calls
it al-gass and isfidāg al-gass ("ceruse of plaster").

MEYERHOF: Dioscorides V, 116; Serapion 291; Ghafiqi 225; Ibn al-
Beithar 468; ʿAbd ar-Razzāq 206.

Gypsum is found in abundance in the deserts of North Africa, in the
form of crystalline masses of sulfate of lime. The names gibsin and gibs

are Arabicized from the Greek gypsos. Ǧass is the Arabic name for gypsum
or plaster, derived from the Persian term gač. To Kohen (p. 123, first
line), the name isfidāǧ al-ǧass designates crystalline (zaǧāǧi) or transparent gypsum.

79) ǦUNDABĀDUSTUR   Castoreum

MAIMONIDES: It is the testicle of the castor (sammūr). It is husyat
               al-bahr ("testicle of the sea") and al-fāhiša ("the immoral")
                              *
               and qastūra (castoreo in Spanish) and kastórion (in Greek).
               The castor is a marine animal, the "dog of the water" (kalb al mā');
               it leaves the water and searches for its nourishment on land. It
               is not identical with al-qaniliya (conejillo?), as have claimed
               those who do not know al-qaniliya. The people of Maghrib call
               tnis remedy "the fetid" (al-muntina).

MEYERHOF: [Dioscorides II, 24; Serapion 291; Chafiqi 228, Ibn al-Beithar
               516; Tuhfa 103; ʿAbd ar-Razzāq 203; Ducros 225.]

The vocalization in usage is ǧundbādastar; it is the Arabic form of the
Persian name gundbīdastar ("testicle of the castor") (Vullers II, 1036).
The drug is not the testicle but a desiccated excretion of the glands of
the genital apparatus of the Castor fiber L. As these glands with their
contents were often sold in pairs, one mistook them for testicles. Sammūr
originally designated sable, but later castor. According to Dozy (II,414)
and Simonet (129), al-quniliya is the Arabic form of the Castilian conejo
or cuniculus, "rabbit". I also find the Spanish form conejillo. One
would sooner make the comparison (and confusion) with the otter which also
carries the name kalb al-mā' ("dog of the water") in Arabic. Egyptian

* see Simonet 111

druggists sell a castoreum of inferior quality using the Persian name corrupted from manastir. This drug is found in the bazaars of Cairo in the form of a hard, brittle, brownish mass (Ducros). Falsifications are frequent. Castoreum is employed, as in the medicine of our grandfathers, primarily as a stimulant, but also as an antispasmodic and resolutive.

80) GILBĀN   Vetch

MAIMONIDES: (fol. 81ᵛ). It is al-hullar[*]; the wild vetch is al-qarinā (?).

MEYERHOF: [Theophrastus VIII, 3; Serapion 125; Ghafiqi 215; Ibn al-
             Beithar 495; Tuhfa 222; Abd ar-razzaq 211; Issa 105, 9;
             Loew II, 437-442; Ducros 75.]

In dictionaries, the name is vocalized ǧullabān, ǧulubbān and ǧulbān. The popular modern name in Egypt is gilbān. It is the leguminous plant Lathyrus sativus L. The name ǧulbān is half Persian, half Arabic (Vullers 524). The name hullar is the Arabic form of the Persian hular (Vullers 714). Nevertheless, the Semiticists Hrozny and Zimmern derive it from the Assyrian hallūru (Loew 437). Ibn al-Awwām (II, 66-69) describes the cultivation of the vetch in Spain and repeats the assertion of Ibn Gulgul that a person who falls asleep on vetch or its straw may become lame. This is the first description of lathyrism, a type of paralysis of the lower extremities observed following the prolonged consumption of this leguminous plant. Al-qarinā is undoubtedly an incorrect reading for al-qarsinā; it is probably the Castilian name alcarceña (bitter vetch) which is itself derived from the Arabic al-kirsanna. See Renaud-Colin in Tuhfa.

[*] reconstituted name; it is completely distorted in the text

81) ǦIDWĀR   Zedoary

MAIMONIDES: One also says zidwār. It is a type of zerumbet (zurunbād)

which possesses the same virtue as the donoricum (darawnaǧ);

al-antula is one of its species.

MEYERHOF: [Serapion 544; Ghafiqi 205; Ibn al-Beithar 174, 467 and 1479;

Tuhfa 110; ʿAbd ar-Razzāq 282; Issa 63, 4; Loew III, 498-499;

Dymock III, 399-402.]

The name of this drug in lexicons is rendered zadwār and ǧadwār; the
form zidwār is popular. It is the root of the zingiberaceous plant Curcuma
Zedoaria, ROSC. which grows in   oriental India.. The name zadwār is
Persian (Vullers II, 123). Antula is an ancient Spanish name of the plant
that one identifies as the aconite anthora (Aconitum Anthora L.). The
Spanish Arabs found it in the mountains near Cordova and considered it as a
species of zedoary (ǧadwār andalusi "andalusian zedoary"). The Spanish
name antora is perhaps a corruption of the Greek anti-phthorâ (Simonet 18),
because this species of aconite is not poisonous, and was considered as an
antidote against the poison of the wolfsbane and certain venomous animals.
It is for this reason that it also carries the name aconito saludable in
Spanish. From the botanic point of view, this ranunculaceous plant has
nothing to do with zedoary.

82) ǦAWZ   Diverse nuts

MAIMONIDES: a) The edible nut (al-ǧawz al-maʾkūl) is well-known.

b) The cypress nut (ǧawz as-sarw) is also well-known; it is
a nut which is as if split into triangular cones which re-
unite in a spherical form.

c) The metel nut (ǧawz māta) is also called ǧawz mātil, and in
Persian ǧawzaraq(?); it is a small nut with soporific properties.

d) The elkaya nut (ǧawz ar-raqʿ) is another species; it is
the "vomic nut" (ǧawz al-qayyʾ); ar-raqʿ is a tree of large
stature.

e) The Sudanese nut (ǧawz as-Sūdān) is the one which the
Maghribians call ǧawz aš-širk ("nut of the association").
It is larger than a hazelnut, oblong and flabby, and in its
interior there is something resembling seeds.

f) the cocoa nut (ǧawz al-hind, "Indian nut") is an-narǧil,
as we will mention in chapter nūn.

MEYERHOF: a) [Theophrastus III, 6; Dioscorides 197; Serapion 337; Ghafiqi 197;
Ibn al-Beithar 525; ʿAbd ar-Razzāq 199; Issa 102, 8; Loew II,
29-59.]
It is the common nut (i.e. walnut), fruit of Juglans regia L.
The name ǧawz is Persian. The walnut tree was cultivated in
Spain (Ibn ʿAwwām I, 271-277).

b) [Theophrastus II, 2,6; V, 4,1 etc.; Dioscorides I, 74; Ibn
al-Beithar 1168; ʿAbd ar-Razzāq 198; Issa 62, 19; Loew II,
64 and III, 26-33.]
It is the fruit of Cupressus sempervireus L.; the name sarw
is perhaps of Persian origin.

c) [Serapion 288; Ghafiqi 218; Ibn al-Beithar 527; Tuhfa 100;
Issa 68, 14; Loew III, 359; Dumock II, 585.]
The "metel nut" is the fruit of certain solanaceous plants,
notably that of Datura Metel L. and of Datura fastuosa,
a known soporific remedy. The Arabic names mātā and mātil
are derived from the Sanskrit unmatta ("alienated") and
māthula, and passed through Persian. The Persian name

(ğawzaran?) seems corrupted; Ibn al-Beithar orthographs it

ğuzarab but none of these names is found in the dictionaries.

d) [Serapion 338-339; Ghafiqi 216; Ibn al-Beithar 528-529; Issa

75, 2 and 182, 13; Loew II, 63; Dymock I, 340 and II, 460.]

The identification of this drug has been in doubt for a long

time. Modern botanists wanted to associate it with the vomic

nut of Strychnos Nux vomica L. Nevertheless, Forskal (126),

in the 18th century, established that the ğawz ar-raqʿ of the

Arabs is the fruit of the tree named by him Elcaja jeminsis,

and that one now calls Trichilia emetica VAHL.(meliaceae).

It is a large tree that grows in tropical Africa and southern

Arabia. Its seeds,which have emetic properties,are known in

European commerce by the name of "Mafureira seeds".

e) [Ghafiqi 196; Ibn al-Beithar 535; Tuhfa 99; ʿAbd ar-Razzāq

214; Issa 13, 9 and 54, 1; Ducros 55.]

The denomination and the description of this drug differs so

much among the Arabic writers that an identification has not

yet been possible. Nevertheless, one can accept that the ğawz

aš-šark of the Arabs includes the fruit of different species

of the zingiberaceae Aframomum, above all Aframomum Melegueta

K. SCHUM. The seed contained within this fruit is known as

"pepper of Ethiopia" and more commonly as "maniguetta pepper".

See the critical study of this drug by Renaud and Colin (Tuhfa).

The druggists of Cairo always sell the seed by the name tin

el-fil ("elephant fig"). One uses it as a tonic and astringent.

Ducros has provided the description and design thereof.

f) The cocoa nut will be discussed below at number 257 (nārǧil).

83) GAFT AL-BULLŪT   Acorn aril

MAIMONIDES: It is the thin peel which is found on the interior of the shell.

MEYERHOF: [Dioscorides I, 106; Serapion 193; Ibn al-Beithar 493; Tuhfa
109; ʿAbd ar-Razzāq 216; Ducros 42; see above number 42.]

The term gaft is Persian and has the meaning "bark, peel, lining".
One is dealing with the envelop or pellicle just below the shell of the acorn,
called aril by botanists. The druggists of Cairo sell the acorns of the oak
Quercus pedunculata EHRENB. without the cupula, but endowed with the aril,
as a styptic and astringent (Ducros).

84) GAMHŪRI   Concentrated must

MAIMONIDES: It is the juice of grapes boiled until half evaporated. If
it is boiled until only one third remains, after the evaporation of the other two thirds, one calls it "reduced to a
third" (mutallat), and if it is boiled until only one quarter
remains, one calls it maïbahtaǧ.

MEYERHOF: [Ibn al-Beithar 513; Tuhfa 270.]

The Arabic name ǧamhuri means "popular". The dictionary Tāǧ (III,110)
explains it as follows: "because (this cooked wine) is employed by the entire
public or by the majority". Its use was legal for Musulmans. Some authors
(for example Abu ʿUbaida), nevertheless, declared that it was intoxicating,
just as the prohibited fermented beverages. The terms maïbahtaǧ or maïbuhtaǧ
are Arabicized from the Persian maï-puhta meaning "cooked must".

85) GULǦABĪN   Honey of roses

MAIMONIDES: These are rosed confected with honey.

MEYERHOF: Gulǧabin is a mutilation of ǧulanǧubin, Arabicized form of the
Persian gul meaning rose and angubin meaning honey. See Ibn
al-Beithar 504.

CHAPTER DĀL

86) <u>DĀDĪ</u>   Lecanora, Judas-tree, and its types

<u>MAIMONIDES</u>: It is the name of Indian earth that one mixes with honeyed

wine; <u>dādi al-qatrān</u> ("tarred dādi") is its pure species.

It is also said that <u>dādi</u> is a tree.

<u>MEYERHOF</u>: [Serapion 139; Ghafiqi 236; Ibn al-Beithar 843]

As we have seen above, in paragraph 69 (<u>ǧawz ǧundum</u>), <u>dādi</u> is the

Maghribian name of a substance which was considered as earth by Arabs and

Persians but is in reality a plant, the edible lichen (<u>Lecanora esculenta</u>

EV.). This lichen which contains much fecula is utilized in Persia as

nourishment and galactagogue for women (hence one of its Persian names <u>šir-</u>

<u>zād</u> meaning "milk producer"). In Spain one used it as a ferment to make wine

from honey. This is described by Idrisi (p. 81) who states that the best

quality <u>Lecanora</u> was imported from Khorassan (Eastern Persia); however an

inferior quality thereof is found in Spain, in the mountains surrounding

Saragossa. It is gathered when it is dry, and resembles granulated earth

composed of chick peas. <u>Dādi</u> is furthermore the transcription of the Greek

name <u>dādion</u> which signifies a torch or a flambeau of soft wood, from which one

also extracted tar. From there perhaps is derived the name <u>dādi al-qatrān</u>.

As to the remark "it is said that it is a tree", it is well-founded. Ghafiqi

(236) gives us the description of a tree called <u>dādin</u> or <u>dādi</u> that I have

clearly been able to identify as the Judas tree (<u>Cercis Siliquastrum</u> L.) or

sheath maker, that which Clément-Mullet had already presumed to be so.

Ibn ʿAwwām I, 303-304 describes the cultivation of this tree. See also be-

low numbers 114 (<u>dādi rūmi</u>) and 327 (<u>qanbil</u>) and Dymock I, 162. The seed

of this tree was used in Spain as a ferment and aromatic of artificial wine.

It is for this reason that Maimonides here confused <u>ǧawz ǧundum</u> with <u>dādi</u>.

87) DAWSAR   Bastard barley

MAIMONIDES: This is al-hurtāl, a type of cereal resembling (fol. 82$^{\nu}$)

corn; it is counted among its types.

MEYERHOF: [Theophrastus VIII, 7-9; Dioscorides IV, 137; Serapion 143;

Ghafiqi 249; Ibn al-Beithar 969; Issa 183, 14.]

Dawsar is actually a type of corn, Triticum ovatum L., bastard barley
or oval egilope, a wild gramineous plant. In contrast, the name hurtāl designates types of oats (see Tuhfa 338). There is here a confusion in the
popular designation, as one observes frequently. The egilope is a (type
of) corn with small ears that grows in Mediterranean regions and in the
orient. Its seed was used for cataplasma.

88) DĀRŠĪŠA'ĀN   Aspalathus, furze

MAIMONIDES: One also says šīša'ān (for short). There were different

opinions on this subject and (its identity has) not been de-

definitively established. The opinion which prevails among

recent authors is that it is the furze (al-ǧawlaq), and in

Greek saqularūn. One also says that it is the root of the

Indian nard (sunbul hindi).

MEYERHOF: [Dioscorides I, 20; Serapion 142; Ghafiqi 233; Ibn al-Beithar

842; Tuhfa 113; Abd ar-Razzaq 239; Issa 37,4; Loew II, 424-426.]

The Arabic name is a partially corrupted transcription of the Persian
name dār šišagān, which is probably half Turkish, and designates the "flowering
wood". The plant in question is the aspalathus of Dioscorides which the
Moorish-Spanish pharmacologists, and above all al-Ghafiqi (No. 233), identify
as the furze, particularly Cytisus spinosus LAM. However, Spain abounds with
species of Genista, Sarothamnus, Calycotome, etc. and it is quite uncertain
that one was able to identify the aspalathus of the Greeks.

The last "one says" of Maimonides is not confirmed by botanists.
The Greek name seems mutilated (asfālātūs?, aspalathos or sphágnon?).
Gawlaq is the Arabic form of the ancient Castil ian name yulaca (Simonet
617), modern aulaga, derived from the Latin ulex (furze).

89) DIBQ   Bird lime

MAIMONIDES: It is that which the people of Maghrib call al-ʿilk ("sticky").

MEYERHOF: [Dioscorides III, 89; Ghafiqi 245; Ibn al-Beithar 848; Tuhfa
          50; Issa III, 11; Loew II, 216.]

It is the bird lime extracted from the mistletoe (Viscum album L.,
Loranthaceae). The Greek name of bird lime and mistletoe is ixos.

90) DĪS   Rush

MAIMONIDES: As-sammār is one of its types; it is al-asal (in the text
            al-gasal, probably an error of the copyist).

MEYERHOF: [Theophrastus IV, 12; Dioscorides I, 17; Serapion 159; Ghafiqi
          67; Tuhfa 22; ʿAbd ar-Razzāq 85; Issa 102, 10; Loew I, 556.]

All these names are Arabic. Sammār is found in Loew. Samār or
Sumār - it is thus that most philologues spell it - is the name of Juncus
acutus L. Asal is the generic name for "rush"; dis the name of Juncus
arabicus POST. in the Maghrib, and of Typha angustata B. and CHAUB. in Syria.
Clément-Mullet (Ibn ʿAwwām I, 158) identifies dis with the Arundo festucoides
DESF. which was used in Spain to cover the plantations and to place them
under shelter during inclemencies. Guigues (Serapion 159) considers it
Arundo texa VAHL.

91) DIRDĀR   Elm and ash (trees)

MAIMONIDES: It is a known tree which has no fruits; it is the "tree of
            gnats" and in Spanish fresno. In Greek it is phyllon which
            means "the leaf".

- 71 -

MEYERHOF: [Theophrastus I, 8-10; Dioscorides I, 84; Serapion 154; Ghafiqi
235; Ibn al-Beithar 861; Tuhfa 115;ʿAbd ar-Razzāq 241; Issa
84, 20 and 185, 4; Loew II, 286ff; Ducros 102; Dymock III, 415-419.]

Here, Maimonides is speaking of the ash (Fraxinus excelsior L.). Never-
theless, the Persian name dardār designates the elm (ulmus campestris L.).
This divergence is explained by the fact that dardār or šaǧarat al-baqq in
the Orient (Persia, Iraq) is the name for the elm; in the West (Syria, Egypt,
North Africa) it is the ash. Similarly the word baqq in Iraq designates the
gnat, but in Syria, in Egypt and in Morocco a (different) bug (see H.Ducros,
Note Sur le Derdār and M. Meyerhof, Sur le nom dardār (orme et frene) chez les
Arabes; both in the Bulletin de l'Institut d'Egypt, vol. XVIII, Cairo 1936
pp 115-121 and 137-149). It is nevertheless strange that Maimonides states
that the dardār has no fruits, since he himself later gives the name of this
well-known fruit (see number 212 lisān al-ʿasāfir). This enigma is perhaps
explained by the assertion of the botanist Abuʾl-Hair (Ibn ʿAwwām I, 272)
that there existed in Spain a type of sterile ash tree that is reproduced by
off-shoots. The fruit of the ash tree is still sold today in the bazaars of
Cairo (see Ducros number 102 and figure for plate VIIb).

The orientalist R.P.Anastase-Marie has provided a learned article in
Arabic on the šaǧarat al-baqq (in the revue Al-Thaqāfā, Beirut I, 1).

92) DĪBSĀQŪS   Teasel

MAIMONIDES: It is the "thorn of the wool-combers or fullers" (šawk ad-
darrāǧīn) with which one combs woolen garments.
MEYERHOF: [Dioscorides III, 11; Ibn al-Beithar 987; Issa 71, 5; Loew I, 587.]

The word of the title is the transcription of the Greek dipsakos which
the Arabs also translated ʿatšān ("thirsty"). The plant is Dipsacus fullonum
MILL.; it does not grow in Egypt but in Syria (Post I, 611). In Spain the
teasel was cultivated and the heads harvested in August.(Ibn ʿAwwām II, 128).

93) DULB   Plane-tree

MAIMONIDES: It is a reddish tree. Its Arabic name is ʿaitān, and in
            Persian as-sinār. That which is known in the Maghrib is that
            it is the tree with which one dyes into yellow; the people
            there call it as-sufaira' ("the little yellow"), whereas the
            Egyptians call it al-qaisar.

MEYERHOF: [Theophrastus I-IV: Dioscorides I, 79; Serapion 163; Ghafiqi
            234; Ibn al-Beithar 875; Tuhfa 117; ʿAbd ar-Razzāq 240; Issa
            143,11; Loew III, 65-67.]

    The plane-tree (Platanus orientalis L.), in antiquity, was greatly re-
puted for its beauty and for its shade, as it was to the Arabs and Persians
of the middle ages. The name dulb is of Semitic origin (Assyrian dulbu;
Aramean dulbā); in Biblical Hebrew the plane-tree is called ʿarmon. The
Arabic name ʿaitān is ancient and was already mentioned by Abu Hanifa ad-
Dinawari. Sinār or sinnār is the Arabic form of the Persian činar. Concerning the migration of names of the plant tree, see Hehn (217-222). The
wood called sufaira', which gives a yellow dye, cannot be that of the plane-
tree. Actually, Ibn al-Baitar (1403) states that the Arabic-Spanish
botanists who claim that the sufairā' is the plane-tree, are in error.
It is the wood of the buckthorn (Rhamnus Alaternus L.), and its name in
Egypt was ʿud al-qisa; the orthography qaisar in our manuscript is false.
Concerning the cultivation of the plane-tree in Spain, see Ibn ʿAwwām
(I, 373ff), and the commentary of his translator Clément-Mullet (Etudes
sur les noms Arabes de Diverses Familles de Végétaux in Journal Asiatique,
6th series, vol. 15, 1870, pp 122-133).

94) DŪQŪ   Wild carrot and its types

MAIMONIDES: The majority of commentators have said that it is the seed

              of the wild carrot (al-ǧazar al-barrī). Just as one finds

              in the manuscripts of Galen concerning composite remedies

              that "the seeds of the wild carrot and dūqū are identical",

              so, too, it is said that these are the seeds of another type

              of carrot. More recent authors have preferred(to consider)

              that these are the seeds of al-ahilla; this is the plant which

              serves as a toothpick, and is very well known to the inhabitants

              of the West (fol. 82ᵛ) by the name al-muntina ("the fetid"), and

              it is burned in the furnaces.

MEYERHOF: Dioscorides III, 73; Ghafiqi 244; Ibn al-Beithar 983; Tuhfa

              114; ʿAbd ar-Razzāq 257; Issa 69, 5; Loew III, 449; Ducros 21.

    The term dūqū or dawqū is the genetive of the Greek daúkos meaning

carrot. The Arabs applied this term solely to the seeds of Daucus carota L.

(probably variety Boissieri WITTM.) because Dioscorides only speaks of the

properties of the seed. The Arabic name ǧazar barrī was employed for the

plant itself. On this subject, see Tuhfa 114. Besides, the last part of

the paragraph of Maimonides fortunately confirms the opinion of Renaud and

Colin (Tuhfa 353) that the "wild carrot" of Morocco is the "herb with tooth-

picks" (ahilla, Ammi Visnaga LAM.), where the pedicels of the desiccated umbels

serve as toothpicks for the indigenous people of North Africa (including

Egypt). The name muntin,"fetid", seems to us in popular language to signify

simply "odoriferous", because the Visnaga has an adequately agreeable fragrance.

The druggists of Cairo sell the seed of the cultivated carrot (ǧazar afrangi,

Ducros 21) and the seeds and the dry umbels of the Ammi Visnaga (hilla,

Ducros 23).

95) DĀR SĪNĪ   Chinese Cinnamon

MAIMONIDES: This is the cinnamon from China, and not al-qirfa ("the
bark"); I have said that because the Egyptians call
al-qirfa, dār sīnī. It is said that it is dār sīnī and dār
sūs, and it is (also) stated that it is al qirfa.

MEYERHOF: [Dioscorides I, 14; Serapion 141; Ghafiqi 232; Ibn al-Beithar
841 and 1205; Tuhfa 112, 291 and 369; ʿAbd ar-Razzāq 234-235;
Issa 149, 1-41; Loew II, 107-116; Ducros 127 and 181.]

The distinction among the different types of cinnamon is still very
difficult in our times, and was much more so in the middle ages. The Greeks
only knew the bark of the Cinnamomum aromaticum NEES. which comes from China.
It is this type which should carry the name dār sīnī. The names dār sus
and qirfa were in usage for the species considered as inferior such as
Cinnamomum Cassia BL. which is also called saliha. The cinnamon tree of
Ceylon (Cinnamomum Zeylanicum NEES), was not known either to the Greeks or
to the Arabs. Dār sīnī is the Arabic form of dār čīnī (Persian meaning
"wood from China"). Qirfa is Arabic and signifies "bark". In the bazaars
of Cairo both the Chinese cinnamon (salīha, Ducros 127) and the cinnamon
from Ceylon (qirfa, Ducros 181) are sold.

96) DAM AL-AHAWAÏN   Dragon's blood

MAIMONIDES: It is al-qātir ("the distillate"); its most well-known name
in Maghrib is aš-šayyān, its Arabic name is al-aïdaʿ, and in
Persian hunsawasān.

MEYERHOF: [Serapion 149; Ibn al-Beithar 882; Tuhfa 188; ʿAbd ar-Razzāq
250; Issa 72, 11; Loew II, 198ff; Ducros 103.]

Dam al-ahawaïn ("the blood of the two brothers") is a red resin derived
from diverse liliaceae; in the Orient the Dracaena Cinnabari BALF. (Socotra)

and the Calamus Draco WILLD. liliaceae of Malaya are mentioned, and in the
West the Dragon-tree (Dracaena Draco L.) and other Mediterranean liliaceae.
The "Persian" name is a mutilation of the Persian hun-i-siyawuśan meaning
"Dragon's blood". Loew (II, 199) thinks that the name designates the blood
of Siyawus, national hero of the Persian legend (Firdawsi). The resin itself
is nearly unknown in our days in the bazaars of the near Orient. In Egypt
today there is sold by the name dam al-ahwa a type of red polyp (Tubipora
musica). But Ducros twenty years ago still found the true red resin of
Calamus Draco WILLD. at the druggists of Cairo. 'Abd ar-Razzāq (number 134)
states that Dragon's-blood was employed in Algeria as a substitute for coral
against cardiac and pulmonary ailments.

97) DAND   Croton

MAIMONIDES: There is a Chinese one which resembles the grains of ricin,
               and there is a Spanish one which is called tartago in Spanish.
               The Spurge (māhūbadāna) is one of its species.

MEYERHOF: Serapion 150; Ghafiqi 251; Ibn al-Beithar 886; Tuhfa 122;
               Issa 60, 19; Loew I, 594; Ducros 78 and 105.

   Dand is the Persian name and hirwa' sini ("Chinese ricin") the Arabic
name of the tropical euphorbiacea Croton Tiglium L. ("small Indian pignon"),
drastic purgative well known to physicians. Dand is derived from the Sanskrit
danti (Laufer 503); this name today designates the seeds of the euphorbiaceae
Baliospermum montanum MUELL. ARG. (Chopra 567), which has properties similar
to those of the croton. Māhūb-dāna is the Persian name of the spurge
(Euphorbia Lathyris L.); its Spanish name is tartago (Simonet 534). The
Arabic name of its seeds in Algeria and in Morocco, was and still is habb
al-mulūk ("seeds of kings"). This last denomination is given to the seeds
of croton in the bazaars of Cairo as a result of confusion by Ducros (78)

who thinks incorrectly that this name signifies "seed of the Moluccas".
The Spanish "croton" of which Maimonides speaks must be another type of
euphorbium employed in Spain, as for example Euphorbia Cyparissias L. The
druggists of Cairo today sell under the name dand barrī ("wild croton") the
seeds of the "large Indian pignon" or "bean of hell" (Iatropha Curcas L.)
(Ducros 105), an American euphorbium which is originally from Brasil and
which consequently was unknown to the Arabs of the middle ages. This plant
is now cultivated in the Indies and in other tropical lands; its seed is,
like that of the croton, a violent and dangerous drastic. See also below,
at number 396 (hirwaʿ).

98) DULLĀʿ   Watermelon

MAIMONIDES: It is the Palestinian melon (al-bittīh al-filastīni) and one
                also calls it the Syrian melon (al-bittīh aš-šāmi) and the
                Indian melon (al-bittīh al-hindi); the people of Egypt call
                it "the green melon" (al-bittih al-ahdar).

MEYERHOF: [Serapion 58 and 164; Ghafiqi 239; Ibn al-Beithar 304; ʿAbd ar-
                Razzaq 171; Issa 50, 12; Loew I, 550-553; Laufer 438-445.]

    It is the watermelon (Citrullus vulgaris SCHRAD.) and its varieties which
are very numerous. In Egypt today one calls it simply battih. Its diuretic
properties having been known for a long time, it was employed above all
against dropsy. See above number 55. The origin of the watermelon is
attributed by botanists to South Africa (Engler), and by philologists to
Indiα (Laufer). The names bittīh hindi in Arabic, and hinduvāna in Persian
argue in favor of the latter hypothesis. See ʿAbd al-Latif p. 34ff and our
number 54 above (bittih), and the note to article 332 (qarʿ) below.

99) <u>DIFLĀ</u>   Rose-laurel

<u>MAIMONIDES</u>:   It is <u>ar-rūdūd</u> and in Persian <u>harzahraǧ</u>, that which, it is

said, signifies the "poison of the donkey".

<u>MEYERHOF</u>:   Dioscorides IV, 81; Ghafiqi 248; Ibn al-Beithar 873; ʿAbd ar-

Razzāq 246; Issa 124, 11; Loew I, 206-212.

<u>Diflā</u> is an Arabic transcription of the Greek <u>daphné</u>, and <u>rudud</u> an abbre-

viated corruption of the Greek name <u>rhodódaphné</u> which is the rose-laurel

(<u>Nerium Oleander</u> L.).   The Persian name - deformed in the text to <u>hūrahraǧ</u> -

was reestablished by me according to the Persian <u>har</u> ("donkey") and <u>zahra</u>

("poison").   It is known that the leaves of the rose-laurel contain a poison

which may be harmful to beasts of burden.   The orientalist J.G.Wetzstein re-

lates how his horse died in Palestine at the bank of the Jordan after having

eaten about thirty rose-laurel leaves (in the introduction of the botanic

work of K. Koch, <u>Die Bäume und Sträucher des alten Griechenlands</u>. 2nd edition,

Berlin 1884, p. XVII).   Hehn (309-311) attributes the origin of the rose-

laurel to Asia Minor.   Its cultivation in Spain is mentioned by Ibn ʿAwwām

(I, 374ff).

100) <u>DUHN AL-HALL</u>   Sesame oil

<u>MAIMONIDES</u>:   It is the oil of non-decorticated sesame (<u>simsim</u>); the oil of

decorticated sesame is known by the name <u>sīraǧ</u>.

<u>MEYERHOF</u>:   Dioscorides I, 34; Ibn al-Beithar 963; <u>Tuhfa</u> 120.

The first name should better be pronounced <u>duhn al-hill</u>; <u>Tuhfa</u> also

gives the form <u>hall</u> ("vinegar"), which is even less correct.   The term <u>sirag</u>

is of Persian origin (<u>sira</u>, Vullers II, 498).   Maimonides here gave a plausible

explanation of these two names concerning which there is some confusion in the

dictionaries.   Ibn al-Beithar gives a contrary explanation, according to the

Arabic-Christian physician Masih (8th century).

101) DUHN AL-KALĀNAǦ   Coconut oil

MAIMONIDES: One also says kalkalānaǧ; it is the oil of the coconut (ǧawz
hindī).

MEYERHOF: [Ibn al-Beithar 931; Dymock III, 516.]

This oil is mentioned by Ibn al-Beithar by the name duhn an-nārǧil·
The word kalānaǧ is not found in the dictionaries; it is perhaps derived
from the Sanskrit kulanga which designates the root of galanga. Kalkalānaǧ
is (according to Vullers II, 869) the Persian name of an electuary against
diarrhea and dysuria. Mahzan (I, 276-278) gives a long exposition on the
preparation of these electuaries (kalkalānaǧāt).

102) DUHN AZ-ZIFT   Pitch oil

MAIMONIDES: It is of pitch (zift)and whale's oil (zaīt madās)

MEYERHOF: [Dioscorides I, 72; Ibn al-Beithar 1114.]

This substance thus does not completely correspond to the pissēlaion
of Dioscorides which constitutes a pure extract of pitch. See number 138.

103) DŪSĀB   Date honey

MAIMONIDES: It is the honey of dates ('asal at-tamr) in particular.

MEYERHOF: [Ibn al-Beithar 819, 850, 981 and 2211.]

Date honey is mentioned for the first time by Pliny (XIX,91). Dūsāb
is a Persian term for "honey of grape or dates" (Vullers I, 932); its
Arabic equivalent is dibs (Ibn al-Beithar 850), which today in Syria only
designates the honey or syrup of dried grapes (Berggren 330ff).

104) DAWǦ   Buttermilk

MAIMONIDES: It is the cream of cow's milk turned sour.

MEYERHOF: [Ibn al-Beithar 977 and 2097.]

The word dawǧ is Persian; the Arabic term for buttermilk is mahīd.

105) <u>DAYĀSARŪN</u>   Nut rob

   <u>MAIMONIDES</u>: It is the confection of nuts (<u>rubb al-ǧawz</u>).

   <u>MEYERHOF</u>:   Probably an error of the copyist for <u>diyāqārūn</u>, (<u>dia karyón</u>

                   meaning "preparation of nuts" in Greek).

106) <u>DUHN AL-ǦUL</u>   Oil of roses

   <u>MAIMONIDES</u>: It is the oil of roses (<u>duhn al-ward</u>).

   <u>MEYERHOF</u>:   [Dioscorides I, 43; Ibn al-Beithar 911.]

   <u>Ǧul</u> is the Arabicized form of the Persian word <u>gul</u> meaning rose.

107) <u>DUHN AL-HINNĀ</u>   Henna oil

   <u>MAIMONIDES</u>: It is <u>al-farfūs</u>.

   <u>MEYERHOF</u>:   [Dioscorides I, 55; Ibn al-Beithar 899, 719; <u>Tuhfa</u> 174.]

   <u>Farfūs</u> is certainly a mutilation of <u>qifrūs</u>, Arabic transcription of

   <u>kypros</u> meaning henna (<u>Lawsonia inermis</u> L.), instead of <u>kyprinon myron</u> meaning

   perfume or oil of henna. There was prepared, and one still prepares today

   in the Orient, an oil from the flowers of this plant. See below number 149

   (<u>hinnā</u>).

108) <u>DIYĀMARŪN</u>   Mulberry rob

   <u>MAIMONIDES</u>: It is the confection of mulberries (<u>rubb at-tūt</u>).

   <u>MEYERHOF</u>:   The word of the title is the transcription of the Greek <u>dia moron</u>

                   meaning "preparation of mulberries". See Simonet 175.

   (fol 83^z). On this page of the original manuscript, the copyist

   Ibn al-Beithar forgot to insert the titles of the paragraphs which he had

   the habit of writing in red ink. I have filled these blanks in as much as

   possible but in brackets.

109) ⌈DIYĀQUDĀ⌉   Poppy syrup

MAIMONIDES: It is the syrup of poppy (šarāb al-hashās).

MEYERHOF: ⌈Ibn al-Beithar 988.⌉

One also finds the forms diyāqūd and dyāqūdūn, transcription from the Greek dia kódyón. It is a soothing and soporific remedy prepared with the heads of poppy. It is the predecessor of our syrup of morphine (diacode syrup). See Simonet 174. Ghafiqi ms. (fol 135b) states: "Diyāqūd is the syrup of poppy. It is called diyāqūdiyūn in Romaic and in ancient Greek, and diyāqūdā in Syriac".

110) ⌈DARĀSAĠ⌉   Chondrilla

MAIMONIDES: A red plant that one eats; it is one of the species of
           chicory (hindabā') and is also called at-tarhūn.

MEYERHOF: ⌈Theophrastus VII, 7 and 11; Dioscorides II, 133; Ibn al-
          Beithar 824, 366 and 2315; Issa 47, 16; Loew I, 433ff.⌉

Darāsaġ is Persian, tarhūn (see number 173) probably also. I think that tarhūn here is a faulty reading for tarahšaqūn, because the chondrilla and the dandelion Taraxacum officinale WIGG., belong to the same genus of compositae (Chicoraceae). The Arabic name of the chondrilla is ya'did. See numbers 114, 173 and 175.

CHAPTER HĀ'

111) ⌐HILYAWN⌐   Asparagus

MAIMONIDES: It is al-yaramī in Arabic, māsunaǧ in Greek and isfāraǧ in
            Spanish; and one also says safāraǧ.

MEYERHOF: ⌐Dioscorides III, 151; Serapion 227; Ibn al-Beithar 2260;
            Tuhfa 27, 123; ʿAbd ar-Razzāq 256; Issa 24, 4; Loew II, 195-197.⌐

It is Asparagus officinalis L. The alleged Greek name is mutilated;
as to mārsubaǧ (for this is the correct reading), it is an Arabic form of
the Persian name mār-ĉuba ("serpent wood" meaning asparagus) Vullers II,
1115). Isfāraǧ is the Arabic transcription of the Castilian esparrago and
Catolonian esparrech (Simonet 192). Nevertheless, Serapion already knew
the form asfāraġ as Arabic transcription of the Greek name asparagos.
Hooper and Field (p. 88) found the name mār-ĉuba (used) in Hamadān, Persia
for Asparagus adscendens ROXB. However, Asparagus officinalis N., Asparagus
sarmentosus and Asparagus racemosus WILLD, are also in medical usage (as
diaphoretics) in the near Orient. Its popular name in Egypt, Syria and
Persia is halyūn.

112) ⌐HALĪLAǦ⌐   Myrobalan

MAIMONIDES: It is called hārsar in the language of the Indians; and it is
            al-mufarfah(?).

MEYERHOF: ⌐Serapion 71 and 226; Ibn al-Beithar 2261; Tuhfa 43 and 126;
            ʿAbd ar-Razzāq 253; Issa 178, 16 and 179, 1-2; Dymock II, 1-5;
            Laufer 378; Ducros 13-15.⌐

The title of this paragraph is also lacking and was supplied by us;
furthermore, the last name has neither diacritical points nor vowels. I
suppose that one is here dealing with the well-known drug halīlaǧ (also

ahlīlag or ihlīlag). It is the Arabicized Persian name halīla, itself
derived from the Sanskrit haritāki. The term hārsar given by Maimonides
is probably a corruption of the Sanskrit name which is still preserved
today in the dialect of Bengal. In Hindustani, myrobalan is called harrā
or haryā. Ghafiqi MS. (fol. 144b) cites among the synonyms for myrobalan
chebula the mutilated Indian names hāzari, hāriqun and hārut, all taken from
Hāwī Kabīr of ar-Rāzī. It is one of the species of myrobalan, laxative fruits
of the combretaceae Terminalia Chebula RETZ. (or citrina ROXB.). They were
unknown to the Greeks - who termed myrobalanoï the fruits of Moringa aptera
GAERTN. (in Arabic ban). The Indians reaped the fruits of these trees which
grew everywhere in   India and in Burma. They greatly appreciated the
astringent qualities of the unripe fruit and laxative (qualities) of the
ripe fruit. The drug was imported into Persia by way of Afghanistan (from
whence the name "myrobalans of Kaboul"), and from there to the Arabic-
speaking countries. See the commentary of Renaud-Colin in Tuhfa, and the
remarks of Sir George Watt on the commerce of the drug (The Commercial
Products of India, London 1908, pp. 1072-1076). Ducros found three types
of ahlīlig myrobalans in the bazaars of Cairo, one of which, the smallest,
is called hindi ša'fri ("Indian Hordeiform"). It is used as an intestinal
astringent and as a tanning material. Al-mufarfah is probably a mutilation
of al-'arfag, name of another Indian drug (Malabathrum).

113) [HARNAWA]   Indian pepper

MAIMONIDES: It is that which is called al-fulaïfala in Spain.

MEYERHOF: Serapion 208; Ibn al-Beithar 1701 and 2253; Tuhfa 394;
           'Abd ar-Razzāq 258; Loew 358ff.

The correct vocalization is fulaïfila. Leclerc and others have con-
ceded the identification of this name by the Arabs as the fruit of the

agalloch tree (Aloexylon Agallochum LONR.), because they thought that
"Indian pepper" or pimento (Capsicum TOURN) and its varieties, were derived
from India, but Schweinfurth proved that certain of its varieties are originally from Africa, and that their fruits may have been known to the Arabs.

114) [HINDABA']   Diverse chicoraceae

MAIMONIDES: It is in Greek antūbiyā, and there are many types. The type
               which is widely known and reputed in Maghrib is the one which
               is called tifāf in Berber and sarrāliya in Spanish. Its name
               in Arabic is ya'dīd and aš-šarqīn.   /

               There is another type, wild, which is called talahšaqūq,
               at-talahšaqūn and at-tarahšaqūn in medical books; its name in
               Greek is āmīrūn, and its name in Arabic is al-'alat; it is the
               "bitter vegetable" (al-baqla al-murra).

MEYERHOF: [Dioscorides II, 132; Serapion 165; Ibn al-Beithar 2253; Tuhfa
               124; 'Abd ar-Razzāq 254; Issa 48, 11-12 and 177, 12 and 172, 8;
               Loew I, 415, 433-439.]

Hindaba-' is the Arabic form of the Syriac antubiyā, term derived from
the Greek name intybos, which is like seris, the generic name of several
chicoraceae. Here one is dealing first with chicory (Cichorium Endivia L.), then
Cichorium divarticatum SCHOUSB. (alat), and finally wild chicory or dandelion
(Taraxacum officinale WIGG.). Amirun is not Greek but Latin (amarum). The
affirmation of Loew (I, 436) that such a Greek name exists is not confirmed
in the dictionaries. Šarrāliyā is the transcription of the ancient
Castilian sarraja, modern cerraja, in Portuguese cerralha, and designates
the sow-thistle (Sonchus oleraceus L.). All these plants were designated by

* in the text antuniyā, the copyists' error

Maimonides in his other works by Arabic names. They are part of the
"bitter herbs" (maror) consumed by Jews on the festival of Passover.
The name sarqin is found nowhere else (poor reading for galawin, modern
Egyptian name. See our numbers 110, 173 and 175). For the description
of the cultivation of chicory in Spain, see ʿIbn Awwām (II, 146-149).

115). [HAYUFĀRIQŪN]   Hypericum

MAIMONIDES: It is that which is called ad-dādīʿar-rūmī; its most well-
            known name to the people of Maghrib is al-munsiyya ("forget-
            ful"), and in Spanish baniyūla (vinuela). It is the "heart
            herb" (ʿušbat al-qalb), and it is also called nusa (perhaps
            Castilian . nuez mearing nut?).

MEYERHOF: [Dioscorides III, 154; Ibn al-Beithar 2205; Tuhfa 125; Issa
            96, 14; Loew I, 655-657.]

        The name of the title is the transcription of the Greek hyperikon.
The plant in question is St-John's wort (Hypericum perforatum L., Hypericaceae)
which furnishes a red and cordiform fruit. The name dādī-rūmī ("Greek dadi")
was given by Hunain Ibn Ishaq. Munsiyya is a name which is self-explanatory
("forgetful") but was not found in other books of synonyms. Issa gives,
among others, the name muʾnis al-wahs ("which appeases grief") which has
the same apparent sense as the former. The last name, markedly distorted,
should perhaps also be read muʿnisa ("calming"). The Spanish name vinuela
designates a small vine (Simonet 62); the form given by Simonet (p.2) is
abobriella, and later (613ff) yerba corazonera, whereas the name of St-John's
wort in modern Spanish is corazoncillo. Both names signify "heart herb",
undoubtedly because of the shape of the fruit. The reading nusa is as uncertain as its explanation.

116) ⌐HĀL⌐   Cardamom

MAIMONIDES: It is the small al-qāqulla; one calls it hāl-bawwā and ğar-
          bawwā; it is aš-šamšīr.

MEYERHOF: ⌐Serapion 260 and 265; Ibn al-Beithar 1722; Tuhfa 342; ʿAbd ar-
          Razzaq 739; Issa 74, 25; Loew III, 499ff; Dymock III, 428-436;
          Ducros 80.⌐

    It is the small cardamom (Elettaria Cardamomum WHITE and MATERN,
Zingiberaceae), an Indian drug whose Persian names hāl and hil are derived
from the Sanskrit ēlā. Buwwā is the Persian word for "aroma"; ğar-buwwā is
probably another reading for hīr-buwwā (Vullers I, 769). Qāqulla appears
to be a word of ancient Semitic origin, because one encounters it in Assyrian
in the form qāqūla (Meissner, according to Loew). Šamšīr is a faulty reading
of the Persian name šušmīr (Vullers II, 479). The small cardamom is sold in
the bazaars of Cairo as a condiment under the name habbehān, derived from
the classical Arabic habb al-hāl (Ducros).

    (fol. 83ˇ)

117) HAYŪFĀQASTĪDĀS   Hypocistus or orobanche juice

MAIMONIDES: One also says hūfaqtīdās. This name is applicable to the juice
          of the orobanche (at-tarātīt).

MEYERHOF: ⌐Dioscorides I, 97; Ibn al-Beithar 2266; Tuhfa 199; ʿAbd ar-Razzāq
          407.⌐

    Ibn al-Beithar contests the explanation given above by certain authors,
for example, Ibn Sina, and repeated by Maimonides. He tries to apply the
name hayūfāqistīdās (derived from the genitive of hypokistis) to the true
hypocistus (Cytinus Hypocistis L.), plant of the cytinaceae family. Idrisi
(number 261) divides his opinion. For the orobanche, see below at number
174 (tarātīt).

118) HARTAMĀN   Oats

MAIMONIDES: It is al-qartamān, one of the types of cereals (qatānī); its origin is al-hurtal.

MEYERHOF: [Theophrastus VIII, 4; Dioscorides II, 94; Serapion 127; Ibn al-Beithar 775; Tuhfa 338; 'Abd ar-Razzāq 753, Issa 28, 10; Loew I, 686-690.]

The grain in question is oats (Avena sativa L.). The names hartamān and qurtumān - it is thus that dictionaries vocalize them - seem actually to be derived from hartal. This word is Arabic, and not Persian, as some Arabic authors have claimed.

119) HAYY AFSURAĞ   Quince confection

MAIMONIDES: It is the confection of quinces (safarğal).

MEYERHOF: This name is the Arabicized form of the Persian bihī-afsura (bihī meaning quince; afsura meaning expressed essence, juice, confection); it is one of the numerous confections known to the Oriental pharmacopeia.

120) HADABA   Woodlouse

MAIMONIDES: It is the worm (Crustacean) which is found beneath filtering jars, and which contracts and coils itself up. Its Arabic name is himār-qabbān.

MEYERHOF: [Dioscorides II, 35; Serapion 244; Ibn al-Beithar 2250.]

It is the woodlouse (Oniscus asellus) which sometimes served as a remedy against jaundice and fevers, as the earthworms that we encounter later on at number 402. The Arabic names designate "the donkey which rolls itself into a ball", and are the translation of article II, 35 of Dioscorides ("the donkeys which are found under water jars"). Woodlouses were officinal in Europe under the name Millepedae until the beginning of the nineteenth century.

CHAPTER WĀW

121) **WARD**   Rose

       MAIMONIDES: It is al-ğul to physicians, although the Arabs only applied

                 this name specifically to its white variety.

       MEYERHOF: [Theophrastus VI; Dioscorides I, 99; Serapion 393; Ibn al-

                 Beithar 2274; Tuhfa 137 and 278;ʿAbd ar-Razzāq227 and 260;

                 Issa 156-157; Loew III, 193-211; Ducros 116.]

      Gul is the Persian word for "rose". Muhassas (XI, 196, line 2) has

the orthography gull. Gulnasrīn (is the name) for a small white rose (dog-

rose. Vullers II, 1312). The Coptic (overt), Arabic (ward), Persian (gul),

Greek (rhodon) and Portugese (guedre) names, and the name of the rose in

the languages of central and western Europe are all derived from the Iranian

form varda (Loew II, 194).

      Rose leaves were in use by the Musulman peoples to prepare rose water,

and above all ocular remedies. The dried buds of the red rose (Rosa gallica

L.) are still sold in the bazaars of Cairo under the name zirr ward (Ducros).

122) **WASAH AL KŪR** ("Filth of the hive")   Propolis (bee-glue)

       MAIMONIDES: It is al-ʿağar.

       MEYERHOF: [Dioscorides II, 84; Serapion 526; Ibn al-Beithar 1576 and 2289;

                 ʿAbd ar-Razzāq 262.]

      The name of the title designates the propolis of Dioscorides, a type of

resin with which the bees at first obstruct the apertures of their hives.ʿAğar

is certainly a mutilation of ʿikbir. Ghafiqi (according to Ibn al-Beithar)

contests the identify of propolis and ʿikbir, and states that this latter sub-

stance is the pollen gathered by the bees. The "dirt of the hives" was used

as a remedy against a cough and ailments of the skin. The translation "dirt

of baths" presented by Guigues (Serapion 526) is erroneous.

123) <u>WARS</u>   Diverse

    <u>MAIMONIDES</u>: This name designates a herb which grows in Yemen and which

                produces a yellow color. In addition, it is applicable to a

                concretion in the bile of cattle and which is formed like

                calculi in the kidneys and in the bladder. People in Egypt

                call it "the pearl of cattle" (<u>harazat al-baqar</u>). *

    <u>MEYERHOF</u>: [Serapion 518; Ibn al-Beithar 2283; <u>Tuhfa</u> 133; ʿAbd ar-Razzāq

                268 and 350; Issa 117, 7; Loew II, 26-67; Dymock I, 420-423

                and III, 298.]

The Arabic physicians and botanists described the name <u>wars</u> as a red
coloring material derived from India and from Arabia. European botanists
thought that it was the product of <u>Memecylon tinctorium</u> WILLD. It is only
recently that it was discovered that <u>wars</u> is the product of the leguminous
(plant) <u>Flemmingia rhodocarpa</u> BAK. which grows in India, in Southern Arabia
and in Abyssinia (red exterior glands of the shells). It forms a red-
pomegranate powder ("Adrianople red") which serves to replace or adulterate
the <u>kamala</u>, product of the "rottlerin of dyers" (<u>Mallotus philippinensis</u> MILL.).
This latter material in Arabic carries the names <u>wars hindī</u> and <u>qanbīl</u>
(see below number 327).

As to the other substance, it is the biliary calculus of cattle called

* In the text: <u>gazarat al-baqar</u> or "carrot of cattle", a curious error of
the copyist, Ibn al-Baitar. The celebrated French naturalist Pierre Belon
in <u>Les Observations de Plusieurs singularitez</u> etc., Paris 1554, p. 205,
describes the "gallstone of cattle" that the butchers of Cairo in his epoch
sold as a drug esteemed primarily by the Oriental Jews; he gives it the
Arabic name <u>Haraczi</u>, equivalent to <u>haraza.</u>

wars in Morocco (Renaud-Colin. In Egypt I have not heard the name indicated by Maimonides (harazat al-baqar meaning "pearl of cattle"), but
it was well known to Kohen who mentions it (p.158, line 26), with a
description of the drug, to allow it to be verified and to guarantee against
adulteration.   Dāwud (I,234) also knew this drug as well as the name
harazat al-baqar; he explains it as haǧar al-baqar ("calculus of cattle")
and also gives it the name warsīn (?faulty reading gor wars). 'Abd ar-Razzāq
(number 350) designates it with the names haǧar marārat al-baqar ("biliary
calculus of cattle"), haraza, harazat al-būmiya (unexplained name), harda
(term already found in Ibn Biklāris, according to Dozy I, 271) and wars'.
This last name is undoubtedly a faulty reading for wars.

124) WAŠAQ   Gum ammoniac

MAIMONIDES: One also says ašaq, ašaǧ and wašaǧ. It is lizāq ad-dahab
           ("chrysocolla") and "gum of ferula" (samġ al-kalah);one calls
           it al-ġatta (guta) in Spanish. There is also a type of kalah
           which has a gum whose properties are similar to those of the
           ašaq; this species is the one which one calls "suicide" (qātil
           nafsihi).

MEYERHOF: [Dioscorides III, 84; Serapion 414; Ibn al-Beithar 83; Tuhfa
          29 and 135; 'Abd ar-Razzāq 28; Issa 71, 18; Loew III, 457;
          Dymock II, 156-160; Ducros 174.]

The gum ammoniac mentioned by Dioscorides was undoubtedly an African
product derived from Ferula marmarica ANHS. and TAUB. or from Ferula
tingitana L. (Umbellifereae). The Arabs identified this gum-resin with
ussaq or wuššaq, product of the Persian umbelliferous plant Dorema Ammoniacum
DON. The name which is written in ten different manners is the Arabic form
of the Persian word uša; a second Persian name of gum ammoniac is andarān

(Vullers I, 129). The other gum is perhaps the product of Dorema glabrum
FISH and MEY (Aitchison), and is called "suicide" because it loses weight
by evaporation. The Spanish name, probably guta, today designates gamboge.
Gum ammoniac was utilized for fumigations and entered into the composition
of certain remedies, particularly ocular remedies. Gilders used it in their
work, from whence comes the name "chrysocolla". The Egyptian druggists,
at present, sell particularly the "false gum ammoniac" (fasūh) derived from
Maghrib. This drug presents itself in voluminous irregular masses, brownish
yellow (in color); its taste is sour, pungent, bitter and nauseating (Ducros).
The one which is sold in Cairo is probably derived from Ferula tingitana L.,
Ferula communis L. (both mediterranean plants) and from Ferula orientalis L.
which grows in Armenia, in the Caucasus and on the mountains of Greece.
The fasūh is administered in Egypt as a mild purgative and abortifacient,
and serves for the incantation of the festival of 'asūra (the tenth day
after the new year).

125) WAGG   True sweet rush

MAIMONIDES: It is that which is called asbatānna (espadana) in Spanish;
it is that which one calls "the flower" (az-zahra); its Greek
name is akoron.

MEYERHOF: [Dioscorides I, 2; Serapion 512; Ibn al-Beithar 2270; Tuhfa
129-130 and 349; 'Abd ar-Razzāq 259; Issa 5,6; Loew I, 697; Dymock
III, 539-542.]

The drug in question is the rhizome of the araceae Acorus calamus L.,
a Chinese and Indian plant, later renowned in the West. The name wagg is
the Arabic form of the Persian wag, and this name is derived from the
Sanskrit vacā (Laufer 583). The Arabs confused this drug with the kalamos
of Dioscorides which is another Indian root (see below number 329, qasab ad-
darīra). The Spanish name is, more correctly, asbatila, in Castilian

espadilla (Simonet 193). Ašbatāna (Castilian espadana) designates
"the mass of water" (Typha latifolia L.). Both of these names are derived from the Latin spatula and designate plants with sword-blade leaves
(Renaud). The rhizome of Acorus is sold in the bazaars of Cairo by the
name qasab ad-darira (Ducros 189) or 'irq ēkar, this latter name is evident
derived from akoron. The root serves as a carminative and enters into the
preparation of certain aphrodisiacs called manzūl.

126) WASMA   Isatis and indigo

MAIMONIDES: It is al-hatr; these are the leaves of the indigo plant
             (an-nīlag) and it is al-'izlim; it is (fol. 84^i) that which
             the people (in Egypt) call an-nīl and which one uses to dye
             into black.

MEYERHOF: [Dioscorides II, 184; Serapion 157 and 517; Ibn al-Beithar
           2291; Tuhfa 182; 'Abd ar-Razzāq 267, 400 and 588; Issa 101,
           1 and 98, 14; Loew I, 493-505; Ducros 34.]

The Arabic name wasma is applicable in the first place to the leaves of
woad (Isatis tinctoria L., cruciferous plant), but also to those of the indigo
plant (Indigofera tinctoria L., leguminous plant). The Isatis is renowned
in Mediterranean countries. The Indigofera, native of   India, was later
introduced in Persia, in Egypt, etc. The continual confusion which existed
between these two plants caused them to indiscriminately have the same names
(wasma, 'izlim, hitr; nīla, etc.). Ducros (34) around 1910, still found in
the bazaars of Cairo seeds of indigo (habb en-nila) and leaves of isatis
(henna magnūn). Today one only finds the artificial indigo of European
manufacture. Ibn 'Awwām (I, 125-126) describes, according to the botanist
Abu'1-Hair, the cultivation in Spain of woad which he calls as-samāwī ("sky
colored, azure"). See below articles 159 (habb an-nīl) and 249 (nila).

127) WADAʿ   Cowry

MAIMONIDES: It is the shell of a worm (mollusc) which is found in the

sea; one calls it al-kawda in the Indies.

MEYERHOF: [Ibn al-Beithar 2272; Tuhfa 130, 459; ʿAbd ar-Razzāq 261; Hobson-

Jobson (Cowry) 269-271.]

It is cowry, shell fish of a well-known gastropod mollusc (Cypraea

moneta). The Indian name is kawrī. In medicine, the Arabs pulverized it

and used it in dry collyria.

128) WARAŠĀN   Wood pigeon, ring-dove

MAIMONIDES: It is a type of pigeon (al-hamām).

MEYERHOF: [Ibn al-Beithar 2284; Tuhfa 134; ʿAbd ar-Razzāq 271.]

One is dealing with the columba ring-dove (Columba palumbus). The

blood of young doves was employed for collyrium pastes(šiyāf) against

ocular ecchymoses. Idrisi (134) gives the popular Arabic name dalam for

the ring dove, which is also found in Dozy I, 458.

129) WARAL   Varan and scincus

MAIMONIDES: One says that it is the young of the crocodile (timsāh).

It is a type of scincus lizard (saqanqūr); this is confirmed

by the fact that those who eat the flesh of the crocodile

state that they experience a strong erection.

MEYERHOF: [Dioscorides II, 66; Ibn al-Beithar 2285 and 1197; Tuhfa 131

and 385; ʿAbd ar-Razzāq 265.]

Waral - in modern Egyptian dialect waran - is the saurian Varanus

(niloticus, arenarius, griseus),of quite large stature (up to one meter),

which is very well-known in the deserts of Egypt and North Africa. The

Bedouins eat its flesh. It has nothing in common with the crocodile.

The scincus is a small desert lizard (Scincus officinalis); it is

also very well-known in Egypt where it is sold dry in the drug bazaars
as an aphrodisiac remedy. The famous explorer and naturalist G.Schweinfurth
(died in 1925) told me that around 1880 he saw live scincuses promenading
in the shop windows of certain druggists in Cairo. The flesh of all these
saurians was considered as an aphrodisiac, which is what the relevant note
in Maimonides explains. In his treatise _On Coitus_ composed for the
Sultan ʿUmar ibn Nur ad-Din (1179-1192), Maimonides mentions once the flesh
of the scincus and twice the salt that one finds in the intestines of this
lizard, as well-known aphrodisiacs. The editor of the Arabic text of this
treatise incorrectly translated the passages in question (H. Kroner,
Eine medizinische Maimonides - Handschrift aus Granada. in _Janus_, Leyden
1916; 226, 6 and 228, 5).

CHAPTER ZĀ᾿

130) **ZAITUN**   Olive and olive tree

   MAIMONIDES: There is a wild type which grows in the mountains; its tree

   is called al-ʿatm, in Spanish al-laśtira (olivastro, oleastro)

   and az-zabnūǧ. The people of Maghrib call it az-zanbūǧ, and

   the fruit of this tree, that is the wild (type), is called

   ad-daʿaǧ by the Arabs.

   MEYERHOF: [Theophrastus I-II; Dioscorides I, 105; Serapion 95; Ibn al-

   Beithar 1140; ʿAbd ar-Razzāq 273 and 305; Issa 127, 12-14;

   Loew II, 287-295.]

   All the names cited here by Maimonides designate the wild olive tree

(Olea Oleaster L.K.). The first is generally vocalized ᾿utm. Zabbūǧ or

zanbug (originally a Berber word) is preserved in modern Spanish in the

form acebuche, meaning wild olive tree. Daʿaǧ has the sense of "blackness",

but I suppose that we are here dealing with an error of the copyist for

zaġbaǧ (Freytag I, 240) or zaġbuǧ (Issa) which is a known Arabic name for

the fruit of the wild olive tree. Ibn al-ʿAwwām (I,207-225) speaks at

length of the cultivation of the olive tree in Musulman Spain. The name

of the olive in Spanish (aceituna) is derived from the Arabic.

131) **ZAÏT**   Olive oil (omphacine)

   MAIMONIDES: Zaït al-infāq is that which is expressed from green olives.

   Az zaït ar-rikābī (transported oil) is the well-known oil.

   The Arabs so call it because they only know it as being im-

   ported to them from Syria on the backs of beasts of burden

   (rikāb, "pack-saddle" of a camel, etc.).

MEYERHOF: [Dioscorides I, 30-34; Serapion 94; Ibn al-Beithar 184 and 1141;
Tuhfa 155; 'Abd ar-Razzāq 297-298.]

Infāq or unfāq is the Arabic transcription of the Greek omphakion which
designates the oil extracted from olives before their maturity ("omphacine").
Tuhfa gives it the name zaït al-Filastīn ("oil of Palestine"). Arabia and
Egypt were always obliged to import olive oil because their desert lands do
not lend themselves well to the cultivation of the olive tree. Kohen (p.133)
states specifically that rikāb means "camel", and that this oil was transported on the backs of camels from Syria and Palestine to Egypt. Ghafiqi
(M . fol 177b) says the same thing: "Zaït rikābï This is zaït al-infāq
(omphacine); that is oil obtained from non-ripened olives. The inhabitants
of Iraq call it rikābi because it is imported from Syria on the backs of
beasts of burden (rikāb) which are camels (ibl). The Egyptians call it the
oil of Palestine (az-zaït al-filastīnī)". The oil in Spain is always
called aceite, name derived from the Arabic.

132) ZA'RŪR   Azarole, medlar

MAIMONIDES: It is the "plum of winter" (al-iggās aš-šitiwï) and "the
appetizing" (al-muštahā); it is said that it is the fruit of
the "bear tree" (šagarat ad-dubb). The name of the medlar tree
is an-nulk (nilk).

MEYERHOF: [Serapion 532; Ibn al-Beithar 1112; Tuhfa 152; 'Abd ar-Razzāq
38 and 296; Issa 59, 5; Loew III, 244-256.]

This drug is the desiccated fruit of the azarole tree (Mespilus
Azarolus ALL. or Crataegus Azarolus L.). Za'rūr is an Arabic name of
Semitic origin; the Spanish (acerola) and French (azerole) names are de-
rived therefrom. The name nulk in our text lacks diacritical points. It

is found as an Arabic name (nalk, nilk, nulk) in Issa and Freytag (IV,336),
and as a Persian name (tilk) in Vullers (I, 458). Suwaidi (fol 95b) af-
firms that this name is written with a nun. The name mustahā in Maghrib
also designates the radish (Issa 154, 2). Šağarat ad dubb designates both
the azarole tree and the medlar tree (Mespilus germanica L.)as well as the
strawberry tree (Arbutus Unedo L.). Ibn ʿAwwām has described the cultivation
of the azarole tree (I, 250ff).

133) ZARĀWAND   Aristolochia

MAIMONIDES: There is one type which is round and another long; both exist
            in the Maghrib, but the round one which is imported from ʿIrāq
            (Mesopotamia) is more efficacious; it is this one which one
            employs. The name of the zarāwand in Greek is (fol 84)
            aristolokhia, in Spanish qalabğula (calabazuela) and in Berber
            masmaqura (Spanish masmacora). It is "the tree of Ibn Rustum"
            (šağarat Ibn Rustum) or ar-rā'iza. The name of the long
            species is also "the tree of swallows" (šağarat al-hatātīf).
MEYERHOF: [Theophrastus IX, 13-15; Dioscorides III, 4; Serapion 531;
            Ibn al-Beithar 1099; Tuhfa 140; ʿAbd ar-Razzaq 272; Issa 21,4;
            Loew I, 222ff; Ducros 114.]

The name zarāwand is Persian. The two plants Aristolochia rotunda
and longa L., grow in the mediterranean countries and in central Asia.
The Greek name was given to signify the emmenagoguic action of the root.
The first Spanish name of round aristolochia is the Castilian calabazuela
("small calabash", because of the round tubercles of the rhizome). (Simonet
72). Masmaqūra is not Berber but also Spanish (masmacora, Simonet 342). I
think that the name ar-rā'iza is also Spanish (raiz means root). Finally,
Suwaidi (97a) recognizes a fourth Spanish name for round aristolochia, bubra

(buebra redonda). The origin of the name šaǧarat Ibn Rustum (mutilated in
popular Moroccan to burustam, etc.) is unknown. The unique manuscript of
Idrisi gives (p.143) the Berber name the form burūsiyā.

One still sells the two aristolochias in the bazaars of Cairo (Ducros)
(zarāwand medahrag and tawil).

134) ZANGAFR   Cinnabar

MAIMONIDES: It is said that this is incorrect, and that the true name is
            sanǧafr; it is al-fasrīqūn (psorikon in Greek).

MEYERHOF: [Dioscorides V, 94; Ibn al-Beithar 1132; Tuhfa 147; ʿAbd ar-
          Razzāq 284.]

The Arabic names are corruptions of the Persian šangarf (Vullers II,
471) which designates the cinnabar (sulfur of mercury). See the discussion
of the representation of kinnabari by the Greeks in Colin-Renaud. Psorikon
of Dioscorides (V,99) was not cinnabar but a combination of vitriol (see
number 140, zāǧ) and calamine.

135) ZAʿFARĀN   Saffron

MAIMONIDES: It is al-ǧādīʾ and one also calls it kurkum.

MEYERHOF: [Theophrastus I, 6; Dioscorides I, 26; Serapion 528; Ibn al-
          Beithar 1110; Tuhfa 151; ʿAbd ar-Razzāq 275; Issa 60, 6;
          Loew II, 7-25.]

The three names are Semitic. Kurkum is derived from the Hebrew and
Aram   karkom, and later designated not only the stamens of the saffron
(krokos, Crocus sativis L.) but also the rhizome of curcumin (Curcuma Longa L.,
Zingiberaceae), because both drugs give an intense yellow tint. See number
205 (kurkum). The saffron was always a precious material and consequently
subjected to falsification. True saffron is only found rarely in the bazaars
of Cairo. ʿIbn Awwām has given a detailed description (I, 115-118) of the
cultivation of the saffron near Seville, and the harvesting of the precious stamens.

136) ZŪFĀ RATB   Suint (Grease of wool; sandiver)

MAIMONIDES: It is the grease of wool (dasam as-sūf). The Greek (Zūfā) is
without any relationship toward (suint), and without relation
to any characteristic (thereof); it is a known herb.

MEYERHOF: [Loew II, 84ff.]

As Leclerc (Ibn al-Beithar 1136-1137) and Renaud-Colin (Tuhfa 141,142)
have remarked, the Arabs confused the two Greek terms of Dioscorides (II,74
and III,25): oisypos, "suint", and hyssopos, "hyssop", which were both
transcribed zūfā. One distinguished them by the adjectives reading zūfā
ratb ("moist zufa") for squint, and zūfā yābis ("dry zuba") for hyssop.
That also caused much confusion in the Latin translations of the middle ages.
The hyssop (Hyssopus officinalis L., a labiate) grows in the Mediterranean
region and in middle Asia. Its leaves and its flowery summits were employed as pectoral stimulants and as a condiment. Dymock (III,116) declared
that the plant called zūfā yābis in   India is a type of Nepeta (Nepeta
ciliaris, a Labiate). See also Serapion 137 and 469 (commentary of Guigues)
and ʿAbd ar-Razzāq 277-278 (commentary of L. Leclerc).

137) ZARNAB   Uncertain

MAIMONIDES: It is al-falanga and "crow's foot" (riǧl al-ġurāb) and
"grasshopper foot" (riǧl al-ǧirād).

MEYERHOF: [Serapion 181; Ibn al-Beithar 1098; ʿAbd ar-Razzāq 288; Issa 178,
4; Loew I, 364-366; Dymock III, 374-375.]

The name zarnab is Arabic; it has not yet been identified, up to the
present. The identification adopted by Issa that it is the common yew
(Taxus baccata L.) does not seem to be justified. The association with the
Indian bixin Flacourtia Cataphracta ROXB. is discussed by Leclerc (Ibn al-Beithar),
Dymock, and Loew. It thus seems better to leave the question in abeyance. As

to the name falanǧa, it is Persian and, according to Idrisi (146) and
Dozy (aflanǧa I, 29), identical with zarnab. According to Vullers (II,
690), it is a red seed which enters into the composition of perfumes.
Dozy is inclined to identify falanǧa, according to Ibn al-Gazzār, with the
Spanish falaǧa or helecho meaning fern, whereas Clément-Mullet (Ibn al-ʿAwwām)
identifies it as cuscuta. Forskal heard the name riǧl al-ǧurāb in Arabia
used for a type of horned poppy, Chelidonium dodecandrum or Roemeria
dodecandra STAPF. Kohen speaks of this plant in two locations: first
(p. 132 line 11) by the name riǧl al-ǧurāb which he identifies as ātiririllāl
(in Berber meaning "bird's foot") of Ibn al-Baitar, adding that it was the
latter who introduced this remedy against white leprosy (baras) in Egypt;
and afterwards (p. 133, last lines) he states that, according to Ibn al-
Gazzar, the zarnab was a large tree of Mount Lebanon having leaves like those
of the willow and an odor of citron. However, he adds (p. 134, first lines)
that the name zarnab is also used for two types of yellow flowers with
aromatic odors imported from ʿIrāq which he himself had seen. Dāwud (I,346)
raises (his voice) against identifying zarnab as a Lebanese tree and claims
it is a herb not taller than one third of an arm's length. According to
him, it grows in Persia and in Syria, but the last type lacks aroma and
tartness.

138) ZAFT   Pitch

MAIMONIDES: Liquid pitch (az-zaft ar-ratb) is called al-qīr; it is
            asphalt (al-asbant). Dry pitch is also called al-qār.

MEYERHOF: [Dioscorides I, 72; Serapion 166; Ibn al-Beithar 1114; Tuhfa
            150; ʿAbd ar-Razzāq 276 and 758; Ducros 178.]

   The word meaning "pitch" in Arabic is usually vocalized zift and not
zaft. Qār and qīr are derived from the Greek keros, "wax". It is possible

that these names originate from the Akkadian kir-ra which has the meaning

of "bitumen, asphalt", according to E. Forrer in his analysis (Orientalistische

Literaturzeitung, 40th year, 1937, p. 675) of the remarkable work of R.J.Forbes

Bitumen and Petroleum in Antiquity, (Leyden 1936). "Bitumen", asbant, de-

rives from the Greek asphaltos. Ibn Ganāh cites this name in the form

asbalt (Dozy I, 24). Renaud and Colin (Tuhfa) have provided a tableau of

the confusion which reigned among the Greeks, and even more so among the

Arabs, concerning the different species of bituminous vegetables and minerals,

and which seemed inextricable. The druggists of Cairo sell asphalt under

the name qār al-yahūdiyya (bitumen judaicum) (Ducros).

See above the "oil of pitch" at number 102 and below number 168 (humar).

139) ZAĪBAQ   Mercury

MAIMONIDES: It is also called zāwuq, and the people of Maghrib call it

az-zawq.

MEYERHOF: [Dioscorides V, 95; Serapion 529; Ibn al-Beither 1143; Tuhfa

149; ʿAbd ar-Razzāq 287.]

Zaïbaq or ziʾbaq is the Arabic form of the Persian name jiva or giva,

meaning quicksilver or mercury. ʿAbd ar-Razzāq and Renaud-Colin (Tuhfa)

give the popular Maghribian term zāwaq. The name az-zawq (pronounced az-zöq)

is preserved in Spanish in the name azogue, meaning mercury.

140) ZĀG   Vitriol

MAIMONIDES: There are numerous types: one of these is al-qalqand, and

one also says al-qalqant; another is al-qalqadis and yet

another is al-qalqatār which is also called al-halqatār.

The "vitriol of Cyprus" (az-zāg al-qubrusī) is the green one;

the "vitriol of shoemakers" (zāg al-asākifa) is the yellow one.

MEYERHOF: Dioscorides V, 98-99; Serapion 535; Ibn al-Beithar 1080;

Tuhfa 144; Abd ar-Razzāq 283; Ducros 133.

The word zāg is Arabicized from the Persian zāg meaning vitriol or copperas. Qalqant is the Greek khalkanthon; qalqadis is khalkitis, and qulqutār - thus it is vocalized in the dictionaries - derives perhaps from (the Greek) khalkokrâton. These are all impure vitriols, above all iron sulfates; one employed them particularly in collyria against eye maladies. The "vitriol of shoemakers" is the melanteria of Dioscorides (V, 101); atramentum sutorum of the Latins. In the bazaars of Cairo, one sells by the name sahira or zāg ahdar ("green vitriol") an impure iron sulfate (Ducros), the qalqant of the Arabs, and the "green copperas" of the European druggists. According to Ibn al-Beithar (1080 and 1313), šahira is an ancient name for vitriol, but also (ibid. 2129) that for a substance employed to purify gold. These are black crystalline masses which form in the waters of copper mines.

141) ZABAD AL-BAHR   Diverse

MAIMONIDES: This name ("meerschaum" or sea foam) is applied to the sponge,
            as we have already mentioned. And this (name) is applied to
            the gravelly, light substance that one finds on the volcano
            of Sicily and which the people of Maghrib call "the scraper'
            (al-hakkāka) and the people of Egypt "the foot brick" (tubat
            ar-rigl).*

* Simonet in his Glosario p. 541 attempts to derive the word tuba from
  the Latin tophus, Low Latin topus, tufus, etc., German tuffstein,
  Portugese and Italian tufo. But here we are dealing with the Arabic
  word tuba meaning brick because knowledge of the Latin name in Egypt
  is inadmissable. The stone for scraping corns, even today, has the form
  of a brick.

There are two types (fol. 85$^{\check{a}}$): one is black and very rough, and one is white and less rough; it is this (latter) one that is used to scrape horses. It is well-known in Egypt where physicians call it al-qa'isūr; one also says al-qafsūr. As to the black type, it is the one the Greeks have called abārīqā.

People were of a very different opinion regarding the names we have just mentioned but the above is what recent authors have verified.

MEYERHOF: [Dioscorides V, 118; Serapion 534; Ibn al-Beithar 1086; Tuhfa 153;'Abd ar-Razzaq 285 and 717.]

The name zabad al-bahr ("meerschaum") is the translation of halkyonion of Dioscorides which designated a mixture of sponges, algae and polypiers rejected by the sea. The druggists of Cairo and Morocco (Tuhfa 153) identified it, in our times, as lisān al-bahr ("tongue of the sea") which is the bone of the cuttle-fish. It served, and still sometimes serves, as an ingredient in the dry collyria against specks in the cornea of the eyes. See below number 214.

The white stone of which Maimonides here speaks is the pumice-stone, qa'isūr or better qa'isūr, Arabic transcription of the Greek kiseris. In Egypt, the people use a black rock that one calls hagar haffaf ("rasing stone"). One uses it to scrape callosities of the feet.

R.P.Bovier-Lapierre obligingly informed me that he gathered several rare light-colored foot scrubbers, evidently made of pumice-stone in the ruins of Fostāt, the city where Maimonides lived. These specimens are no longer sold today in the bazaars of Cairo. On the other hand, he was able to amass in Fostāt a large number of black foot-scrubbers made of bubbly basalt from Hawrān (Gebel ed-Drūz, Syria), a material which resembles a coarse sponge which has turned to stone. One finds much of it

in the bazaars of Cairo. It is very likely that these are the two types
of "foot bricks" described by Maimonides.

The "foam of the sea" ("meerschaum") known in Europe has nothing in
common with zabad al-bahr; it is a mineral (natural hydrosilicate of mag-
nesium).

As to the Greek name abārīqā, it is perhaps a mutilation of the term
kata Besbikon (halos akhnê, "foam of salt" of the Island of Besbikos)
given by Dioscorides who enumerates five types of halkyonion.

142) ZAHRAT AN-NUHĀS   "flower of copper" (scoria)

MAIMONIDES: It is the sediment which forms in the water in which one ex-
            tinguished molten copper.

MEYERHOF: [Dioscorides V, 77; Ibn al-Beithar 1134 bis; Tuhfa 161; 'Abd ar-
            Razzāq 301.]

The Arabic name is the translation from the Greek khalkou anthos of
Dioscorides, which one should not confuse with khalkanthon (vitriol) which
we encountered in number 140. Leclerc (Ibn al-Beithar) translated it as
"verdigris"; however, the latter in Arabic is called zingār. One has not
yet established which copper salt corresponds to khalkou anthos (flos
aeris of the Latins).

143) ZAWĀN   Darnel

MAIMONIDES: It is as-sailam and ad-danqa and in Spanish bišta (piste).
            The people of Maghrib call it az-ziwāl; it is al-hasar.

MEYERHOF: [Dioscorides II, 100; Serapion 453 and 538; Ibn al-Beithar
            1139 and 1370; Tuhfa 156 and 448; 'Abd ar-Razzāq 228, 299 and
            944; Issa 111, 6; Loew I, 723-729.]

Zawān or zuwān is the intoxicating darnel (Lolium temulentum L.
Gramineae), a plant which grows with the cereals. Its seed, mixed into
bread, causes dizziness. The Greeks designated the plant by the name aîra
and they knew the toxicity of its seeds. Schweinfurth (Annales du Service
des Antiquités d'Egypte, V, 187, Cairo) found ears of darnel (var.
macrochaeton A. Br.) in Egyptian tombs of the 3rd millenium before the
common era. Zawān is an Arabic word; the Syriac is zizānā. From this
name is derived the Greek name zizania and from the latter which is found in the
New Testament, the French zizanie. See the philologic commentary of the oriental names of darnel in Loew (I, 728). Kohen (p.133 line 11) saw darnel seed
used in Egypt as a constituant of collyria against corneal leucoma in the eye.

The names danqa and hasar are probably Arabic but of unknown origin.
Sailam(and salmak) are Persian names for the enebriating darnel. ʿAbd ar-
Razzāq also cites the names barrāqa and gulāf. As to the Spanish name
bišta which is found in Simonet (p. 446) in the form pixt, it is derived
from the Latin pistum, and today in Morocco designates the seed of Phalaris
canariensis L. or "alpist of canaries" (canary grass) that one gives to
birds (Renaud-Colin in Tuhfa, 772 at the top). The name alpiste is
Castilian as well as Portuguese and French (Simonet p. 446).

144) ZAĪT AS-SUDĀN   Argan oil

MAIMONIDES: It is argan oil (zaīt al-hargān). It is the oil well-known
            to us in Maghrib by the name zaīt urgān. Urgān is a type of
            known tree; one cooks the pips of its fruits and one extracts
            this oil, which is also called "liquid manna" (al-mann as-sā'il).

MEYERHOF: [Ibn al-Beithar 1145; Issa 20, 8; Loew III, 154]

The usual orthography is argān. This name designates the argan tree
(Argania orientalis VIREY or Argania Sideroxylon ROEM. and SCH., Sapotaceae), a

spinescent Moroccan shrub which has an ovoid fruit whose seeds are rich in oil. This oil is employed in Morocco for the same usages as olive oil. The Moroccan author of Tuhfa didn't mention this oil, probably because it is too well-known in his country.

145) ZURUNBĀD   Zerumbet (ginger)

MAIMONIDES: It is that which the people of Egypt call 'irq al-kāfūr ("root of camphor").

MEYERHOF: [Serapion 544; Ibn al-Beithar 1097; Tuhfa 139; 'Abd ar-Razzāq 282; Issa 192, 1; Dymock III, 399; Ducros 115.]

The name is Persian (zarunbā or zurunbāha, Vullers II, 130). In Arabic it is sometimes vocalized zarunbād, zaranbād, etc. The drug is the root of Zingiber Zerumbet ROSC. (Zingiberaceae). One sells it in slices, even today, in the bazaars of Cairo, always by the name 'irq al-kāfūr, as Maimonides indicated it, or kāfūr el-ka'k ("camphor of cakes"). This tubercle is used as a carminative, excitant, sudorific and tonic (Ducros).

146) ZUGĀG   Glass

MAIMONIDES: The antique white glass is the one which one calls "the glass of Pharaoh" (az-zugāg al-fir'awnī); it is also "the Syrian and Pharaonic bottles" (al-qawarīr aš-šāmiyya w'al-fir 'awniyya).

MEYERHOF: [Serapion 543; Ibn al-Beithar 1094; Tuhfa 146; 'Abd ar-Razzāq 286.]

One is here dealing with the antique glass that one finds in great quantities in the ancient historic sites of Egypt and Syria. It is green, blue or white. As Maimonides states, the latter was preferred. It was mixed crushed into dry collyria for making blemishes disappear from ailing eyes. Still in our times, the people of Egypt attribute a particularly salutary property to mineral residues of antiquity.

CHAPTER ḤĀ'

147) HANDAQŪQĀ   Lotus (trefoil)

MAIMONIDES: It is an-nafl, ad-daraq, al-ǧābur, and (fol 85ᵛ) al-'urqusān;
            one also calls it habāqā; it is al-kurkumān and in Spanish
            turbila.

MEYERHOF: [Dioscorides IV, III; Serapion 236; Ibn al-Beithar 718; Tuhfa
          170; 'Abd ar-Razzāq 66, 335, 491 and 612; Issa 183, 2-4; Loew III,
          481 and 522.]

   Handaqūqā is a Syriac name (Fraenkel 141); the Arabs took it for
Nabathean. It designates the fragrant lotus (Trigonella coerulea SER.),
and handaquqā barri (similar to lótos agrios of Dioscorides), the wild
lotus (Trigonella elatior SIBTH.). The other names are in agreement with
the designations given by Issa, except for ǧābur which is lacking in the dictionaries. The names nafal and habaq are applicable to other plants, and
Colin-Renaud are correct in speaking "of the confusion which prevails amongst
the Arabs concerning the three principal types of leguminous fodder plants:
trefoil, lucern and melilot". The Spanish name turbila (tribilo, Simonet 547)
corresponds to the modern Spanish trebol (from the Latin trifolium): the
reading turnila meaning trigonella is not excluded. Ibn Biklāris and
Ibn al-Beithar give the Spanish synonym triflun (triphyllon). Today in
Egypt the name handaqūq designates Trigonella hamosa L. (Schweinfurth 64).

148) HUDAD   Lycium juice

MAIMONIDES: This name is applied to the juice of a plant. The plant it-
            self, whose juice is al-hudad, is fīlazahraǧ, and the Greek
            name of this juice is lykion. It is the "collyrium of Hawlān"
            (kuhl Hawlān).

MEYERHOF: [Dioscorides I, 110; Serapion 205; Ibn al-Beithar 680; Tuhfa
          166; 'Abd ar-Razzāq 314; Issa 112, 15; Loew III, 133ff; Ducros 168.]

Hudad or hudud is the Arabic equivalent chosen by Hunain for the Greek
lykion. In Renaud and Colin (Tuhfa 166) one finds discussions on the
nature of this thorny plant which modern botanists have made into the rham-
naceous Lycium afrum L. (synonym is Rhamnus infectoria L.). The name
filazahrağ or fallazahrağ is derived from the Persian fil-zahra meaning
"elephant bile" (see below number 315). The concentrated juice of this
plant was sold by the druggists of the middle ages as an ingredient for
collyria. Freytag (I, 538) states that Hawlān was the name of an Arabic
tribe from Yemen to which one ascribed the derivation of the name of this
collyrium. This interpretation seems logical because, for a very long
period, the commerce of Indian drugs passed through the ports of Southern
Arabia. The druggists in the bazaars of Cairo today sell, under the name
hudad yamānī ("Yemenite lycium"), the thorny branches ofthe Lycium europaeum L.
(Ducros), which we will encounter again below (number 294) under the name 'awsig.

149) HINNĀ'   Henna

MAIMONIDES: It is al-yarna* and "the fruit of the henna" (tamrat al-
              hinnā') which is called al-fāgiya;** it is ar-raqūn and
              ar-riqān ("tinted red or yellow").***

MEYERHOF: [Dioscorides I, 95; Serapion 262; Ibn al-Beithar 719; Tuhfa
             174 and 319; ʿAbd ar-Razzāq 312 and 700; Issa 106, 10; Loew II,
             218-225; Ducros 91.]

This plant is the lythrariaceous plant Lawsonia alba LAM. whose green
leaves, when pulverized, furnish the well-known coloring material of the
Orient, and which still today plays a very large role (in the lives of) the
peoples of Egypt and neighboring countries. It was known in ancient Egypt

*   in the text al-yarta

** in the text al-fa'iya or "the flowery one"

*** Issa writes raqqun and riqqān, Kohen p. 132 raquq, obvious error of the
    copyist.

by the name kupre, in Coptic kouper, in Greek kypros, in Hebrew kofer etc.
The name tamr al-hinnā ("fruit of henna") designates, strangely, the
flower of henna, and this not only in Egypt, but also in Syria and Arabia
(Loew). One employs the juice of its macerated leaves as an astringent
(Ducros). The cultivation of henna in Spain was described in detail by
Ibn ʿAwwām (II, 118-122).

150) HUMMĀD   Rumex, sorrel

MAIMONIDES: It is the "vegetable of Khorassan" (al-baqla al-hurāsāniyya)
and "the wild beast" (as-silq al-barrī). It is very well-
known in Spain under the name of al-lābāssa and is also called
in Spanish rabanil (?), in Berber tāsamāmt and in Greek lapathon.
It is al-qitfa, and the Arabs call this herb al-qataf. Ar-ramat
is a type of rumex and it is called hūšān.

MEYERHOF: [Theophrastus VII, 1-6; Dioscorides II, 114; Serapion 273; Ibn
al-Beithar 698; Tuhfa 171 and 397; ʿAbd ar-Razzāq 142 and 313;
Issa 132, 3 and 158, 9; Loew I, 358-360; Ducros 90.]

The Arabic name hummād is derived from the root h.m.d., "to be sour,
acid", and generally designates plants of the groups Rumex (acetosa) and
Oxalis (acetosella). The Spanish name labāssa is the Castilian lapato,
derived from the Greek lapathon (Simonet 294). The other Spanish name is
mutilated and should correspond to the Castilian acederilla (Simonet 4).
The Berber tāsmāmt is derived from the root asemmūm meaning sorrel (communication of M.H.-P.J. Renaud). Qataf is an Arabic name which better designates
species of orache (for example Atriplex hortensis L., chenopodiaceae), and
hūšān or haušan is another name for this plant. Ramat or rimt (Issa 90, 16)
is the name of another chenopodiaceae, Haloxylon articulatum BGE. Another

type of this rimt exists in the Egyptian deserts (Haloxylon Schweinfurthii ASCHERS., Ramis p. 71). The druggists of Cairo sell, under the name hummēda, the fruits of Oxalis (sorrel) which are used as blood depuratives and stomach tonics (Ducros). Concerning the cultivation of sorrel, see Ibn ʿAwwām (II, 169-171). For the Spanish name rabanil (doubtful reading), we found an equivalent rabanilla in Simonet (477), but this name designates cruciferous plants and is derived from the Latin raphanus.

151) HASAK   Terrestrial tribulus

MAIMONIDES: It is ġallu ǧiġu (gallo ciego) in Spanish, which signifies "the
               one-eyed cock" (ad-dik al-a'war). It is the "spine of camels"
               (šawk al-ǧimāl), and in Persian šākawhaǧ.* It is that which in
               Maghrib is called himmas al-amir ("chick-pea of the emir").
               Al-faqʿa is a type of tribule (hasak).

MEYERHOF: [Theophrastus VI, I etc.; Dioscorides IV, 15; Serapion 247;
               Ibn al-Beithar 669; Tuhfa 168; Abd ar-Razzāq 103 and 316;
               Issa 182, 12; Loew III, 512-513; Ducros 83.]

* This name, mutilated from the Persian sakarhang, is perhaps derived from
  the Sanskrit goksura (Chopra 408). Kohen, in addition, on p. 134, gives
  the Arabic names sagarat ad-dik al-a'war meaning "herb of the one-eyed
  cock", and hisn al-ʿasākir meaning "fortress of soldiers"; furthermore
  on p. 123, adrās al-kalb meaning "teeth of the dog" and adrās al-ʿaguz
  meaning "teeth of the old man". Fleischer, in his Studien ueber Dozy's
  Supplement aux dictionnaires arabes in Ber. d. phil. hist.-Klasse d. Kgl.
  Saechs. Akademie der Wissensch. 1884, p. 16, explains the Persian name as a
  composite of the Persian sih meaning "three" and guhang meaning "tips" or "buds".

The Arabic name hasak designates several types of thorny plants, and in this chapter, the tribule terrestre of the Greeks (Zygophyllaceae). The name "spine of camels" was given to it because its fruits attach themselves with their prickles to the feet of beasts of burden. The strange Spanish name "blind cock" (Ibn Biklāris correctly translates gallo ciego as "blind cock" dik a'mā, and not "one-eyed") is not explained (Simonet 241ff). Faq'a is probably an erroneous transcription of qutba which is another Arabic name designating thorny plants (in Hebrew qoteb meaning "spiny"), and in particular four types of tribule (Issa and Loew). The Arabicized Persian name sakuhag, sukuhang, etc., is derived from the Persian sakuhang or sakarharg (faulty reading; Vullers II, 444 and 454). The Egyptian druggists sell the fruit of the terrestrial tribule under the name dirs al-ʿaguz ("molar of the old man") and zafirat al-ʿaguz "nail of the old man") as an antispasmodic (Ducros).

152) HAZĀZ AS-SAHR   Orchil and diverse (mosses)

MAIMONIDES: It is a type of moss (tuhlub) which grows under rocks. Its name in Latin (Spanish) is urǧalla (orchilla), in Greek leikhénos. One uses it to give wool a wine-colored hue.

MEYERHOF: Dioscorides IV, 43; Serapion 258; Ibn al-Beithar 664; Tuhfa 184; Abd ar-Razzāq 337; Issa 186, 13; Loew I, 24; Ducros 92.

The Arabic name has the meaning "scurf or lichen of rock" and is encountered in many forms. The majority of Arabic authors have not determined the species of lichen whose name was translated from the Greek of Dioscorides (Peri leikhenos tou epi ton petron). Maimonides explains here that one is dealing with a coloring lichen, probably the orchil, orchilla in Spanish (Roccella tinctoria DC., Simonet 407). One should remark that Ibn al-Beithar gives the name hinnā, Quraiš to this lichen

("henna of the Qurai̇š Arabs"), and that this name is still known in the
bazaars of Cairo, as a synonym for hazāz sabġi ("coloring lichen").
Ducros identified this lichen with a Lecanora, probably Lecanora circummunita
NYL. This plant, brought from Maghrib and subjected to the same procedures
of ammoniacal fermentation as the orchils, furnishes a red dye (Ducros)
(fol. 86^{r}).

153) HULBA   Fenugreek

MAIMONIDES: It is al-farīqa.

MEYERHOF: Theophrastus III, 17,2; Dioscorides II,102; Serapion 405;
Ibn al-Beithar 682; Tuhfa 175; ʿAbd ar-Razzāq 336; Issa 183,5;
Loew II, 475-481.

Hulba is the best known Arabic name of the seeds of fenugreek
(Trigonella Foenum graecum L., Leguminous plants), in Greek télis, in
Hebrew tiltan. The name farīqa is Arabic-Syrian (Abu Hanifa ad-Dinawari;
see Dozy II, 260). The plant is cultivated in Mesopotamia, in Syria and in
North Africa, as fodder for animals, and its seeds are used as a condiment
and remedy. In Egypt (where one calls them helba) the seeds are germinated
and eaten as "hors-d'oeuvre". The Arabic name is preserved in the modern
Spanish alholva meaning fenugreek.

154) HURŠUF   Artichoke

MAIMONIDES: It is al-kankara and al-ʿakkūba (in the text al-ʿaluba, faulty
reading); it is that which one calls al-qannāriyya in Spain,
and the Maghribians call it afzān al-maqlūb.

MEYERHOF: Theophrastus VI, 4,11; Dioscorides III, 14; Serapion 203 and
415; Ibn al-Beithar 658; Tuhfa 213; ʿAbd ar-Razzāq 318, Issa
64,19; Loew I, 407-412.

The plant is the artichoke (<u>Cynara Scolymus</u> L., Composeae). It is
described by Maimonides (in his commentary on the Mishnah, Seder Tohoroth, ed.
Derenbourg Berlin 1887, p. 269) under the Hebrew name ʿakkūbit, Arabic-
Spanish <u>hāršaf</u> and Maghribian <u>afzān al-maqlūb</u>. The name <u>afzān</u> seems to be
Berber, but one could read <u>aqrān</u> (Arabic meaning "horns", because of the
horned form of the shells. Renaud). ʿAkkūba is derived from the Aramaic
and designates numerous thistles (Dozy II, 155). The original form of the
Persian name is <u>kangar</u> (Vullers II, 901); as the "Spanish" name <u>qannāriyya</u>
(Simonet 87), it seems to be derived from the Greek <u>kinara</u>. The denomination
<u>qannāriyya</u> is still in usage today in Morocco (Colin-Renaud), whereas in
Egypt the artichoke is called <u>al-haršūf</u>, and in Spanish <u>alcachofa</u>, name
derived from the Arabic, as is also the (name) "artichoke" (itself). See
IbnʿAwwām (II, 291-292) regarding the cultivation of the artichoke in Spain.

155) <u>HABB AR-RĀS</u>   Staphisagria

<u>MAIMONIDES</u>: It is <u>habb as-sabib</u> ("seed of nits") and <u>zabīb al-ǧabal</u>
                   ("dry grape of the mountain"), and in Persian <u>mayūbazaǧ</u>.

<u>MEYERHOF</u>:   [Dioscorides IV, 152; Serapion 19; Ibn al-Beithar 1085 and 2201;
                   <u>Tuhfa</u> 258; ʿAbd ar-Razzāq 304,326 and 534; Issa 69, 13; Loew III,
                   115ff; Ducros 113.]

The Arabic name <u>habb ar-rās</u> ("seed of the head") still today designates
the seed of the renonculaceous plant <u>Delphinium Staphisagria</u> L., employed
since antiquity as an antivermin remedy ("the herb of lice"). The name <u>habb as-
sabib</u> is perhaps a faulty reading for <u>habb as-siʾbān</u>("seed of nits").
<u>Mayūbazaǧ</u>, <u>mayufizaǧ</u>, <u>miwizaǧ</u>, etc., are transformations of the Persian
name <u>mawizak</u> which signifies "small dry grape" (i.e. raisin). The drug
is still sold today, by the aforementioned names, in the bazaars of Cairo. It
is employed in powdered form or in a decoction for external use for pedicular
affections, scabies and scurfs (Ducros 113).

156) HABBA HADRĀ'   Fruit of the false pistachio tree

MAIMONIDES: It is the fruit of the terebinth (butm); the wild species is

ad-darw, and in Spanish one calls it bīna raštaqa (pino rustico).

MEYERHOF: [Theophrastus III, 15; Dioscorides I, 71; Serapion 59; Ibn al-

Beithar 302 and 570; Tuhfa 178; 'Abd ar-Razzāq 322; Issa 141,14;

Loew I, 192-193.]

It is the fruit of the terebinth or the false pistachio tree (Pistacia

Terebinthus L.) and other anacardiaceae. Dioscorides had already mentioned

that the fruit of the terebinth is edible. The Arabic name signifies

"green seed" (granum viride of the middle ages). Darw is the Arabic name

of the lentisk (Pistacia Lentiscus L.), whereas the Spanish name pino rustico,

in reality, designates the wild pine (Pinus silvestris L.). The "green seeds"

are still used in alimentation in Mesopotamia (Guigues XXXIX); in our times

they are sold all over in the bazaars of Cairo, and it is astonishing that

Ducros does not mention this well-known drug. See above at number 66 (butm),

and Ibn 'Awwām (II, 368ff).

157) HĀSĀ   Thyme

MAIMONIDES: It is one species of savory (sa'tar); its name in Greek is

thymbron, and in Spanish tumila (tomillo).

MEYERHOF: [Theophrastus I, 12 and others; Dioscorides III, 36; Serapion

249; Ibn al-Beithar 548; Tuhfa 163; 'Abd ar-Razzāq 309; Issa

180, 23; Loew II, 104-106.]

The name hāsā is Aramaic (hās'ā in Judeo-Aramaic, Loew), and the

equivalent of thymos (not thymbra, Dioscorides III, 37) which designates

thyme (Thymus capitatus LK. and HOFFM., Labiates) and the varieties of the

same genus (serpolet or Thymus Serpyllum L., etc.). Its other Arabic names

are sa'tar barrī ("wild savory") and sa'tar al-hamīr ("savory of donkeys").

Tomillo (Simonet 550) is today the Castilian name of the common thyme

(Thymus vulgaris L.). In Egypt, there are two types of thyme designated

by the name za'tar (Thymus capitatus and Thymus bovei BENTH., Ramis 164).

The herb is sold in the streets by the Bedouins. In modern medicine one

makes use of the red and white oil extracted from the common thyme for

distillation. It is, for example, the essential ingredient of pertussin,

known remedy against whooping-cough and bronchitis.

158) HANZAL   Colocynth

MAIMONIDES: It is murrār as-sahrā' ("the bitter of the desert") and it

              is called al-hadag̃ and al-kabasa; it is also called habbat

              al-habid.* It is aš-šara. Some have claimed that it is

              al-ʿalqam, but this is not accurate.

MEYERHOF: [Dioscorides IV, 176; Serapion 304; Ibn al-Beithar 714; Tuhfa

              177; ʿAbd ar-Razzāq 257,311,558,632 and 688; Issa 509; Loew I,

              537-542.]

One is dealing with the curcurbitaceous herb Citrullus colocynthis SCHRAD.,

kolokynthis or kolokyntha agria of Dioscorides IV, 176, whose branches lie

flat on the ground and whose round and very bitter fruits ("coloquintes

officinales") are very well-known in the deserts of North Africa. Hanzal

is its most widely known Arabic name; the other Arabic names are vocalized

hudg̃, sary and habad. Kabast is a Persian mame (Vullers II, 791). As to

the Arabic ʿalqam, it is in usage for the colocynth, but in Spain and in

Maghrib, the "donkey cucumber" (Ecballium Elaterium A. RICH.) which is also

a bitter curcurbitaceous plant, was designated by this name; from there

comes Maimonides' observation. The pulp of the colocynth was, and con-

tinues to be, employed as a drastic purgative. Ducros (93) only mentions

* according to Issa and the dictionaries, this name designates the seeds of

  colocynths

the leaves of the colocynth as a drug of the Cairo bazaars. However, one can still observe everywhere, even in our times, the dried fruits which are given in milk as a purgative. It seems that the colocynth was cultivated in Spain in the Middle Ages (Ibn ʿAwwām, II, 226).

159) <u>HABB AN-NĪL</u>   Seed of kaladana

MAIMONIDES: It is "the Indian safflower" (<u>al-qirtim al-hindī</u>): it is
that which one calls <u>habb al'aǧab</u> in Maghrib ("miracle seeds").

MEYERHOF: [Serapion 199; Ibn al-Beithar 557; ʿAbd ar-Razzāq 408 and 588;
Issa 99, 19; Loew I, 463; Dymock II, 530-532; Ducros 79.]

The Arabic name designates the seed (called in French by the Persian name <u>kaladana</u>) of a beautiful Indian convolvuleous plant <u>Ipomoea hederacea</u> JACQ. ("star of the morning", in English "blue morning glory"). It is a species which is today found in all warm countries and which is cultivated in the gardens of Egypt. The triangular and blackish seeds were officinal in the Indo-English pharmacopoeia of 1868, and were extolled as a mild purgative. One always sells them in the bazaars of Cairo (figure in Ducros, plate VIII, 28). See above, number 126 (<u>wasma</u>) and below, number 249 (<u>nilag</u>).

160) <u>HARMAL</u>   Harmal

MAIMONIDES: There are two types, one of which is called <u>isfand</u> in
Persian, and <u>basus</u> in Greek; the name of harmal is also
<u>zari'at al-basus</u> ("seed of basus").

MEYERHOF: [Dioscorides III, 46; Serapion 243; Ibn al-Beithar 650; <u>Tuhfa</u>
176; ʿAbd ar-Razzāq 94 and 315; Issa 135, 24; Loew III,
507-511; Ducros 22 and 67.]

It is the "wild rue" of Dioscorides, the plant <u>Peganum harmala</u> L. that one classifies today among the zygophylleae. The name <u>harmal</u> is perhaps, and basus certainly, of Aramaic origin (bassosa, Loew III, 509). In

Kohen p. 133, line 24, one reads zari'at as-sarir; in Ibn al-Beithar,

according to Dozy I, 586, zari'at al harir ("seed of silk"). Isfand is

the Arabic form of the Persian ispand (Vullers I, 91 derives the name from

pehlevi spenta meaning white, pure). The fruits and seeds of harmal are

sold in the bazaars of Cairo as emetics and soporifics (Ducros). At the

same time they serve for purposes of magic, particularly in Algeria ('Abd

ar-Razzāq) and in Morocco (Colin-Renaud). The roasted seed, subjected to

chemical transformations through the use of sulfuric acid, is the base for

an "Andrianople rouge". The cultivation of the harmal in Spain is mentioned

by Ibn 'Awwām (II, 306).

161) <u>HABB AZ-ZALAM</u>   Edible galingale

    <u>MAIMONIDES</u>: These are the small roots which resemble the galingale of

                Koufa (as-su'd al-kūfī) that people eat. Its name is

                "Sudanese pepper" (fulful as-Sūdān).

    <u>MEYERHOF</u>: Theophrastus IV 8,2,6,12; Dioscorides I, 4; Serapion 201;

              Ibn al-Beithar 559; Tuhfa 189; 'Abd ar-Razzāq 319; Issa 66,2;

              Loew I, 558-559; Ducros 74.

The tubercles of the edible galingale (Cyperus esculentus L.) are im-

ported from upper Egypt into Cairo and sold by the name of habb al-'azīz;

these are white, amylaceous, olivary tubercles with yellowish radicles.

Su'd kūfī is probably a name of the rhizomes of the round galingale

(Cyperus rotundus L.). The name "Sudanese pepper" simultaneously designates

the fruits of Xylopia aethiopica R. RICH. (anonaceae), a totally different

drug, and this has provoked confusion in certain Arabic works of synonyms.

The tubercles of the round galingale are also sold in Cairo (see below

number 274, Su'd). Ibn 'Awwām (II,202-203) describes the plant and its culti-

vation in Spain.

162) HAYY AL-'ALAM   Orpine

MAIMONIDES: In Greek it is aeizoon (fol 86ᵛ), in Spanish ubila raštaqa

(uvilla rustica) and in Persian hamīsaqūs. There are two

types, one of which has oblong seeds filled with liquid like

the pulp of the fruits of the pine (sanawbar); this type is

the one that in Maghrib is called "grape of terraces" ('inab

as-sutūh)because it grows on the terraces of houses.

The other has round leaves like those of the chestnut tree

(qastal), and is also filled with liquid; this type is the one

that is called anbūb ar-rā'ī ("flute of the shepherd"), and

the people of Maghrib call it zalā'if al-mulūk ("bowls of kings").

MEYERHOF: [Theophrastus VII, 15, etc; Dioscorides IV, 88-92; Serapion 67;

Ibn al-Beithar 732; Tuhfa 187 and 277; 'Abd ar-Razzāq 308; Issa

166-167, 1; Loew I, 467ff.]

One is here dealing with numerous plants of the family of crassulaceae,

all of which have pulpy stems and leaves. The first type most probably

corresponds to the arborescent sempervivum (Sempervivum arboreum L.) or

the houseleek (Sempervivum tectorum L.). Uvilla rustica ("wild grape") is

the Spanish name of certain species of orpine (sedum) (Simonet 558. The

latter cites on p. 440 another Spanish synonym: pinuela). Hamisak (and not

hamisaqūs) is the Persian name for Sempervivum in general (Vullers II, 1475).

The Arabic name "bowls of kings" is found in Tuhfa (277) in the form sahifat

al-muluk or musa'ifiqāt ("small cymbals"). It may designate certain species

of Cotyledon. I nevertheless think that the Arabic name is in good accord

with the description of the orpine of Spain (Sedum hispanicum). This plant

has pulpy leaves which feign the shape of the small bowls or castanets

which surround the stem. In Syria one called this plant udn al-qasis

("Priestly ear") because of the shape and thickness of the leaves
(Suwaidi 107a). 'Abd ar-Razzāq claims to have heard the name udna in
Rosette (Lower Egypt) as designating the large species of Sempervivum.
Comparison with the leaves of the chestnut tree is not correct. One
should rather compare the leaves of the Sedum to the shape of the chestnut.
The juice of this plant served in the preparation of collyria.

163) HURF   Garden-cress

MAIMONIDES: This is at-tufā and habb ar-rašād and one calls it al-maqalitā.
            When one speaks of hurf abyad ("white hurf"), hurf bābilī
            ("Babylonian hurf"), hurf madanī ("hurf of cities" or "from
            Medina"), one refers to the garden-cress which exists in Spain.

MEYERHOF: [Dioscorides II, 155; Serapion 403; Ibn al-Beithar 653-655;
            Tuhfa 167;'Abd ar-Razzāq 310, 556 and 901; Issa 107, 9 and 124,1;
            Loew I, 506-511; Ducros 72.]

Hurf is the Arabic name of several species of pepperwort (Lepidium) and
cress (Nasturtium, Cruciferaceae). Here one is dealing primarily with the
garden-cress (Lepidium sativum L.) and the water-cress (Nasturtium officinale
R. Br.). Habb ar-rašād are the red seeds of the garden cress that one sells
in the bazaars of Cairo (Ducros). The first name should be vocalized tuffā'
(Suwaidi, Tuhfa, Issa). Maqalitā (Arabicized muqlayātā) is the Syriac name
of the roasted seeds (Guigues p. 25 and Loew I, 509) from (the Hebrew) qali
meaning roasted. Hurf abyad, according to Issa (104,7) is the speckled dead
nettle (Lamium maculatum L.); hence a labiate, a totally different plant. Hurf bābilī
is the name of several species of Lepidium. Kohen(p. 126 s.v. tālasfi meaning
Thlaspi and p. 128) says that hurf bābili is hurf as-sutuh ("terrace-cress")
or girgir al-kalb ("dog cress"); it is the cress of the fields (Lepidium

campestre L.). The seeds are used as a diuretic, and externally for cataplasms against scrofulous ulcers (Ducros). Concerning the cultivation of
garden-cress in Musulman Spain, see Ibn ʿAwwām (II, 248ff).

164) HAǦAR YAHŪDĪ   Judaic stone

MAIMONIDES: It is the one called "the striated stone" (al-haǧar al-muṣuttab);
            it is the one also known as mudarrib al-hasāt ("stone sharpener").

MEYERHOF: [Dioscorides V, 137; Serapion 219; Ibn al-Beithar 601; ʿAbd ar-Razzāq
            388, Ducros 122.]

    This stone which is always sold in the bazaars of Cairo and the near-East,
was well described and illustrated (plate IX, 8) by Ducros. The Lapis
judaicus that one finds in Egypt is the prickling of a fossil echinid (Cidaris
glandiferus) which originated in Syria and in Palestine. "This drug presents
itself in the form of olivary buds 1 to 4 centimeters long, one of whose
extremities shrinks into a type of collar...The surface of this bud (radiate)
is traversed....by equidistant and fine striations." Gentle to the touch,
this stone is readily reduced to an impalpable powder; it is always used as
a lithontriptic and diuretic (Ducros). Its popular name in Egypt is zaĪtun
Benī Isrāʾil ("olives of the children of Israel").

165) HIRBĀʾ   Chameleon

MAIMONIDES: This name is employed for a type of small animal which re-
            sembles the lizard (stellion) hirdawu; it is the one which
            the Greeks call khamaileon.*

MEYERHOF: [Dioscorides II, 79; Ibn al-Beithar 662; Tuhfa 188; ʿAbd ar-
            Razzāq 348.]

* In the text, the word lubahnitis refers to a Greek name of the plant
  longhkitis or lychnitis; it is an error of the author or the copyist.

I have nearly nothing to add to the commentary of the learned editors
of the Tuhfa. The common chameleon of North Africa is Cameleo Vulgaris DAUD.
Chameleon blood, by local application, is recommended by Dioscorides and the
Arabs to hinder the eyelashes which grow therein (trichiasis of the eyelashes), and to repulse them once they become detached. A similar application of the blood of frogs and bats was already recommended in the Ebers
papyrus (Ancient Egypt, circa 1650, B.C.E.).

166) AL-HĀǦ   Alhagi

MAIMONIDES: It is a shrubby tree whose name is also al-ʿaqūl, upon which
            falls the manna (at-taranǧabín).

MEYERHOF: Serapion 360 and 497; Ibn al-Beithar 408 and 553; Tuhfa 194
          and 259; ʿAbd ar-Razzāq 875; Issa 8, 17; Loew II, 414-416.

This plant is the thorny leguminaceous plant Alhagi Maurorum TOURNEF.
(Alhagi manniferum DESV.), very well-known in the deserts of North-Eastern
Africa, Arabia and the West of Asia. It produces a sweet exudate (tar
angubín "honey of dew", Persian word), the "manna of Persia" which has a
great reputation in the Orient as a mild laxative. As to the use in
agriculture of the dried Alhagi, see Ibn ʿAwwām I, 458.

167) HABBA SAWDĀʾ   Nigella; here "chichm"

MAIMONIDES: It is that which one calls "dry collyrium of the Sudan"
            (kuhl as-Sūdān); it is not nigella (as-šuníz). One also calls
            it at-tašmízaǧ, aš-šašmaq and aš-šišmaq.

MEYERHOF: Serapion 521; Ibn al-Beithar 415 and 573; Tuhfa 454; Issa 42,8;
          Loew II, 514; Ducros 134.

Habba sawdāʾ, "black seed" in Arabic, is the name both of the nigella
(Nigella sativa L.), the "black cumin of the Orient", and the seed of the
Cassia Absus L., a wild leguminous plant of the Sudan, Arabia and southern

Persia. These seeds bear the Persian name čašm (tchachm), "eye" or čašmak

(tchachmak), "little eye", because they have the shape of small, black and

brilliant lentils, like the eyes of little animals. From these are de-

rived the other names mentioned by Maimonides. The seeds which are called

šišm (chichm) in Egypt, are used as dry collyria against all sorts of ophthal-

mopathies. The Persian word suniz also designates nigella (see Nr. 365).

See M. Meyerhof, Histoire du chichm, remède ophtalmique des Égyptiens, in

Janus 1914, p. 261ff. One still sells this drug in the bazaars of Cairo.

One should note, in passing, that Suwaidi (101a) also gives the name habba

sawdā' to the "Abyssinian cumin" (kammum habasi) which is bishopswort or

stonewort (Carum copticum BENTH., Ombelliferaceae).

168) HUMAR   Asphalt (Bitumen of Judea)

MAIMONIDES: It is "the pitch of the sea" (zaft al-bahr) and "the black

             of the Jew" (kufr al-Yahudī) (fol 87ʳ); one also says qufr

             al-Yahūd ("bitumen of Jews").

MEYERHOF: [Dioscorides I, 73; Serapion 209; Ibn al-Beithar 705 and 1818;

           Tuhfa 150; ʿAbd ar-Razzāq 476; Ducros 178.]

     It is the mineral or asphalt bitumen, extracted from the Dead Sea in

Palestine; hence the names mentioned by Maimonides. The names humar and

qufr al-Yahud were already mentioned by the Arabic geographer Ibn Hurdādbih

at the beginning of the (3rd)-9th century (Kitāb al-Masālik Wa ᴶ l-Mamālik,

auctore Abu ᴶl-Kasim Obaidallah...Ihn Khordadbeh, in Bibl. Geographorum

Arabicorum. Edit, M.J. deGoeje. Vol. VI, p. 79 of the Arabic text). The

root h.m.r. already designated bitumen or asphalt in biblical Hebrew (hēmar);

q.f.r. means bitumen; in Hebrew (qofer), Accadian (kupru), Aramaic (qupra),

Armenian (kupr), etc. See the exposé by Renaud and Colin in Tuhfa l.c.

In Egypt, to this day, one still sells this raw asphalt in the bazaars under

the name q̄ar al-yahūdiya ("bitumen of Judea"). It is utilized as a
dressing for contusions and ulcers, as a maturative and cicatrisant and,
by internal use, as an expectorant (Ducros).

169) HAǦAL   Partridge

MAIMONIDES: It is al-qabaǧ.

MEYERHOF: [Ibn al-Beithar 644 and 1736]

The name haǧal denotes several species of partridge; in Palestine, for
example, Caccabis Chukar, and in Arabia and Egypt Ammoperdix HEYI. Qabag is
the Arabic form of the Persian name kabaǧ or kapak (Vullers II, 791).
According to Damiri (I, 509), the name qabaǧ denotes the male partridge;
but Sawaidi (102a) makes no mention of such a difference in the name.
The gall of the partridge, used as a collyrium, was recommended as a remedy
for a cataract (Idrisi).

CHAPTER TĀ'

170) TUHLUB   Water lentil

    MAIMONIDES: It is "the water lentil" ('adas al-ma') and "the hair of

        spinners" (ša'ar al-guzzāl).

    MEYERHOF: [Theophrastus IV, 10 (ikme); Dioscorides IV, 87 (phakos telmaton);

        Serapion 488; Ibn al-Beithar 451; Tuhfa 201; Abd ar-Razzaq

        391; Issa 106, 15; Loew I, 16.]

    This drug is the "water lentil" (Lemna minor L.), an aquatic plant well-
known on the stagnant waters of Europe and of certain warm lands. It was
employed exteriorly in compresses and as a hemostatic, as well as in the preparations of collyria.

171) TABĀŠĪR   Bamboo concretion

    MAIMONIDES: It is the "ash of the serpent" (ramād al-hayya)

    MEYERHOF: [Serapion 445; Ibn al-Beithar 1447; Tuhfa 195; Abd ar-Razzaq 390;

        Issa 29, 14; Loew I, 591 ff; Ducros 148]

    Tabāšīr is a Persian word (Laufer 350 supposes that the word is derived
from the sanskrit tavak-ksīra, meaning vegetable juice) which designates
"bamboo manna", crystalline concretions that one extracts from the internodes
of bamboo. They are composed of silica, potash, lime and organic substances.
Renaud and Colin (Tuhfa 195) declare that the name tabāšīr is also used for
ivory or calcinated bone with which one falsifies the true bamboo manna. It
appears that the name designated by Maimonides refers to something comparable.
In Egypt, one still sells the true Indian product under the name tabāšīr hindī,
and it is utilized for the preparation of dry collyria, as a tonic, astringent, etc.
(Ducros). Popularly, the name tabāšīr designates chalk in Egypt and in Syria.

172 TĪN   Clay, argil

    MAIMONIDES: a) Sigillate earth (tīn mahtūm) is that which one also calls

        "sigillate earth of Lemnos" (hawātīm lamniyya) and "sigillate earth of Bohaira"

        (hawātīm al-Buhaira). One also calls it "lacquered rubric" (magra lakkāniyya) and"the seal of Yemen" (al-hātim al-yamanī).

b) As to the species of argil which is called "cimolite earth"
(tīn Qīmūliyā), it is identical to the "saponaria earth of Toledo"
(tafl tulaītulī), according to the unanimous opinion of physicians.

c) The species which is called "Armenian earth" (tīn arminī) is a
red and viscous argil which is imported from Armenia. One also calls it
"Romaic earth" (tin rūmī) and "Cyprus earth" (tīn qubrusī) because it is
the same argil, in spite of the difference of the land of its origin. It
is the earth which we in Magrib call al-ingibar.

d) The "earth of Nichapour" (tin naīsabūrī) is the one one calls
"edible earth" (tin al-akl); it is a white argil that one transports
(through the streets).

e) When physicians speak of "Eve's earth" (tin Hawā) and of
"Khouzistan earth" (tin hūzī), they refer to the viscous argil, free of
gravel and comparable to that which the Egyptians call iblīz (balīz).

f) The species that one calls "Samos earth" (tin Sāmūs) is the
"star earth" (tin al-kawkab).

MEYERHOF: [Dioscorides V, 151-156; Serapion 496-499; Ibn al-Beithar 1488-1495;
Tuhfa 50, 196-198; Abd ar-Razzaq 393-399; Ducros 150-151]

These are nearly all the medicamented earths introduced into medicine by
the Greeks. The Arabs faithfully preserved the names, although it was impossible
for them to procure the earths of the Greek island.

a) Sigillate earth of Lemnos was the best known (terra lemnia), even
in European medicine. It is a hydrated peroxide of iron which served
as an antitoxin.

b) The identity of cimolite earth and saponaria earth of Toledo is
more than doubtful. The latter had an excellent reputation in Musulman
Spain. It was a saponaria earth. See Tuhfa No. 198.

c) Armenian earth, like its equivalents, was viscous and served for compresses on fractures which required reduction. Hence, its Arabic name inǧibar ("reduction").

d) In the Musulman world there were several types of edible earths of which the most famous is that of Nichapour (Oriental Persia). The custom of eating one type of earth still persists in Afghanistan (B.Laufer, Geophagy in Field Museum of Natural History; Anthropol. Series 18 No. 2, Chicago 1930).

e) We have nowhere else encountered the first two names indicated in this paragraph. Khouzistan was the province in the southwest of Persia. Tin iblīz is the ancient name of the (sour) lime of the Nile which one still uses today in compresses against certain eruptions of the skin. Suwaida (117 a) calls it tin misrī meaning "Egyptian earth".

f) Samian earth, as that of Lemnos, was very well-known in European medicine, above all, to arrest hemorrhages (according to the prescriptions of Galen).

Armenian bole is still sold in Cairo under the name tin armallī or tin rūmī ("Greek earth"). It is a clay earth tinted red by iron oxide. The terra sigillata or that of Lemnos which one sells in the bazaars of Cairo to the present times, is a silicate of alumina or magnesia, poor in iron oxide but rich in silica and alumina (Ducros also gives an analysis made in Cairo).

173) TARHŪN   Tarragon, wild celery

MAIMONIDES: It is said that these are Pyrethrum leaves ('āqir qarhā), but this has not been confirmed (fol 87[v]) by recent authors. They state, on the contrary, that it is one of the types of celery (karafs, wild celery).

MEYERHOF: [Ibn al-Beithar 1459; Tuhfa 200; Abd ar-Razzaq 418; Issa 22,5; Loew I, 380]

Tarhūn is the Arabic form of the Persian name tarhūn (Vullers I, 433) which
is perhaps derived from the Greek drakōn or drakontion. Today this name designates the tarragon (Artemisia Dracunculus L., composite) but in the middle ages,
this name was applied to other plants, as the words of Maimonides indicate.
See also the commentary of Renaud-Colin (Tuhfa) and our numbers 110 and 114.
Suwaidi (121a) distinguishes two types, one Babylonian and one Greek.

174) TARĀTĪT   Cynomorium, broom-rape

    MAIMONIDES: It is the plant which is called "goat's beard" (lihyat attaīs);
                  it is zubb rubbāh and mard (nāridin).* Its name in Spanish is
                  fuššala (husillo). We have explained above that the juice of this
                  plant is called hayufāqastīdas.

    MEYERHOF: [Ibn al-Beithar 1460; Tuhfa 174; Abd ar-Razzaq 407; Issa 65, 10;
               Loew I, 44 and II, 299-301.]

The Arabic name tarātīt is in use for the "mushroom of Malta" (Cynomorium
coccineum L., cynomoriates), parasitic plant of Mediterranean regions which is
also found in the deserts of Egypt. Because of its resemblance to a penis,
it is called zibb al-ard ("rod of the earth") in Egypt. The Bedouins (call it)
zubb rubbāh (monkey penis). The Spanish name fuššala, according to Dozy
(II, 269) and Simonet (236), is derived from the Latin fusellus ("small spindle"),
and in modern Castilian is husillo. The cynomorium was much in use under the
name fungus melitensis as a hemostatic.

One also calls other parasitic plants tarātīt and zubb al-ard and, from
an obscene point of view, certain orobancheates such as Phelipaea (Cistanche)
lutea DESF. (See Issa 50, 1 and 138, 6). It is their juice which was called
hypocistidos. See our number 117.

175) TARAHŠAQŪN   Dandelion

    MAIMONIDES: It is the "lettuce of donkeys" (hass al-himār)

---

* In the text naridis, error of the copyist.

MEYERHOF: [Ibn al-Beithar 1469 and 2263; Abd ar-Razzaq 405 and 846; Issa 177,15; Loew I, 434 ff; Ibn 'Awwam II, 357.]

This plant is the well-known composite plant called dandelion or pissenlit (Taraxacum officinale VILL. or WEBER). The Arabic name is trans-formed from the Persian talh šukūg ("bitter purslane") which is found in various corrupted forms talahsaqūg, talahšaqūn, tarahšaqūq, etc. It is strange that Maimonides does not mention the other well-known Arabic synonyms of Taraxacum, such as hass barrī ("wild lettuce"), hindība' barrī ("wild chicory"), murāir, etc. The dandelion was used at all times as a vegetable, and as an external and internal remedy. Its juice served for the preparation of collyria. See above our numbers 110 and 114.

176) TAL'   Bunch of young dates

MAIMONIDES: It is the first fruit that the palm tree (nahl) produces each year when the sheath opens.

MEYERHOF: [Dioscorides I, 109; Ibn al-Beithar 1473; Abd ar-Razzaq 401; Loew II, 333-336; Ibn 'Awwam I, 323.]

The name tal', which is still in usage in Egypt, and many other Arabic names (Schweinfurth 229), designate a young bunch with or without the bract (sheath) within which is enclosed the inflorescence ("spadice"). This part of the date tree (Phoenix dactylifera L.) has always been recommended as an astringent and calming tonic. According to Ibn 'Awwam, one also made bread therefrom. See above the cabbage-palm (No. 68, ǧummār), and below at number 204 (kufarrā) and, above all, 206 (kāfūr), where we will furnish details concerning the designation tal'. Muhassas (XI, 119 ff) has an entire chapter on tal'. Kohen (p. 137, line 16 ff), describes a resin of the spathe of the palm tree (samǧ tal' an-nahl) which, according to the authority of the furnisher of this drug, can only be produced by the old trees.

177) TALQ   Talc, mica, steatite, etc.

MAIMONIDES: It is "the star of the earth" (kawkab al-ard), and one also

              calls it hasīmā.

MEYERHOF: ⎡Dioscorides V, 138; Ibn al-Beithar 1472; Tuhfa 203;

            Abd ar-Razzaq 381 and 404.⎤

As Leclerc has already remarked (Ibn al-Beithar 1472, note), the Arabs
confused the asbestos of Dioscorides with talc. In addition, by the name
kawkab al-ard ("which shines on the earth like a star"), they understood mica
and flaky gypsum. Talq is the Arabic form of the Persian talk (Vullers II, 547).
Hasima (variants in Ibn al-Beithar are qasīmā, hasamītā, etc.) is a Syriac
name which is not found in the dictionaries. Suwaida (119b) has the form
hasīmā.

CHAPTER YĀ'

178) YUTTỤ̄' (SIC!)   Latex plants

MAIMONIDES: There are numerous types of these plants that one calls al-
            yuttū'āt, all of which have in common the property of pro-
            ducing a milky juice (labaniyya, latex) which is viscous and
            very sour and cauterizes the body on contact. If one takes a
            small quantity internally, it produces diarrhea and emesis.

            Among the latex plants, one can enumerate aš-šubrum, al-kawba,
            al-lā'iya, al-māzariyun, al-māhūbdāna, al-māhīzahra and al-'ušar.
            That which one calls sukkar al-'ušar (sugar of Calopropis) is
            a dew which flows cn the shrubby tree of Calotropis.

MEYERHOF: ⌈Theophrastus IX, 11-15; Dioscorides IV, 164; Serapion 522; Ibn
            al-Beithar 2302; Tuhfa 210; Issa 79-80; Loew I, 602-627.⌉

Yattū' (as the Arabic philologues write it) is derived from the Syriac
yattū'ā and from the verb n.t.' which signifies "oozing, transuding" (Loew I,605).
It is the translation of the Greek tithymallon which, according to Theophrastus
and Dioscorides, is the generic name of latex plants. Dioscorides enumerates
seven varieties, and the Arabic physicians follow his example. They are the plants
of different species: šubrum is the name of Euphorbia Pithyusa L. Kabwa is the
name of a euphorbium mentioned by Rhazes (Ibn al-Beithar Arabic IV, 207, line 7)
and which is impossible to identify. Māzariyūn is Daphne Mezereum L., Thymelaceae.
Lā'iya is perhaps Euphorbia triaculeata FORSK. (But see below, number 215);
mahubdana is Euphorbia Lathyris L.("caperspurge, spurge"). Mahizahra is a
Persian name which signifies "fish poison" and it is the cocculus or "shell of
the East" (Anamirta paniculata COLEBR., Menispermaceae); and 'ušar is the Ascle-
piad Calotropis procera R.BR. The "sugar" of Calotropis is an exudation of
inflorescences, not yet well-observed and examined. In Dymock (II, 428-437)
one finds a historic and pharmacologic analysis of this plant and of its latex.
Ibn 'Awwam (II, 374 ff) enumerates six species of tithymals (yattū'āt) found

in Spain. On this subject, see the commentary of his translator J.J.Clément-Mullet (Études sur les noms arabes de diverses familles de végétaux. Journal asiatique. 6th series, vol. 15, p. 55-90)

179) YABRŪH   Mandragora (mandrake)

MAIMONIDES: It is al-luffah, the "apple of the devil" (tuffah al-ǧinn).
             In Persian one calls it šābīzak and also šabīzaǧ, and in Spanish
             ubalita (see the commentary). One also says al-maqad and al-azaǧ,
             and its Greek name is Khamaïmêlon.

MEYERHOF: [Theophrastus IX, 8-9; Dioscorides IV, 75; Serapion 276, 343 and
             525; Ibn al-Beithar 2034 and 2300; Tuhfa 207; Abd ar-Razzaq
             180 and 890; Issa 114, 13; Loew III, 363-368.]

The Arabic name yabrūh is derived from the Syriac yabrūhā (in Hebrew
duda'im), name of the anthropormorphic root of Mandragora officinarum L.
(Solanaceae). Luffāh and tuffāh al-ǧinn are Arabic names; šābīzak and šābīzaǧ
are Persian names (Vullers II, 181 and 378) of the fruit of the plant which
resembles a small apple. The Arabic names maqad and azag are lacking in the
treatises and dictionaries. The Greek name khamaïmêlon ("earthly apple") which
designates the camomile is introduced here by error. The other Arabic authors
render the Greek name correctly mandragoras. The Spanish word in our manuscript
is mutilated and is found in Idrisi (206) in the "Latin" form arǧbalīta, which
Simonet (22) explains, according to the Mozarabic form archo-bellitho, as
derived from belladona. In Egypt, mandrake root was formerly imported from
Palestine. Today,one no longer sees it in the bazaars of drugs. See also our
number 216 (la'ba).

180) YANBŪT   Anagyris (bean-trefoil)

MAIMONIDES: It is the Nabathean carob-tree (al-harrūb an-nabatī) and in
             Spanish (fol. 88ʳ) hina qazqūna (see the commentary); it is
             "the greyish thorn" (aš-šawka aš-šahbā')

- 126 -

MEYERHOF: [Dioscorides III, 150; Ibn al-Beithar 2320; Tuhfa 9, 182 and
204; Abd ar-Razzaq 243; Issa 14,16; Loew II, 418 ff; Ducros
76 and 224.]

The identification of yanbut was in doubt for a long time (see Ibn al-
Beithar), because this name was often employed to designate thorny shrubby
trees in general, primarily by the Jewish writers Sa'adya and Ibn Ganah.
However, the researches of Loew and the investigations in the bazaars of the
Near-East leave no doubt that this name, like the two aforementioned names,
designates the leguminous plant Anagyris foetida L.("offensive wood"). This
one has many other Arabic names (see Issa). The Spanish name appears distorted;
it should perhaps read espino hediondo ("offensive thorn") or something
similar. One finds no explanation thereof in either Dozy or Simonet. (Dr. Renaud
was kind enough to inform me that the manuscript of the 'Umda has gina (?cento)
and adds qunuza (konyza) as the Greek name; qazquna is therefore perhaps a
mutilation of qunuza.)

Another possible reading is yichia gascuna (Simonet 565 and 256), equivalent
to the modern Castilian veza de Gascuna, which in French is vetch of Gascogne
(a parent type of Anagyris). Kohen (136 line 13) uses the name šawka šahbā' to
designate epithyme.

In the bazaars of Cairo, one still sells the leaves of the anagyris under
the name el-muntina ("the offensive") as a purgative and emmenagogue (Ducros
224). The seeds are also sold, under the name habb al-kila ("kidney seeds")
as an emetic and diuretic (Ducros 76).

181) YĀSIMĪN (SIC!)   Jasmine

MAIMONIDES: It is al-'arif.

MEYERHOF: [Serapion 290; Ibn al-Beithar 2298; Tuhfa 138 and 205; Abd
ar-Razzaq 421-422; Issa 101, 10; Loew III, 396 ff.]

The Arabic name is derived from the Syriac, and is ordinarily vocalized

yāsamīn. In popular Egyptian dialect it is yasmīn. The drug is the flower
of the well-known plant Jasminum officinale L.(oleaceae). In Egypt, one
sells above all the "Arabian jasmine" (full, Jasminum sambac AIT). The Arabic
name 'arif is not found in the dictionaries. I propose to translate it "odorous",
derived from the word 'arf meaning "odor".

CHAPTER KĀF

182) <u>KAZBARAT (SIC!) AL-BĪR</u>   Capillary (Maiden-hair)

<u>MAIMONIDES</u>: These are the "hair of Medusa" (<u>ša'ar al-ġūl</u>), the "hair of Orion"
(<u>ša'ar al-ġobbār</u>), the "hair of the devil" (<u>ša'ar al-ġinn</u>) and
<u>maqāyir</u>.

It is that which is called <u>as-saniqa</u>* and its name in Spanish
is <u>arġaqīl</u> and <u>qaršaqīla</u> (<u>carrasquilla</u>). Its Greek name (<u>sic!</u>)
is <u>baršīyawusān</u>.

<u>MEYERHOF</u>: [Theophrastus VII, 14, 1; Dioscorides IV, 134-135; Serapion 75;
Ibn al-Beithar 254; <u>Tuhfa</u> 65 and 450; Abd ar-Razzaq 126, 517,
729 and 953; Loew I, 7: Ducros 200.]

<u>Kuzbarat al-bi'r</u> is the usual orthography. This name signifies "coriander
of wells" and is the Arabic designation of the graceful little fern <u>Adiantum
Capillus Veneris</u> L. (Pteridiae). The other Arabic names have, in part, been
translated from the Greek. The classic Greek name is <u>adianton</u>. The name which
Maimonides thought was Greek is Persian: <u>parr-i-siyawusan</u> which means "hairs
of (Persian heros) similar to Siyawus". <u>Maqāyir</u> is certainly a faulty reading
for <u>dafā'ir</u> (<u>al-ġinn</u>) (Issa) meaning "braids (of demons)", or <u>dafā'ir al-aqūz</u>
meaning "braids of the aged" (abd ar-Razzaq). The Mozarabic - Iberic name for
capillary, <u>arachoquil</u>, is mentioned by Simonet (19); the other name, <u>carasquilla</u>
(Simonet 106), is obsolete. The modern Castilian name <u>Adiantum Capillus Ven.</u> is
<u>culantrillo de pozo</u>. The herbaceous part of the plant is still sold in the bazaars
of Cairo, as a remedy (Ducros).

183) <u>KAZBURA (SIC!)</u>   Coriander

<u>MAIMONIDES</u>: It is <u>an-naqda</u> and one also calls it <u>an-na'da</u>. Its most well-
known name to the people (? of Maghrib) is <u>al-kasbura</u> with <u>sin</u>.

* in the text <u>as-sabiqa</u>; the name <u>saniqa</u> or <u>sanikin</u> is Persian. See Vullers II,
195. Kohen, 134 line 11 has the faulty reading <u>salifa</u>

When physicians speak of dry coriander (kazbura yābisa) they
do not, by this name, designate the seeds of the coriander with
which one seasons foods, as most physicians think. Rather what
is meant are the dried leaves of this coriander.

MEYERHOF: [Theophrastus VII, 1-5; Dioscorides III, 63; Serapion 329; Ibn
al-Beithar 1933; Tuhfa 230; Abd ar-Razzaq 429; Issa 58, 3;
Loew III, 441-447; Ducros 199]

The usual orthography is kuzbara or kusbara. This name was derived from
the sanskrit kustumbārī, but coriander is also found in Assyria under the name
kusibirru (Meissner in Loew III, 441) and in Aramaic kūsbaretā. From this
last name are derived the Arabic and Persian names. Vullers (II, 1009) mentions another Persian name gišnīz. We found the name naqda (na'da is a corruption)in Dozy (II, 709), according to Ibn Biklaris. (Freytag I, 194-195 gives
the names taqda and taqra which also seem to be curruptions. They are not
Persian, as Ducros claims). The plant Coriandrum sativum L. (ombelliferaceae)
is cultivated in all of North Africa, in Syria and in Palestine. One sells the
small well-known fruit in the bazaars of Cairo as a condiment, and also as a
carminative and stomachic. The cultivation of the coriander in Spain is
described by Ibn Awwam (II, 253-255)

184) KURUNB   Cabbage (and cauliflower)

MAIMONIDES: It is baqlat al-andār.

The Syrian cabbage (al-kurunb aš-šami) is the cauliflower
(al-qannabīt). It is the one the people in Egypt simply call
al-kurunb, because they have no other cabbage except cauliflower.

MEYERHOF: [Dioscorides II, 120; Serapion 131; Ibn al-Beithar 1909; Tuhfa
224; Abd ar-Razzaq 445; Issa 33, 3-4; Loew I, 482-487; Ibn
'Awwam II, 156-165.]

The kitchen cabbage (Brassica oleracea L.var. capitata, Crucifereae) is

called kurunb in Arabic, the name evidently derived from the Greek krambê. The
cultivation of cabbage appears to have commenced in Italy. The other Arabic
name is found in Ibn al-Beithar (321) under the form baqlat al-ansar ("vegetable
of the partisans of the Prophet"). The orthography amsar, printed in the Arabic
edition, is erroneous.

The names qannabit or qinnabit and qarnabit are also derived from the
Greek. (In Byzantine and modern Greek konopidi, kounoupida, etc. see Langkavel,
Botanik der spaeteren Griechen, Berlin 1866, p. 27 and Fleischer, Etudes sur le
Supplément aux Dictionaires arabes de Dozy, in Berichte der K. Saechs. Gesellschaft der Wissenschaften, Phil. Hist. Klasse 1885, p. 394). They designate
the cauliflower (Brassica oleracea L. var. Botrytis L.) which Suwaidi (148a
also calls kurunb mawsili ("cabbage of Mossoul") and kurunb hamadâni ("cabbage
of Hamadan"). Ibn 'Awwam (II, 155-165) describes in detail the cultivation of
cabbage and cauliflower in Spain. It is interesting to note that the kitchen
cabbage was unknown in the middle ages, not only in Egypt, but also in
Palestine (Loew 438). Today, one grows it everywhere in both countries.

185) KARSANA   Bitter vetch

MAIMONIDES: It is al-kasnâ.

MEYERHOF: [Theophrastus VII, 5 and VIII, 11: Dioscorides II, 108; Serapion
           261 and 316; Ibn al-Beithar 1912; Tuhfa 222; Abd ar-Razzaq 472
           and 499; Issa 188, 18; Loew II, 481-491.]

The plant in question is the bitter vetch (black vetch; black pea; Vicia
Ervillia WILLD., Leguminous plants). The Arabic name karsana, better karsanna,
is derived from the Hebrew karšina or from the Aramaic karšinnâ, which seems
to be derived from the sanskrit root kršna meaning "black" (Schrader, according
to Loew II, 485). This name passed into the Persian vernacular (kašnak, kušnak,
kušna, kašnâ, kasnak, etc.) (Vullers II, 835 and 845 ff). One should not confuse
karsinna with qarsa'anna (see our no. 190). The cultivation of vetch and related
leguminous plants in Spain is described by Ibn 'Awwam (II, 94-97). Even today,

vetch still carries the name <u>alcarcena</u>.

186) KAŠŪT   Dodder

MAIMONIDES: One also calls it <u>al-kušut</u> and <u>kušūtā</u>. It is the "rabbit
sorrel" (<u>hummād al-araab</u>) and <u>aš-šitābard</u>, and one also calls
it <u>zahmūd</u> and <u>satmūn</u>. Greek dodder (<u>al-kašūt ar-rūmī</u>), on
the other hand, is the absinth <u>(afsintin)</u>, as we have mentioned.

MEYERHOF: [Dioscorides IV, 177; Serapion 116; Ibn al-Beithar 1940; <u>Tuhfa</u>
32 and 226; Issa 63, 8; Abd ar-Razzaq 443; Loew I, 453-461.]

The Arabic name <u>kašūt</u> is derived from the Syriac <u>kašūtā</u> (<u>kaša</u> means
accumulate) and designates the parasitic dodder plant or epithyme (<u>Cuscuta</u>
<u>Epithymum</u> MURR; <u>Cuscuta Epilinum</u> WEIT.,etc., Convolvulaceae) which attaches
itself to the nourishing plants with the aid of suckers. The last three names
are Persian. The first should probably read <u>šitāband</u> meaning "rapid current"
(Vullers II, 411); the second is corrupted in the manuscript and should read
<u>zagmūl</u> meaning dodder seeds (Vullers II, 117); the third name <u>šatmūn</u> or <u>šašmūn</u>
is lacking in the dictionaries. See above No. 23 (<u>afītīmum</u>).

Regarding <u>kašūt rūmī</u>, see No. 3 (<u>afsintin</u>, wormwood).

Fresh dodder juice was used as a constituent of hepatic and gastric remedies, and for the preparation of collyria.

187) KUMATRĀ   Pear

MAIMONIDES: It is that which the people of Maghrib call "the plum"
(<u>al-iggās</u>).

MEYERHOF: [Theophrastus I, 2 and IV, 14; Dioscorides 116; Serapion 274;
Ibn al-Beithar 1963; <u>Tuhfa</u> 221; Abd ar-Razzaq 37; Issa 151, 13;
Loew III, 235-240.]

Renaud and Colin (<u>Tuhfa</u>) already found in Ibn Biklaris the designation
<u>ingās</u> for the pear, next to the classic name <u>kummatrā</u> which is of Syriac origin.

'Abd al-Latif (36) states that, in his times, the pear was also called i̇g̈g̈ās
in Syria (today in̆g̈ās or nag̈ās) (Post I, 454). In Yemen, one also calls it
in̆g̈ās. On the cultivation of many types of pear trees in Spain, see Ibn
'Awwam (I, 240-242).

(fol. 88ᵛ)

188) KUNDUR   Incense

MAIMONIDES: It is al-lubān.

MEYERHOF: [Theophrastus IX, 4-11; Dioscorides I, 68; Serapion 323; Ibn

al-Beithar 1974; Tuhfa 214; 'Abd ar-Razzaq 430; Issa 32,4;

Loew I, 312-314; Ducros 204.]

The two names kundur and lubān are derived from the Greek khondros
libanon ("clots of incense"). It is the product, known since time immemorial
and represented in the reliefs of the Egyptian temples, Boswellia (Burseraceae),
above all Boswellia Carterii BIRDW. It is a tree of Arabia and of Somalia.
The name kundur was considered Persian, and was employed by physicians. The
name luban, as the Greek libanos, is derived from the Semitic; Assyrian lubanu,
Hebrew lebona, Aramaic lĕbottā, etc. The root l.b.n. signifies "to be white";
it is the color of the fresh resin, not yet solidified. That which I was
shown in the bazaars of Cairo as true incense (liban dakar or bahūr 'arabī)was
only debris. Ducros also found translucent incense drops which served for
fumigations. The Arabic name al-lubān is in fact found in French: oliban
(Devic and Lammeus).

189) KAMĀDURIYŪS   Medicinal Germander

MAIMONIDES: It is the "oak of the earth" (bullūt al-ard) and in Latin

burnutqa (bertonica).

MEYERHOF: [Theophrastus IX, 9. 5; Dioscorides III, 98; Ibn al-Beithar 1966;

Tuhfa 218; 'Abd ar-Razzaq 452; Issa 179,4; Loew II, 104.]

The name kamāduriyūs is the Arabic transcription from the Greek khamaidrys,
and ballūt al-ard is the literal Arabic translation of this name ("oak of the earth").

I think that the "Latin" name burnutqa is a faulty reading for bertonica, name
of the germander in the vicinity of Saragossa, according to Simonet 46 and 453.
(Idrisi 226 has the faulty reading alinunturaqa). It is the medicinal germander ("small oak") Teucrium Chamaedrys L., (Labiates). The leaves of this
plant were used as a stomachic, diuretic and antiscrofulous agent.

190) KAMĀFĪTŪS   Ground-ivy(and eryngium)

MAIMONIDES: One also says hamābītūs. In Spanish one calls it ǧalla
qrišta (galli crista) and also ǧānat qabta (centumcapita)
and qardālla barbāta (cardiello piperito?), which signifies
"peppery thorn" (aš-šawk al-mufalfal). One also calls it
banuāla (pinuela).

Many have said that this plant is the eryngium (al-qarsa'anna). Būškarāna is one type of eryngium. Botanists in
Spain have noted that "the Jewish thorn" (aš-šawka al-
yahūdiyya), the plant which is called "the black thorn"
(aš-šawka as-sawdā), is ganat qabta and al-qarsa'anna, and
not at all al-kamāfītūs. This plant, al-qarsa'anna, is
not used by us, except for its root.

MEYERHOF: [Theophrastus VI, 1, 3; Dioscorides III, 158 and III,21;
Ibn al-Beithar 1965 and 1754; Tuhfa 217 and 322; 'Abd
ar-Razzaq 453; Issa 7, 23 and 77, 19; Loew II, 71 and I,
439 ff.]

In this paragraph, Maimonides deals with two different drugs whose Spanish
names seem to have been frequently confused by Arabic physicians. The first is
the khamaipitys of Dioscorides which one identifies with the ground-ivy
(Ajuga Chamaepitys SCHREB, Labiates). Its Arabic name kamāfītūs is a
transliteration of the Greek name. In Spanish it carries the name gallocresta
("cock's comb"), which however designates other labiates, such as the hormin
(Simonet 242). Today in Spain one calls it pinillo oloroso. This drug is

no longer in use.

The other plant is an ombelliferaceous, and greatly resembles thistles.
It is the eryngion of the Greeks, which one identifies with Eryngium
campestre L., or with Eryngium creticum LAM. (panicaut), a Mediterranean
plant with blue flowers which has many small capitula. It is for this reason
that its Latin name is centum capita ("hundred heads", in Castilian ciencabezas)
(Simonet 159). The doubtful Spanish name cardiello piperito is perhaps a
faulty reading for cardiello borriquero (Simonet 103). One Spanish name is
corrupted and lacks diacritical points; I have reconstituted it in the form
banuōla according to Ghafiqi (ms. fol. 101b). It is pinuela, name wnich in
ancient Castilian designates both the chamaepitys as well as the houseleek
(Sempervivum tectorum L.). Būskaranna or baškarān (Dozy 1, 90) is a mutilated
Spanish name which designates the eryngium. According to Simonet (569), it is
derived from the Latin viscarago. The Arabic names of eryngium, qarsa'anna,
qirsa'anna, etc.(one should not confuse this name with karsanna. See No.185),
are derived from the Syriac qersa'annā. Eryngium creticum in Syria today has
the name qursa'anni (Post I, 507). Its leaves are consumed in Palestine as a
salad, hence the Arabic name baqla yahūddiya ("Jewish legume"). The root
served as a remedy against hydrops and as an antirabies agent.

191) KATĪRĀ   Tragacanth gum

MAIMONIDES: It is the gum of the herb al-qatād. The name al-qatād is
                also as-sahāğ; and this gum is also called halūsiyā.

MEYERHOF: [Theophrastus IX, 1 and 8; Dioscorides III, 20; Serapion 320;
                Ibn al-Beithar 1889; 'Abd ar-Razzaq 435 and 639; Issa 26, 7;
                Loew II, 419-424; Dymock I, 479-482.]

The plant tragakantha of tne Greeks, katād to the Arabs, was identified
with many (13 altogether) species of the leguminous plants Astragalus. In
Syria it is called the Astragalus gummifer LAB., in Mesopotamia Astragalus
kurdicus BOISS., in Persia Astragalus heraticus BUNGE which furnishes the

officinal resin which is extracted by incisions in the roots of the plants.
One still sells this gum (katīrā, Syriac name) in the bazaars of Cairo as a
pectoral and diuretic. The name sahāǧ is lacking in the dictionaries, whereas halūsiyā is also found mentioned by Ibn al-Beithar (694) as a name for
the tragacanth; it is undoubtedly Syriac. The Hebrew Biblical name nekāt
most likely designates tragacanth gum (Loew II, 420).

192) KAM'A   Truffle

MAIMONIDES: The people of Maghrib call it al-kama. It is al-futr.

MEYERHOF: [Theophrastus I, 1-6; Dioscorides II, 145; Serapion 409; Ibn
          al-Beithar 1964; Tuhfa 220 and 320; 'Abd ar-Razzaq 440 and
          704; Issa 184, 7-13; Loew I, 26-39.]

   Kam'a is the Arabic name of truffle, especially the white truffle
(Tuber album SOW.) and Tuber Micheli. Futr is the Arabic generic name for
"mushroom". One finds much of it in the deserts of Syria and Northern Arabia
after the winter rains. The two names are Semitic (Assyrian kamtu; Hebrew -
Michnic kemēha and fetūri). For the other Arabic names, see the commentaries
of Renaud-Colin in Tuhfa, and Ibn 'Awwam (II, 433) with the remarks of
Clément-Mullet.

193) KAMMŪN   Cumin and types

MAIMONIDES: The wild cumin (al-kammūn al-barri) is the black cumin
            (al-kammūn al-aswad). It is the one which is called "royal
            cumin" and the "cumin of Kirman" (al-kammūn al-mulūkī, al-
            kammūn al-kirmānī). It is al-bāsaliqūn ("royal").

MEYERHOF: [Theophrastus VII, 3 - VIII, 8; Dioscorides III, 59-61; Serapion
          97; Ibn al-Beithar 1967; Tuhfa 229 and 454; 'Abd ar-Razzaq 426-
          427; Issa 62, 18; Loew III, 435-439; Ducros 202-203.]

   Kammūn is the Arabic name of the fruit of the cumin (Cuminum Cyminum L.,
Ombelliferaceae). The Semitic (words are): Assyrian kamūnu, Hebrew kammōn,
Aramaic kammōnā, etc. Kammūn barrī and kammūn aswad are the two names for
black cumin (Nigella sativa L., see our No. 365), whereas kammūn kirmānī designates

Carum nigrum ROYLE; and kammūn mulūkī or basilikon (refers to) bishopswort
or stonewort (Carum copticum BENTH; see at No. 259). Today the druggists
in Cairo call cumin kammūn and sanūt; nigella (they call) kammūn iswid and
habba sōda (Ducros). Regarding the Maghribian names, see the commentaries
of Renaud-Colin in Tuhfa. Concerning the cultivation of cumin in Spain,
see Ibn 'Awwam (II, 241-224).

194) KABBĀBA   Cubeb

MAIMONIDES: It is "the seed of the bridegroom" (habb al-'arūs) and
             harkus.

MEYERHOF: [Serapion 133; Ibn al-Beithar 1879; Tuhfa 190; 'Abd ar-Razzaq
           428; Issa 141, 2; Loew III,62; Ducros 195; Dymock III, 180-183.]

     The name kabāba (in Arabic one writes kabbaba) is Persian. The drug
itself is a product of the Sunda Islands. It is the petiolated fruit of
Piper Cubeba L. (Piperaceae). One finds it at all the druggists in the
Orient. In Cairo, one sells it under the name kabbāba hindi ("Indian cubeb"),
drug strongly mixed with earth and debris of other plants (Ducros). It serves
in a decoction as a disinfectant for the urinary tract. Harkūs is a word of
Persian origin. However, the word hargūš designates a totally different
plant, the large plantain (Plantago major L.)

195) KARAWIYYA (SIC!)

MAIMONIDES: One also calls it (fol. 89ʳ) "Armenian caraway" (al-kammūn
             al-arminī) and garunbād and garīgād (?). Al-qardamānā is the
             wild caraway (karāwiya).

MEYERHOF: [Dioscorides III, 57; Serapion 103; Ibn al-Beithar 1774 and
           1913; Tuhfa 340; 'Abd ar-Razzaq 745; Issa 41, 2; Loew III,
           437-440; Ducros 118 and 179.]

     Maimonides first writes karawiyya as the author of Tuhfa (340), but then
karāwiya, as all the other authors. This latter orthographic form is undoubtedly derived from the Syriac, and both names are transcriptions from the Greek

karô or karyia. It is <u>Carum carvi</u> L. (Umbelliferous plants). Qurunbād is
the Persian name of the wild caraway (Vullers II, 723). Qarīgād, qarīgān,
qaranfār (Ibn al-Beithar) etc., are mutilations made by the copyists. It
was known to the Latins under the name Carnabadium (Loew).

The name qardamānā (Syriac) is the result of numerous confusions of
Syriac translators who thought the kardamômon of Dioscorides is the kardamon
agrion (see <u>Tuhfa</u> and Loew). <u>Karāwiyā barrī</u> ("wild caraway") or <u>karāwiyā</u>
ǧabalī ("mountain caraway") is the bastard caraway (<u>Lagoecia cuminoides</u> L.,
Umbelliferaceae). Under the name qardamānā or hurf el-murūǧ or hurf zarīf,
one still sells the fruits and summits of the Cruciferous plant <u>Cardamine
pratensis</u> L. in the bazaars of Cairo. Caraway and the bastard caraway were
cultivated in Spain (Ibn 'Awwam II, 244-246).

196) <u>KARAFS</u>   Smallage, celery, parsley and types

MAIMONIDES: There are six types of <u>karafs</u> (celery), among which is the
parsley (<u>al-maqdūnis</u>) which is called "celery of Sarakhs"
(<u>al-karafs as-sarahsī</u>). It is "Romaic celery" (<u>al-karafs
ar-rūmi</u>) and some say it is <u>petroselinon</u>.

That which is known to the physicians of Maghrib under
this name are the seeds of the mountain celery (<u>al-karafs
al-ǧabalī</u>). These are black and large seeds resembling
stavesacre seeds (<u>habb ar-ra's</u>). The name of mountain
celery seeds in Greek is <u>seseli</u>, and that of wild caraway
(<u>karafs barrī</u>) in that language is <u>samarniyun</u> (<u>smyrnion</u>).
As to the species of carvi which is called <u>karafs al-mā'</u>,
it is that which the Berbers call <u>kariyūnaš</u>.

MEYERHOF: [Theophrastus VII, 6, 3; Dioscorides III, 64-68; Serapion 102
and 308; Ibn al-Beithar 1902 and 2161; <u>Tuhfa</u> 82, 200 and 337;
'Abd ar-Razzaq III, 180, 432 and 495; Issa 19, 5; 89, 4; 41, 5;
171, 3-4; 170, 11; 137, 6; Loew III, 423-435.]

Karafs, in Hebrew karpas, is the generic name for umbelliferous plants
called selinon by the Greeks. The types mentioned by Maimonides are:(1) karafs
meaning celery, smallage (Apium graveolens L.); (2) karafs rūmi or karafs sarahsi
or maqdūnis, meaning parsley (Carum Petroselinum BENTH. and HOOK.). The name
maqdūnis is derived from Makedonion, because this plant is supposed to have
originated from Macedonia. In Egypt one calls it baqdūnis and its seeds are
sold in the bazaars (Ducros 33); (3) karafs ǧabali meaning mountain smallage
(Peucedanum Oreoselinum MONCH.). The Greek name of this plant is oreoselinon;
(4) karafs barri meaning maceron (smyrnium perfoliatum L., and smyrnium olusa-
trum L.,); (5) karafs al-mā' meaning aquatic smallage, water smallage or water
parsnips (sium latifolium L.). The Berber name karnūnaš or qarnīnaš seems to
have designated types of Sium; today gernūneš is the popular Maghribean name
for water-cress (Nasturtium officinale L., Cruciferaceae) (Renaud-Colin in
Tuhfa 337).

One should mention that today the druggists of the bazaars of Cairo sell,
under the name bizr el-karafs el-ǧabali ("seeds of mountain smallage"), the
diachain fruit of the lovage (Levisticum officinale KOCH.) (Ducros 31). Celery
and parsley were cultivated in Musulman Spain (Ibn 'Awwam II, 295-297).

197) KABAR   Caper-bush

MAIMONIDES: It is al-qabar and al-lasaf and one also says asaf.

MEYERHOF: [Theophrastus VI-VII; Dioscorides II, 173; Serapion 99; Ibn
al-Beithar 1877; Tuhfa 223; 'Abd ar-Razzaq 43, 425 and 956;
Issa 38, 13; Loew I, 322-330; Ducros 30.]

The caper-bush (capparis spinosa L. and varieties) grows in the wild state
in Egypt, Syria and Palestine. The Arabic names kabar, kabbār, etc. are derived
from the Greek and are conserved in Spanish (alcaparra). The other names are
derived from Hebrew and Aramaic ṣělāf. The caper is not the fruit but the floral
bud of the plant which, in Egypt, also carries the names lassāf (Schweinfurth 11)
and šok el-homār ("donkey thorn", Issa). 'Abd ar-Razzaq gives the name asaf.

The seeds are sold in the bazaars of Cairo under the name bizr el-kabar; they
serve as a carminative and aphrodisiac (Ducros). In Spain, the caper-bush was
cultivated in gardens (Ibn 'Awwam II, 316 ff).

198) KURRĀT   Leek and varieties

MAIMONIDES: It is bulbos and one says balābis. The Syrian leek (al-
             kurrāt aš-šāmī) is the culinary leek (al-kurrāt al-bustānī)
             that people eat as a seasoning and which is called al-qaflūt.

             The one which is called "Nabathean leek" (al-kurrāt
             an-nabatī) is the "mountain leek" (al-kurrāt al-ğabalī).

             The wild leek (al-kurrāt al-barrī) is called tītān.

MEYERHOF: ⌠ Theophrastus VII, 1-5; Dioscorides II, 149; Serapion 136;
           ⌊ Ibn al-Beithar 1910; Tuhfa 83, 408; 'Abd ar-Razzaq 441 and
             470; Issa 9, 6 to 10, 2; Loew II, 131-138. ⌉

The Arabic name kurrāt is probably Semitic (Assyrian: karāšu; Aramaic:
kěrětī and kěrěšā, etc.). However, Fraenkel (144) claims that it is a name
borrowed into Greek, and Zimmern (Loew II, 133) thinks that it is perhaps
borrowed into Sumerian qaraš. Bulbus and balābis are drawn from the Greek and
sometimes refer to the asphodel, but often simply to a bulb of a liliaceous
plant. As to the species indicated by Maimonides:

1) kurrāt šāmī, bustānī and qaflūt (from the Greek prason kephalôton)
correspond to the shallot (Allium ascalonicum L., liliaceae).

2) kurrāt nabatī is the name of the "false leek" (Allium Ampeloprasum L.),
kurrāt bustānī may designate the culinary leek (Allium porrum L.) and the white
horehound whose place is not here.

3) kurrāt barrī and tītān (name of Greek origin ? also in Ibn al-Beithar
1487) have been identified with the wild leek or porret (Allium rotundum WIM.
and GRABO). Certain Arabic authors took the name taïtān for Nabathean; it is an
imaginary etymology. Muhassas (XI, 165-166) has the reading at-tītān and considers the name purely Arabic.

Remnants of the leek were found in the tombs of ancient Egyptians. The

Hebrew Biblical name of leek (Allium porrum L.) is hasīr, and is found
mentioned in general by Maimonides himself (in Hilchoth Schechita VII, 19).
Different types of leek were cultivated in Spain in the middle ages (Ibn
'Awwam II, 198-202).

199) KAHRABĀ   Yellow amber, succin

MAIMONIDES: One also says kārabā; it is the resin of the romaic poplar
(al-hawr ar-rūmī).

MEYERHOF: [Dioscorides I, 82; Serapion 283, 300 and 306; Ibn al-Beithar
1982; Tuhfa 216; 'Abd ar-Razzaq 438.]

Yellow amber was considered by the Greeks and Arabs as the solidified
resin of a conifer or of the black poplar (Populus nigra L.). Ibn al-Beithar
arises against this assertion and cites al-Gafiqi who states that one finds
succin in waste lands far from trees. The Arabic name is derived from the
Persian kāh-rubā "straw-stroke" (Vullers II, 787); in Pehlevi kahrupai
(Laufer p. 523). One employed the powder of succin as a hemostatic and stomachic.

200) KAZMĀZIK   Gall of tamarisk

MAIMONIDES: It is the fruit of the tamarisk (at-tarfā') and one also
calls it gazmāzik (fol. 89ᵛ) and gazamāziq. One also calls it
the "savory one" (al-'adba).

MEYERHOF: [Dioscorides I, 89; Serapion 493; Ibn al-Beithar 17 and 1929;
Tuhfa 23, 106 and 228; 'Abd ar-Razzaq 197; Issa 177, 2;
Loew III, 398-402; Ducros 56.]

The Arabic names are derived from the Persian gazmāzak or gazmāzū
(Vullers II, 998). It is not the fruit but the gall of the oriental tamarisk,
as we have expounded in the article on this tree (see our No. 9; atl). These
galls are still sold in the bazaars of Cairo, but under the name 'adba rather
than tamr el-atl ("fruit of the tamarisk"). They are employed as antidiarrheal
agents and for the preparation of astringent collyria. 'Abd ar-Razzaq calls it
gawz at-tarfā'("nut of the tamarisk").

201) KĀKANǦ   Winter-cherry (strawberry tomato)

   MAIMONIDES: It is the "prairie nut" (g̣awz al-marg̣) and its Greek name is

              halikakabon. It is a type of culinary black nightshade

              ('inab at-ta'lab). It is that which one calls šag̣arat al-

              lahw ("tree of joy").

   MEYERHOF: [Dioscorides IV, 71; Ibn al-Beithar 1589 and 1874; Tuhfa 219;

              'Abd ar-Razzaq 378, 488 and 651; Issa 139, 7; Loew III, 375ff.]

   This plant is the winter cherry (Physalis Alkekengi L., solanaceae). Its

fruit is a berry enveloped by an accrescent calyx, inflated and colored; it is

a laxative and diuretic. The name kākanǧ (also kākuna) is Persian, but perhaps

borrowed (Vullers II, 779). I suppose the name kākanǧ is related to the Sanskrit

kākamāčī which, according to Chopra (p. 595) designates the black nightshade

(Solanum nigrum L.). In Egypt, the fruits cultivated in gardens and sold as a

delicacy have the popular name es-sitt fi'n nāmūsiya ("lady in the mosquito

net"). Idrisi (p. 224) calls this plant 'inab at-ta' lab al-kabir "large

black nightshade". See below at number 297 ('inab at-ta'lab).

202) KUSTBARKUST   Helictere (screw-tree)

   MAIMONIDES: It is that which in Egypt is known by the name al-'atfa

              ("convolvulus"), and one also says "right convolvulus" and

              "left convolvulus"

   MEYERHOF: [Ibn al-Beithar 1939; Issa 92,6; Dymock I, 231-233.]

   Kustbarkust is the Arabicized form of the Persian term for "convolvulus"

kašt bar kašt whose meaning is "fold over fold" (Vullers II, 838). The plant

is the sterculiaceous Helicteres Isora L., which originates from southern Asia.

It is a shrubby tree resembling the hazel bush. The five carpels of its fruit

(ovarian sacs) are twisted, from whence its Arabic and Persian names. In the

Indies, one uses the fruits and the rhizomes as astringents. In Egypt today,

the plant is as unknown as its medicinal usage. See also Hooper & Field, p. 124.

203) KĀSĬM   Lovage

MAIMONIDES: It is az-zawfarā and in Spanish taqlīra. As to the species

called romaic lovage (al-kāsĭm ar-rūmī), it is that which

the Greeks call ligystikon and whose seed is called by them

sāsaliyūs (seselios). We will speak thereof under letter sīn.

MEYERHOF: [Dioscorides III, 51; Ibn al-Beithar 1869; 'Abd ar-Razzaq 112,

307 and 439; Issa 108, 14; Loew III, 471 ff; Ducros 32.]

The drug is the umbelliferous plant Levisticum officinale KOCH (lovage).
We have mentioned (at number 196) that the seeds of this plant are for sale
in the bazaars of Cairo under the false designation karafs ǧabali ("mountain
celery") (Ducros). One uses it as a carminative, emmenagogue, etc. The
name kāsĭm is Arabic (Freytag IV, 39), and zawfarā is borrowed into Syriac
(Dozy I, 614). I was unable to locate a Spanish name which might be related to taqlīra, except talictro (Thalictrum, "rhubarb of the poor").
'Umda says tagarro and tagārna (Renaud), our number 283 taqāra. Ghafiqi
(ms. fol. 228 a) has tagara"in Latin". It is said that the semina seseleos
cretici are the product of Tordylium officinale L.

204) KUFARRĀ   Spathe of the palm-tree

MAIMONIDES: One also says ǧufarrā. It is part of the young cluster of the

palm-tree (tal 'an-nahl).

MEYERHOF: [Dioscorides I, 109; Serapion 92 and 331; Ibn al-Beithar 1955;

'Abd ar-Razzaq 458; Loew II, 335-336; Ibn 'Awwam I, 323.]

According to Fraenkel (p. 147), these names are Aramaic: ǧupārā, gupparrā,
etc., and Persian: kupurrā. However, derivation from the Assyrian (giparu)
is possible (Kuchler, in Loew II, 336). The Syrian commentators define
gufarrā as the pollen of the palm-tree, the Arabs as a part of the spathe.
The word is unknown to Egyptian cultivators (see Schweinfurth 229). Compare
also our articles 69 (ǧummār), 176 (tal')and above all number 206 below (kāfūr).
Kohen (p. 127, line 10) has the names ǧufarrā, kufarrā, qufarrā and kāfūrī.

205) <u>KARKUM</u>   Curcuma (and celandine)

    <u>MAIMONIDES</u>: It is <u>al-hurd</u> and "the yellow roots" (<u>al-'uruq as-sufr</u>).

                     Al-māmīrān is one of its types.

    <u>MEYERHOF</u>: [Serapion 313; Ibn al-Beithar 1917 and 1525; <u>Tuhfa</u> 252; 'Abd ar-
                Razzaq 32 and 431; Issa 47, 1 and 63, 2; Loew II, 7-25 and II,
                371-373; Dymock III, 407-414; Ducros 158.]

        The name <u>kurkum</u> is semitic: Assyrian <u>kurkanu?</u> Hebrew <u>karkōm</u>. Aramaic
<u>kūrkĕmā</u>. These names designate the saffron (<u>Crocus sativus</u> L.) (see our number
135), but were later transferred to an Indian drug, the long curcuma or "Indian
saffron" (<u>curcuma longa</u> L., zingiberaceae). This latter carried the Sanskrit
name <u>haridrā</u> ("yellow wood") from which is derived the Arabic-Persian name
<u>hurd</u>. The rhizome of curcuma offers two different aspects: round tubercles,
and cylindrical or fusiform pieces. It is for this reason that Arabs took them
for two different vegetables. They called them <u>kurkum</u> and <u>'uruq sufr</u> ("yellow
roots") and, to add to the confusion, they gave the same name to the celandine
(<u>chelidonium majus</u> L., Papaveraceae) which produces a yellow, caustic juice,
and which carries the Persian and Syriac names <u>māmīrām</u> and <u>kūrkĕmā</u>, (respectively).
Today in Cairo, the names <u>kurkum</u> and <u>'uruq sufr</u> only designate the rhizomes of
<u>Curcuma longa</u>, yellow roots that one sees everywhere in the baskets of the drug-
gists. They are used as an emmenagogue and diuretic (Ducros), but above all
in dyeing.

206) <u>KĀFŪR</u>   Camphor; here spathe of the palm-tree

    <u>MAIMONIDES</u>: One also calls it <u>qāfūr</u>.

    <u>MEYERHOF</u>: One is not dealing with camphor here, whose Arabic-Persian name
is derived from the Sanskrit <u>kappūra</u>, because Maimonides, as he states in the
introduction to this work, did not intend to speak of drugs which have only
one well-known name.

Maimonides here cites a rarer name of the spathe of the palm-tree (see our number 176 and 204). In effect we find the name qāfūr and kāfūr, explained in Freytag (III, 479 and IV, 49) as spatha, florum palmae involucrum, cited according to Qāmūs, and in the works of Arabic philologues of the eighth to tenth centuries (of the Christian era). Al-Asma'i, in his "Book on the palm-tree and vine" (Kitab an-nahl wa'l-karm ed. Haffner. Beirut 1908 p. 6) states: "Al-kāfūr is the vase (wi'ā') of the inflorescence (tal') of the palm-tree; one also calls it qaffur".

Muhassas (XI, 119 ff), in the long chapter on tal', furnishes additional information: "Tal' is the flower (nawr) of the date-tree while it rests in the spathe (al-kāfūr)...and one also says that at-tal' is al-kāfūr." Later, according to Abū Hamīfa ad-Dīnawarī: "One calls at-tal' al-kāfūr and al-kāfir"; and, according to Ibn Duraid: "Al-kafar is the vase (wi'ā') of tal' and the vase of all fruits...and one also says al-qaffur and al-qāfūr". Finally according to an anonymous author: "Kaffārā in singular is kufurrā." It is thus evident that kāfūr and qāfūr or qaffūr have the same meaning as kufarrā and ǧufarrā of our paragraph 204, and that the majority of ancient Arabic philologues are on record as favoring the sense tal' to mean "young cluster of the date-tree", enclosed in the spathe (kufarrā, kāfūr, qaffūr, etc.). The origin of all these names must be Aramaic. See Loew II, 335 ff and Fraenkel 147.

Kohen (p. 127, line 10) gives the name kāfūrī and explains it, perhaps according to a popular etymology: "...because it covers the young cluster (tal') and al-kāfir is as-sātir." These two Arabic participles signify "that which hides or covers".

The great Arabic encyclopedia of Šihab as-Din as-Nawairi (died in Cairo in 732/1332) gives for tal' the synonyms al-kāfūr, ad-dahk, and al-iǧrīd. By these names, the author understands the inflorescence of the date-tree and makes them follow by gradation the seven degrees of maturation of dates (Nihayat al-Arab fi Funun al-Adab, vol. XI, Cairo 1935, p. 119).

CHAPTER LĀM

207) LIBLĀB   Convolvulus and ivy

MAIMONIDES: It is "the cord of the poor" (habl al-masākīn) and qassus
(kissos, "ivy"), and one also calls it "the cold plant" (aš-
šaǧara al-bārida) and "the nerve" (al-'asaba) and rawāsih.
Its name in Spanish is burtuhīla (Latin: buticella), and one
also says qurriyīla (correguela).

MEYERHOF: Theophrastus I, 9-13 and III, 18, 7-8; Dioscorides II, 179 (kissos)
and IV, 39 (helxine); Serapion 333; Ibn al-Beithar 2004 and 1786;
Tuhfa 240, 345 and 209; 'Abd ar-Razzaq 372 and 505; Issa 56, 8
and 91, 2; Loew I, 450 and I, 218-221.

The Arabic name lablāb or liblāb originates from the Syriac hěbilbělā
meaning "to twist". The Arabs designated ivy (Hedera Helix L., Araliaceae) as
lablāb kabīr ("large convolvulus"), and as lablāb saǧir ("small convolvulus"),
our field convolvulus (convolvulus arvensis L., Convolvulaceae). For this
reason, both plants, although different, are discussed by Maimonides in this
same chapter. Habl al-masākīn is a name designating many twining plants.
Šaǧara bārida or baqla bārida ("cold vegetable") and 'asaba are names reserved
for the convolvulus. Rawāsih may designate something which holds fast, or,
with the reading rawāših, creeping plants (Lane III, 1088). The Spanish name
corriola, today correguela, designates Convolvulus arvensis (Simonet 137).
The other name should read butticella (Latin, Simonet 40); today in Castilian
altabaquillo. Ivy is called yedra in Spanish. One employed the juice of the convolv
as a mild purgative. In Egypt, convolvulus overgrows the fields everywhere; one
calls it lebēna or 'ulleq (Schweinfurth 14) and also maddād ("which prolongs
itself", Issa), whereas the name liblāb, in Egypt, is reserved for the leguminous plant Dolichos Lablāb L. (see number 210: lūbiyā). There exist representations
of convolvulus from ancient Egypt (Keimer 45, 102 and 178).

208) **LĀDAN**   Ladanum

    MAIMONIDES: It is the paste (<u>dibq</u>, here resin) that one extracts from the

                    plant which is called <u>kisthos</u> in Greek.

    MEYERHOF: ⌈Theophrastus VII, 1-2; Dioscorides I, 97; Serapion 282; Ibn al-

                 Beithar 1999; <u>Tuhfa</u> 241; 'Abd ar-Razzaq 504; Issa 50, 2-5;

                 Loew I, 362 ff.⌉

    The <u>ladanum</u> is the resin of Aegian plants <u>Cistus creticus</u> L., <u>Cistus</u>
<u>ladaniferus</u> L. and others. The name is Semitic: Assyrian <u>ladunu</u> (Greek <u>ladanon</u>),
Hebrew - Mishnaic <u>lōtem</u>. The exuded resin remains pasty in the hair of goats or
in the strings that one drags over the herb. Today one extracts it by means of
double leather straps that one agitates over the vegetable. The best ladanum is
white, transparent and waxy; it lasts for a long time. One used it as an astringent, antidysenteric agent, and in the preparation of collyria.

209) **LŪF**   Cuckoopint

    MAIMONIDES: It is <u>aron</u> in Greek. There are two types, one has large leaves

                 and the other has narrow leaves. One calls it "the tree of the

                 serpent" (<u>šağar al-hanaš</u>, serpentaria) and in Greek <u>drakontion</u>

                 which means "the eye (fol. 90ʳ) of the dragon" (<u>'ain-at-</u>

                 <u>tinnīn</u>). Its name in Spanish is <u>balīra</u> (read <u>qulībra</u> meaning

                 <u>culebra</u>), and one also calls it <u>falīrīla</u> (read <u>quli brila</u>

                 meaning <u>culebriella</u>). According to one assertion, the root

                 of one of the two types is <u>al-'artanītā</u>.

    MEYERHOF: ⌈Theophrastus VII, 9-13; Dioscorides II, 166-167; Serapion 346;

                 Ibn al-Beithar 2047; <u>Tuhfa</u> 237; 'Abd ar-Razzaq 503; Issa 72, 13:

                 Loew I, 214-216.⌉

    Under the name <u>lūf</u> (derived from Aramaic <u>lūfā</u>), the Arabs understood
numerous araceae, above all <u>Arum italicum</u> L., but also serpentaria (<u>Dracunculus</u>
<u>vulgaris</u> SCHOTT.) and other bulbous plants. See the Arabic index of Issa.

    The Spanish names <u>balīra</u> and <u>falīrīla</u> are faulty readings for <u>culebra</u> and culebriella (see Simonet, p. 145 ff), names derived from the Latin colubrina (meaning serpentaria). The modern Castilian names of Arum are yaro and sarillo. 'Artanītā, as we have seen above (number 55; bahūr maryam), is the Syriac name of the bulb of Cyclamen europaeum L., and has no bearing to Arum; it is probably a faulty reading for ġarġantīya (see number 302).

According to Ibn al-Beithar (2048) and Suwaidi (154a), the Arabs called lufa a crassulaceous plant (Cotyledon lusitanicus LAM.? or Cotyledon Umbilicus L.?), which has nothing to do with luf meaning Arum.

210) LŪBIYĀ   Dolichos and vigna

MAIMONIDES: It is ad-duġur.

MEYERHOF: [Dioscorides II, 146; Serapion 344; Ibn al-Beithar 2042; Tuhfa
            16; Issa 71, 12 and 189, 10; Loew II, 506-512; Ibn 'Awwam II,
            62-66; Ducros 32.]

The name lūbiyā undoubtedly originates from the Greek lobia in passing through Syriac. It is applied in Maghrib to numerous species of kidney-beans and other leguminous plants of which Ibn 'Awwam enumerates a dozen. In Egypt and neighboring countries, the name lūbia baladī designates Vigna sinensis ENDL., small white bean with a black spot at the hilum. Forskal called it Dolichos Lubia, but this name is no longer in use. Lūbiyā 'afin is the name of Dolichos Lablāb L. var. sativa, whose variety hortensis is called liblāb (see above our number 207). The name duġur is Arabic and is found in diverse forms (duġr, diġr, deġr). The seed of lūbiyā 'afin serves not only as an edible, but is also sold by the druggists of Cairo, under the name bizr el-lablāb, as a diuretic and emmenagogue (Ducros). In Spanish, the Arabic name of our plant is still preserved (alubia). Idrisi (248) gives the "Frankish" name fāzūl (faseolo).

211) LISĀN AT-TAWR   Borage

MAIMONIDES: It is al-kuhailā' ("the small black") and al-humāhim and
            one says hamham; it is al-'alīs and one also says 'alas.

MEYERHOF: [Dioscorides IV, 127; Serapion 341; Ibn al-Beithar 2023; Tuhfa

246; 'Abd ar-Razzaq 506; Issa 15, 10 and 32, 1; Loew I,

292-296; Ducros 206.⌋

The Arabic name lisān at-tawr ("bull's tongue") is the translation of

the Greek bouglosson and designates numerous types of borraginaceae, particu-

larly Borrago officinis L. ("borage") and Anchusa italica RETZ ("bastard

borage, beef's tongue"). The name kuha'ilā' was used in Maghrib; hamham (also

himhim and humhum) in the East. The Biblical Hebrew name of Anchus was hallamut.

In Egypt, the druggists sell the leaves of borage (Borrago officinalis L.) under

the name lisán et-tōr, as a sudorific and diuretic (Ducros). The names 'alīs

and 'alas in Arabic designate species of rye and of wheat; their place is not

here (? confusion caused by a copyist).

212) LISĀN AL-'ASĀFĪR   Fruit of the ash-tree

MAIMONIDES: It is the fruit of the ash-tree (dardār). One calls it

tālisfar and it is at-tağakrān (?). Its name in Spanish is

frāšinu (fresno).

MEYERHOF: ⌈Theophrastus I, 8-10; Dioscorides I, 84; Serapion 154; Ibn

al-Beithar 2025; Tuhfa 243; 'Abd ar-Razzaq 241, 507 and 574;

Issa 84, 20; Loew II, 286 ff; Ducros 102.⌋

The Arabic name means "sparrow's tongue"; it is the fruit of the ash-tree

(Fraxinus excelsior L., see above our number 91). It is an oval capsule a

little compressed, ending in a small tongue, from whence its name. See the

figure (plate VIII,6), and description in Ducros. One sells these fruits in

the bazaars of Cairo as diuretic agents. The translations of the medical works

of Maimonides render this name leshon ha-zipporim ("bird's tongue") in Hebrew.

The Persian name tālisfar was identified with lisān el-'asāfir by Ibn Gulgul,

according to the claims of Ghafiqi in Ibn al-Beithar 1443. This is an error,

and the opinion of the other Arabic authors who identify tālisfar with the mace

of the muscat nut is no less erroneous. Ghafiqi himself designates tālisfar as

the roots of an Indian tree. However, according to Dymock (II, 373b), the name originates from the Sanskrit <u>tālīsa pattra</u> and designates the leaves of the

yew (<u>Taxus baccata</u> L., see number 38). Nevertheless, Laufer (584) identifies

<u>tālisfar</u> with the leaves of the bixaceaous plant <u>Flacourtia Cataphracta</u> WILLD.

<u>Taǧakrān</u> must be a Berber term mutilated by the copyist. The most well-known

Berber name of the ash-tree is <u>tāslent</u> and Trabut (L. Trabut, <u>Répertoire des</u>

<u>noms indigènes des plantes spontanées, cultivées et utilisées dans le Nord de</u>

<u>l'Afrique</u>. Algiers 1935, p. 116) gives, in addition, the names <u>tazzult</u> and

<u>tābušišt</u>.

213) <u>LISĀN AL-HAMAL</u>   Plantain

MAIMONIDES: It is the "dog's tongue" (<u>lisan al-kalb</u>) and the "rat's tail"

(<u>danab al-fār</u>). One also says <u>bard wa-salām</u> ("cold and peaceful"),

and its name in Spanish is <u>balantāyin</u> (<u>plantagine, llanten</u>). It

is that which the people in Maghrib call <u>al-massāsa</u> ("tube,

pipette"); it is <u>al-karkūs</u>.

MEYERHOF: [Theophrastus VII, 8-11; Dioscorides II, 126; Serapion 340; Ibn

al-Beithar 2022 and 2027; <u>Tuhfa</u> 242; 'Abd ar-Razzaq 71 and 502;

Issa 142, 23; Loew III, 63 ff; Ducros 207.]

The name <u>lisān al-hamal</u> ("lamb's tongue") is translated from the Greek

<u>arnoglosson</u>. It is the large plantain (<u>Plantago major</u> L.). The curious name

<u>bard wa-salām</u> that one also encounters in 'Abd ar-Razzaq (502) originates from

the property which one attributed to this plant of rendering colder a body

temperature that is too hot. The name <u>karkūs</u> or <u>harkūs</u> is Arabicized from

the Persian <u>hargūš</u> "donkey's ear" (Vullers I, 680). The Spanish name, in

Simonet (449), reads <u>plantain</u>, in modern Castilian <u>llanten</u>. The druggists of

Cairo sell two types of <u>lisān al-hamal</u>; <u>kabir</u> ("large" referring to <u>Plantago</u>

<u>major</u> L.) and <u>sagīr</u> ("small" referring to <u>Plantago media</u> L.). The seed of the

first type serves as an astringent, etc., and the leaves of the second are

utilized as cataplasms (Ducros). The cultivation of plantain in Spain is

described by Ibn 'Awwam (II, 311 ff).

214) LISĀN AL-BAHR   Cuttlefish bone.

> MAIMONIDES: It is aš-šibiyya (sepia).
>
> MEYERHOF: [Dioscorides II, 21; Serapion 534; Ibn al-Beithar 1259 and
>   2029; 'Abd ar-Razzaq 285 and 874.]

The Arabic name signifies "ocean tongue"; the other name is derived from
the Latin sepia (Simonet 515). See above number 141 (zabad al-bahr). One sells
cuttlefish bone in the bazaars of Cairo as an ingredient of dry collyria.

215) LĀ'IYA   Euphorbia (spurge).

> MAIMONIDES: It is al-halablāb and in Spanish lahtariyūla (lactariola). We
>   have mentioned it among the types of latex plants (yuttū').
>
> MEYERHOF: [Dioscorides IV, 164; Serapion 522; Ibn al-Beithar 2001; Tuhfa
>   249; Issa 80, 16; Loew I, 604.]

The Arabic name has a dot over the 'ain and should be read lāġiya as in
Ibn al-Beithar. However, in article 178 concerning latex plants (yuttū'āt)
it is without a point, which is the correct reading. Sontheimer and Issa
identify lā'iya with Euphorbia triaculeata FORSK., whereas in Morocco this
name designates Euphorbia resinifera BERG. (Renaud-Colin). Loew considers
it Euphorbia Paralias L.; Berggren considers it Euphorbia Characias L.; these
two plants are identified with the two corresponding species of tithymallos
meaning yattū' of Dioscorides. Ibn Sina (I,351) mentions that the latex of
lā'iya was poisonous for fish. This argues in favor of its identification with
Euphorbia dendroides L., Euphorbia piscatoria AIT., or Euphorbia hyberna L., all
three of which are used as fish poisons. The latter two plants grow in Spain
and in North Africa. The Spanish name, distorted in the text tahtariyula,
originates from the Latin lactariola. It is preserved in Catalanian lleterola
for certain spurges (Euphorbia belioscopia L., Euphorbia esula L., etc)
(Simonet 290). Renaud (written communication) thinks that halablāb (halab,
halib meaning "fresh milk") has the same sense because of its relationship to
the latex produced by these plants. Halablāb is the name of many different

plants. Halublūb is still the general name for spurge in Syria (Post II,492).

216) LĀ'BA   Mandragora root

MAIMONIDES: It is the "young married" (al-'arūsa), and it is the root of

the mandragora (yabrūh).

MEYERHOF: [See the literature of number 179 above.]

Mandragora root often resembles the form of a human being. It is the
cause of superstitions which are linked thereto by many peoples. Here one
is dealing with the "female" root. The word mandragora is derived, by several
scholars, from the Persian merdumgiyāh meaning "man plant" (Loew III, 336).
The Arabic name of the root, la'ba, is surely related to lu'ba meaning puppet,
human figure (Dozy II, 534). One should note that la'ba barbariyya ("Berberic
puppet"), in Egypt and in Syria, is the name of the two types of Colchicum,
hermodactyl and colchicum (Ducros 209).

217) AL-LAHLĀH   Colchicum, here wild horse-radish

MAIMONIDES: It is the "wild radish" (al-fuǧl al-barrī). Its Arabic name

is al-hadamān and in Spanish labašnā (or labšanā).

MEYERHOF: [Theophrastus VII, 4-6; Dioscorides II, 112; Ibn al-Beithar 1672

and 2267; Issa 154, 1; Loew I, 511-516.]

Lihlāh is the Arabic name of numerous vegetables and above all certain
thistles and colchicum (Colchicum autumnale L.). Nowhere did I find it applied
to the plant which Maimonides is here discussing. This one is wild horse-radish
or wild radish (Raphanus Rapharistrum L., Cruciferae) which has the Arabic names
labsān (see the next article), fuǧl barrī and haidaman (Ibn al-Beithar 2267).
The Spanish (and Greco-Latin) name is lampsana or lapsana; in Arabic labsān
(Simonet 285). The Greek name is rhaphanis agria.

218) <u>LABSĀN</u>   Wild mustard

   <u>MAIMONIDES</u>: It is a type of culinary mustard (<u>al-hardal al-bustānī</u>).

   <u>MEYERHOF</u>: ⌈Dioscorides II, 116; Ibn al-Beithar 2006 and 812; Issa 169, 17;

      Loew I, 516-527.⌉

    <u>Labsān</u> is the Arabic form of <u>lampsane</u> of Dioscorides. One has identi-
fied this plant with wild mustard (<u>Sinapis arvensis</u> L. Cruciferae). It is
the great translator Hunain who rendered the Greek term through the Syriac
<u>hardĕlā dĕdabrā</u> meaning wild mustard. The Hebraic form <u>lifsān</u> was mentioned
by Maimonides himself (Loew I, 520). See the preceding article number 217
and below our number 400 (<u>hardal</u>).

CHAPTER MIM

219) MUĠĀT   Root of glossostemon

   MAIMONIDES: One also says mu'āt. It is the root of the wild pomegranate

                tree (ar-rummān al-barrī), and some say that it is the root

                of the pepper plant (asl šaǧarat al-fulful).

   MEYERHOF: [Serapion 371; Ibn al-Beithar 2147; Tuhfa 271; 'Abd ar-Razzaq

                549; Issa 88, 3; Loew III, 385; Ducros 221.]

      One is dealing with a drug whose origin was unknown for a long time, even-
   though it is still sold in abundance in the bazaars of the near-east and above
   all in Cairo (under the name muġāt). It is the large grey-whitish root of the
   bythneriacea Glossostemon Bruguieri D.C. which grows in the mountains of
   western Persia (Schweinfurth 23). It is sold cut into large portions which are
   crushed, mixed with sugared water and tragacanth gum, and imbibed by women after
   childbirth as a tonic and lactagogue. This same sherbet is offered to visitors
   of the parturient woman. The other names are distorted by orthographic errors
   (mu'āt instead of muġāt, fulful instead of qilqil). The identification of this
   plant by the Arabs with the root of the "wild pomegranate tree", and by modern
   authors with other plants, is equally erroneous. See Meyerhof number 136 note,
   and Hooper and Field, p. 121 ff.

220) MAHLAB   Plum tree of mahaleb (black cherry tree)

   MAIMONIDES: It is also called habb al-ārāk ("seeds of arrack"). The name of

                its tree is al-yusr from which one extracts the wood of yusr.

   MEYERHOF: [Serapion 350; Ibn al-Beithar 2090; 'Abd ar-Razzaq 536; Issa

                149,4; Loew III, 163; Ducros 212; Ibn 'Awwam II, 367.]

      Mahlab is the Arabic name of the fruit of the "cherry-tree of St. Lucie"
   (Prunus Mahaleb L., or Cerasus Mahaleb MILL.) which grows in Europe and in the
   Orient. The name habb al-ārāk is only found in Maimonides; it is perhaps Moorish-
   Spanish. Ārāk is the Arabic name of arrack or mesuak (Salvadora persica
   GAERTN.) whose odoriferous wood is utilized by the Musulmans in place of a
   toothbrush. Yusr is the name of another odoriferous tree, the oil-bearing

East Indian horseradish-tree (<u>Moringa pterygosperma</u> GAERTN.). There is here,
therefore, some confusion. The small cherries of <u>Mahaleb</u> are sold in the
bazaars of Cairo as a bechic, vermifuge and lithotriptic (Ducros). They are
primarily exported to Egyptian Sudan where the negroes use it for perfumed
liniments. See also Anastase p. 42, note 4.

221) <u>MILH</u>   Various salts

(fol. 90^v).

MAIMONIDES: The "salt of naphtha" (<u>al-milh an-naftī)</u> is the brilliant

azure. The "salt of curriers" (<u>milh ad-dabbāga</u>) is the

"plaster of the baker" (<u>ǧir al-farrānīn</u>); it is that which

one calls <u>as-sawraǧ</u>.

MEYERHOF: [Serapion 358; Ibn al-Beithar 1251 and 2165; 'Abd ar-Razzaq 542.]

Maimonides here only mentions two of the numerous species of natural
salts known from the ancients and the Arabs. <u>Milh naftī</u>, according to De Goeje
(in Dozy II, 704), is "a type of salt which comes from the vicinity of Darabgird
(in Persia) and which has the odor of naphte; the rich use it at the table".
The "salt of curriers" was probably a natural impure nitre. This is what is
demonstrated by the name <u>sawraǧ</u>, which is the Arabic form of the Persian name
<u>šūra</u> (Vullers 477) meaning "saline and sterile earth" or "nitre". Kohen
(p. 135, last line) writes <u>šūraǧ</u>.

222) <u>MITNĀN (SIC)</u>   Mezereon, passerine (sparrow-wart)

MAIMONIDES: It is <u>al-azzāz</u>.

MEYERHOF: [Theophrastus IX, 20, 2 (<u>kneoron</u>); Dioscorides IV, 172; Ibn al-

Beithar 2087-2088; <u>Tuhta</u> 234 and 268; 'Abd ar-Razzaq 61, 518 and

528; Issa 68, 5; Loew III, 408-409.]

The Arabic name is in general vocalized <u>matnān</u>; it probably originates
from the Syriac. One has identified it with <u>thymelaia</u> or <u>khamelaia</u> of
Dioscorides and this one with the thymelacaceous plant <u>Daphne Guidium</u> L.
("mezereon"). Today, the name <u>matnān, metnān, metnēn,</u> etc. in Egypt

(Schweinfurth 45) and Syria (Post II, 480), designates Thymelaea hirsuta ENDL. (Passerine), which in Morocco is called ftitisa (Renaud-Colin). The name azzāz (corrupted-awāz in our text)probably only designated the mezereon (Daphne Guidium) which doesn't exist either in Egypt or Syria or Palestine. Dozy (II, 568 ff) and Trabut (Répertoire, p. 90) describe this drug.

223) MAHRŪT   Root of asa foetida

MAIMONIDES: It is al-halī'ūn. It is the root of the asa foetida plant
             (al-hiltīt); we have already mentioned that the leaves of
             this plant are called al-angūdān (see number 18, supra).

MEYERHOF: [Dioscorides III, 80; Serapion 30 and 351; Ibn al-Beithar 2091;
           Tuhfa 255; 'Abd ar-Razzaq 538; Issa 82, 8; Loew III, 452-455;
           Ducros 89.]

     The Arabic name is also written mahrūt with ta at both points. Halī'ūn is perhaps an error of the copyist for silfiyūn (silphion), the Greek name of asa foetida. The druggists in Cairo no longer sell the root of Ferula Asa Foetida L., but they still know the name of samg al-mahrūt ("gum of the root of asa") (Ducros).

224) MAHĀ   Rock-crystal and others

MAIMONIDES: It is the "stone of the sun" (hagar as-sams).

MEYERHOF: [Ibn al-Beithar 2183.]

     Mahā or mahī is a Persian term (? borrowed from Sanskrit), which, according to Vullers (II, 1245), designates a white crystalline stone which was hung around the neck of pregnant women to facilitate their childbirth by a magical force. Dozy (I, 252) explains the name hagar al-mahā as "crystal" or "sapphire", and (I, 251) hagar samsī ("sunrock") as "girasol". This last precious stone is a corundum which casts a great fire, particularly toward the sun. One must consider sapphire or star-stone quartz.

     Al-Beruni, in his Lapidary, writes mahā, mihā, mahāh and mahw and explains these names as a type of rock-crystal (P. Kable, Bergkristall, Glas und

Glasflüssenach dem Steinbuch von el-Beruni, in Zeitschr Deutsch. Morgen l.

Geselschaft, vol. 90. [Leipzig 1936], p. 325-327). This Lapidary was printed

in Haidarabad (East India), through the efforts of Dr. Krenkow, in 1355/1938.

225) MARĪNA   Marine eel

MAIMONIDES: It is the "sea serpent" (hayyat al-bahr).

MEYERHOF: [ʿAbd ar-Razzaq 582; Malouf 165.]

In the text the name is lacking diacritical points, but there is no doubt
that it snould be read marĪna or murĪna which is the Arabicized form of the
Latin Muroena. The marine eel (Muroena helena) is a marine fish which greatly
resembles the eel, and, like the latter, has the Arabic name "marine serpent".
The name of the eel in Egypt even today is teʿbān el-bahr ("sea serpent").
According to Malouf, one calls the marine eel abū marĪnā, and this name is
erroneously given to the lamprey. See Dozy II, 585 and Simonet 378. ʿAbd ar-
Razzaq calls it marmāhĪ (Persian, meaning eel) and marĪn.

226) MASHAQŪNIYĀ   Glass slag

MAIMONIDES: It is the mixture prepared from powders (safāf) and salt

for separating gold from silver. Its most well-known name

in Maghrib is aš-šahira.

MEYERHOF: [Ibn al-Beithar 1313 and 2129; Tuhfa 275; ʿAbd ar-Razzaq 375.]

The word mashaqūniyā is Syriac (mešahqonyā. Brockelmann 407a), which Ruska
(J. Ruska, Al-Razi's Geheimnis der Geheimnisse. Berlin 1937, p. 52) explains
as mešah qunāʿa meaning "blue ointment". However, I would rather accept the
explanation furnished by my teacher the orientalist Enno Littmann: mešah-qonyā
meaning "ointment of ashes" (from the Greek konia). For this last word see
Brockelmann (Syriac Lexicon) 677b. The known Arabic name is zubd al-qawārir
("cream of glasses"). The substance itself is explained by certain Arabic
authors as "glass slag", by others as "glazing or enamel of pottery". Maimonides
here follows the explanation of Ibn Gulgul (in Ibn al-Beithar 2129), who identifies it with šahira which is a mixture of salt and crushed bricks. This mixture

was used to purify gold. In medicine, one used it primarily for preparing
dry collyria against corneal opacities of the eye.

227) MARGĀN   Coral

MAIMONIDES: It is "the arborescent stone" (ḥaǧar ǧaǧarī) and al-qūrāl.*

Al-basad and al-marǧan are the same plant; we have discussed
it (see above number 45).

MEYERHOF: [Dioscorides V, 121; Serapion 56 and 363; Ibn al-Beithar 2122;
Tuhfa 73; 'Abd ar-Razzaq 134, 367 and 555.]

Haǧar ǧaǧarī is the Arabic translation of the Greek lithodendron. Qūrāl
is the transcription of the Spanish coral. Marǧān is the Arabic abbreviation
of the Syriac marganītā (Dozy II, 578), which at first signified "pearl" and
later "coral". Fleischer (Études sur le supplément aux dictionnaires arabes
de Dozy; in Ber. D. K. Sachs, Gesellsch. d. Wiss.,phil.-hist. Kl., 1886, p. 179)
explains the transformation from the Greek name margaritês into margellion,
and in Aramaic margalītā and marganītā from whence is derived the Arabic term
marǧān. See also Anastase p. 88 ff.

228) MAĪ'A   Storax, (benzoin)

MAIMONIDES: It comes as a liquid and as a solid. Liquid storax (maī'a
sā'ila) is the one which is called al-lubnā and also 'asal al-
lubnā ("honey of incense") and lubnā ar-ruhbān ("incense of
monks"). Solid storax (maī'a ǧāmida) is the one which is
called isturk and also satrāhī; it has a red color and penetrating fragrance.

MEYERHOF: [Theophrastus IX, 7, 3; Dioscorides I, 66; Serapion 370; Ibn al-
Beithar 97 and 2196; Tuhfa 58 and 238; 'Abd ar-Razzaq 513 and
529; Issa 110, 4 and 175, 8; Loew III, 388-395; Ducros 226-228.]

* in the text qūrwāl, ? error of the copyist. Simonet 131 gives the Arabic
forms qūrāl and qūrūl of the Spanish name coral.

The Greek name styrax, of Semitic origin, reappeared to the Syrians in
the form asturka and to the Arabs as astarak, isturak, etc. Satrāhī is perhaps
a mutilation of this name. The Arabic name māi'a originates from m.y.' meaning
"to flow, to melt, to liquify", and lubnā is the Semitic name for "incense".

The Arabs distinguished "dry storax", hard resin derived from styrax or
benzoin (Styrax officinale L.), from "liquid storax" which is the resinous
balsamic juice of Liquidamber orientalis MILL. (hamamelidaceae). The latter
is a beautiful tree which reminds one of the plane-tree and which originates in
Asia-Minor and Syria. Its purified product is still in use in Europe against
bronchitis, and externally against scabies. By contrast, dry storax has
nearly been abandoned as a remedy. The storax is a bush which grows spontaneously in Asia Minor and in Greece, and which is sometimes cultivated in Italy
and in Provence. The druggists of Cairo sell as mē'a gāffa ("dry storax") the
dry resin of the storax bush for fumigations; as mē'a nāsfa (also "dry storax")
the bark of the tree from which one extracts the resin, and as mē'a sāila
("liquid storax") the resinous juice of Liquidamber. Ibn al-Beithar and the
majority of Arabic physicians identify stakte of the Greeks with liquid storax.
O. Stever (Myrrhe und Stakte, Vienna 1933) recently refuted this assertion with
undeniable proofs.

229) MULŪHIYA   Corchorus, mallow

MAIMONIDES: One also says mulūkiyā and mulūh. It is the cultivated mallow
(al-hubbāzī al-bustānī)* or the Jewish vegetable. The wild species
is the marsh-mallow (al-hitmī).

MEYERHOF: [Serapion 377; Ibn al-Beithar 2173; Tuhfa 70; 'Abd ar-Razzaq
554; Issa 57, 16; Loew II, 246-248; Ibn 'Awwam II, 289.]

The names mulūhiyā, mulūkiyā, etc. are the Syriac forms of the Greek
names molokhê, molokhion, etc. which designate the mallow. Our plant is the
"corchorus" or "Jewish mallow" (Corchorus olitorius L.), a well-known vegetable

* this adjective is lacking in the text

in Syria, Palestine and Egypt. One eats the mucilaginous fruits thereof. The
seeds are gentle purgatives. The name baqla yahūdiyya ("Jewish vegetable")
originated from the frequent usage of this plant in Palestine. Ibn 'Awwam
speaks thereof as a Syrian plant; he does not state whether it was cultivated
in Spain. It is renowned today in Maghrib (Renaud-Colin).

230) MUQL   False bdellium

MAIMONIDES: This name is applied to the resin of a tree and to a type of
           tree. This type of tree is called al-kur, and it is the
           fruit of this tree that one (fol. 91^v) calls ad-dawn. It is
           a red berry (globule), round and very astringent which is
           called al-waql. The resin of this tree is often encountered
           in medical books. It is this resin that one calls al-muql
           al-azraq ("blue bdellium") and muql al-Yahūd ("Jewish bdellium").

MEYERHOF: [Theophrastus IV, 2,7; Dioscorides I, 67; Serapion 376-378;
          Ghafiqi 238; Ibn al-Beithar 2167-2158; Tuhfa 61, 257 and 439;
          'Abd ar-Razzaq 520; Issa 55, 5: Loew I, 304 ff and II, 303;
          Ducros 145; Dymock I, 310.]

The name muql in Arabic designates: 1) the doom palm (Hyphaene thebaica
MART., in Arabic dawm or dūm), branched fan palm characteristic of Upper-Egypt,
Nubia and Southern Arabia (known to Theophrastus under the name koukiophoron;
its fruit, in Coptic, had the name koukon). In Arabic it was called muql or
waql (Abu Hanifa ad-Dinawari in Muhassas XI, 136). It was thought that this
tree also produced a resin called muql makki ("bdellium of Mecca" meaning
Bdellium aegyptiacum). However, the doom palm does not produce resin, and this
bdellium was probably the resin of the burseraceous plant Balsamodendron africanum ARN. It is perhaps identical with "blue bdellium" and "Jewish bdellium" whose
tree is kur (Ibn al-Beithar 1987). 2) The name muql designates the bdellium
from India originating from Balsamodendron Mukul HOOK., yellow-greenish resin.
One sells both types in the bazaars of Cairo under the name samg al-muql (Ducros).

Qamus (IV,51) states as follows: "Muql with damma (u) is the incense used by
Jews for their fumigations. It is the resin of a tree and there are Indian,
Arabic and Sicilian (types). All these types are used against coughing, snake
bites, hemorrhoids, for the purification of the uterus, etc. Muql makki is the
fruit of the tree ad-dawm; one eats it. It is dry, astringent, cold and stomach
fortifying". Actually, in Upper Egypt, muql is still the name of the fruit; dum
or dom that of the tree. It was impossible for me to determine whether there
is a relationship between the Sanskrit name guggula for Balsamodendron Mukul
(Chopra 287) and the Arabic name muql.

231) MŪ   Spicknel and cornel-tree

MAIMONIDES: It is al-murrān and in Spanish murrāna. It is al-qarāniya
      and it is also yandru (yendro). One says that it is the wood of
      the beech-tree (az-zān).

MEYERHOF: [Theophrastus III, 2-12; Dioscorides I, 3 and I, 119; Serapion
      380; Ibn al-Beithar 2158, 2101, 1753; 'Abd ar-Razzaq 565; Issa
      118,16; 82,2 and 58,7; Loew III, 465 and I, 464 ff.]

Mū is the Arabic name, transcribed from the Greek mêon, for the wild
anet (Meum athamanticum JACQ., spicknel, Umbelliferae). The names murrān and
murrāna originate from the Spanish morena ("black" because of the dark color
of the roots? Simonet 352). The name yendro is old Iberic, and it is still
preserved in the Portugese endro bravo for Meum, whereas the plant has the
Castilian name hinojo de oso (Simonet 64)(and in old Castilian pinillo oloroso,
Laguna 13-14).

In addition, the Arabic-Spanish name murrān, at the same time, also designates the cornel-tree (Dozy II, 585a; Cornus-mas L.) and the beech-tree
(Fagus silvatica L.). The cornel-tree, in Maghrib, has the name qaraniya which
is the Arabicized form of the Greek kraneia (Theophrastus) or krania (Dioscorides).
Thus is explained the juxtaposition of different vegetables in this same paragraph
(Dozy II,339; Simonet 135). 'Abd ar-Razzaq identifies mū with the root of
staphisagria.

232) <u>MASTIKĀ</u>   Mastic gum

    <u>MAIMONIDES</u>: It is <u>al-kiya,</u> and one also calls it "Greek gum" (<u>'ilk ar-</u>
        <u>rūm wa'l-ilk ar-rūmī</u>). There is a black type which is called
        "Nabathean mastic" (<u>al-mastikā an-nabatī</u>).

    <u>MEYERHOF</u>: ⌈Dioscorides I, 70; Serapion 368; Ibn al-Beithar 2139; <u>Tuhfa</u> 251;
        'Abd ar-Razzaq 490, 521 and 674; Issa 141, 12; Loew I, 195-198;
        Ducros 220.⌉

    <u>Mastikā</u> is the Arabic-Syriac transcription of the Greek name <u>mastikhê</u> which
designates lentisk resin (<u>Pistacia Lentiscus</u> L. var. <u>Chia</u> D.C. Anacardiaceae).
The name <u>kiya</u> indicates the principal site of origin of this bush, the island
of Chio in the Greek Archipelago. The drug presents in small drops which are
pale yellow or greenish. It is sold in the entire Orient, in Cairo as well as
the bazaars of travelling merchants. One rarely uses it as a medicament, but it
serves uniquely in the fabrication of paste and varnish. In the Orient, it is
utilized everywhere as a masticatory. It gives a balsamic odor to the breath.

    The "Nabathean mastic", also called "Nabathean gum" (<u>'ilk al-anbāt</u>),is
probably the resin of the pistachio-tree (<u>Pistacia vera</u> L.). Nevertheless,
Ishaq b. Imran (in Ibn al-Beithar 1581) states that this resin was not black
but white. One also extracts mastic from <u>Pistacia Khinjuk</u> STOKES, which grows
in Southern Arabia and in Central Asia. See below at number 301.

233) <u>MIŠMIŠ</u>   Apricot

    <u>MAIMONIDES</u>: It is the "Armenian apple" (<u>al-tuffāh al-armīnī</u>).

    <u>MEYERHOF</u>: ⌈Dioscorides I, 115; Serapion 364 and 372; Ibn al-Beithar 274,
        419 and 2136; <u>Tuhfa</u> 45; Issa 148, 17; Loew III, 155-159; Ibn
        'Awwam I, 313-315.⌉

    <u>Mišmiš</u>(or <u>mušmuš</u>) is the Arabic name of the apricot in Egypt and in Syria
where one dries the pulps of apricots in the sun in order to prepare a flat
paste like leather (called <u>qamar ad-dīn</u>). The preparation of this "leather of
apricots" was described by H. Almkvist (<u>Kleine Beitrage zur Lexicographie des</u>
<u>Vulgararabischen)</u>, in <u>Actes du VIIIe Congrès Intern. des Orientalistes</u>. II (Leyden

1891-1893) p.420 ff. The name mišmiš originates from the Syriac root k.m.s.
meaning "to dry". In Spain and in Maghrib, one calls the apricot barqūq,
name derived from the Latin praecocia (meaning "precocious, early fruit") and
which passed by the Greek of Dioscorides (brekokkia). "Armenian apple" is the
translation from the Greek melon Armeniakon. In Spain, the apricot still carries the
name albaricoque.

234) MŪMIYĀ'Ī   Mummy.

MAIMONIDES: It is the "mummy of the tombs" (al-mūmiya al-quburiyya).

MEYERHOF: Dioscorides I, 73; Serapion 382; Ibn al-Beithar 2190; Tuhfa 263;
'Abd ar-Razzaq 535.

One is here dealing with the real "mummy" of the Middle Ages which was
very famous as a remedy. On this subject see A. Wiedemann Mumie als Heilmittel
("mummy as a remedy" in Zeitschr. des Vereins f. rhein u. westfal. Volkskunde.
III year 1906, fasc.1.) and 'Abd al-Latif (200ff). The latter distinguishes
well the "mineral mummy" which flows from certain mountains from the "mummy
of the tombs", a bituminous mass found in the Egyptian mummies. The former
corresponds to pissasphalte of Dioscorides. The name mūmiyā is derived from
the Persian mūm meaning "wax". Mūmiyā'Ī is the Persian form of the Greek
moûmia (Vullers II, 1231; Dozy II, 635). See the exposition of Hooper and
Field (p.198ff) concerning the different types of mummy known in Egypt. An
old physician in Cairo told me that around 1880 he still received requests
from European pharmacists to furnish them with debris of true Egyptian mummies, as a medicament. The mummy was reputed above all as a remedy which
accelerated the consolidation of fractures. It is for this reason that it
also has the name "bone-setter", ǧabbār (see Steinschneider., Heilm.number 584).

235) MARRŪYA   Horehound and marjoram.

MAIMONIDES: It is "the thyme of old men" (habaq aš-šuyuh), and al-marw,
and aš-šinār, and aš-šarbat, and az-zaǧbar. Its name in
Spanish is mantarašta (mentastro).

MEYERHOF: [Theophrastus VI, 2,5; Dioscorides III, 105; Serapion 177;
Ibn al-Beithar 2108 and 2123; Tuhfa 261; 'Abd ar-Razzaq 697;
Issa 115,7 and 130,4; Loew II, 74ff and 84-101; Ducros 172
and 218.]

In this paragraph, because of the similarity of names, Maimonides confused
two different labiate plants:

1) Marrūya is a Spanish name, marrubium in Latin (prasion in Greek); it is
the white horehound (Marrubium vulgare L.), in modern Castilian marrubio. This
name is preserved in Moroccan dialect as merriyut (Leclerc and Renaud-Colin).
This plant is sometimes called mentastro or mastranza, which is nevertheless the
name of the mint with round leaves (Mentha rotundifolia L.). Šinār or šannār is
an Arabic name of the horehound (Ibn Biklaris according to Dozy I,790). Its
"Persian" name zagbar (in our text ragbar; in Kohen 133 line 13, za'anbar; in
Dawud I,350, za'anir), appears to me to be a mutilation of za'tar meaning
origanum. Šarbāt is perhaps another Persian name (Vullers II,421).

2) Marw is the Syriac-Persian name (Vullers II,1168) of the "Egyptian origanum"
or "wild marjoram" (origanum Maru L.), which is also called marmahuz or
marmahūr in Persian, "thyme of old men" or "basilic of old men" (raihān aš-šuyūh)
in Arabic. The name za'tar (in Issa: zagbar) is also applied to this plant. See
the long article by Loew (with a figure) concerning this plant. It was cultivated in Musulman Spain (Ibn 'Awwam II,285ff). The druggists of Cairo under
the name frāsiyūn sell the white horehound, and under the name marmāhūr the
maritime germander (Teucrium Marum L., Labiates; Ducros).

236) MARZANGŪŠ   Sweet marjoram.

MAIMONIDES: One also says mardaqūš and mardudūš; it is al-'anqar and aš-
šams, as well as the "elephant thyme" (habaq al-fīl) and
al-harak; one also calls it "mouse ears" (ādān al-fār).

MEYERHOF: [Theophrastus VI, 1-8; Dioscorides III, 39; Serapion 365; Ibn
al-Beithar 2100; Tuhfa 252; 'Abd ar-Razzaq 384; 533 and 678;
Issa 130, 2; Loew II, 84; Ducros 216; Ibn 'Awwam II, 277-279.]

Marzangūš is a Persian name which signifies "mouse ear" (Vullers 1161).
In Greek it is myos ôtis, in Arabic ādān al-fār. It was corrupted in Arabic
into mardaqūš, in Spanish into mardadus, etc. It designates the sweet marjoram
(Origanum Majorana L., Labiates). 'Anṣar is one of its Arabic names, whereas
šams is undoubtedly a mutilation of samsaq which is the Arabic form of the Greek
sampsykhon meaning sweet marjoram (Vullers II,322). The name harak today
designates cultivated vetch (Lathyrus sativus L., Issa 105,a). The druggists
in Cairo sell the entire plant of the sweet marjoram, dried, as a panacea
against all illnesses, under the name mardaqūš (Ducros). It was cultivated in
Spain (see Ibn 'Awwam).

237) MĀZIRIYŪN (SIC)   Daphne mezereum.

   MAIMONIDES: It is "the lion of the earth" (asad al-arḍ) and one also calls
                it ṭābimāk and baftīraq and al-mu'īn and "the green one"
                (al-hadrā'); and in Spanish alwaru (lauro) and in ancient
                Greek hamalaun. It belongs to the latex plants (yuttū'āt),
                as we have mentioned.

   MEYERHOF: Theophrastus VI, 2,2 (kneoros); Dioscorides IV, 171-172; Serapion
                369; Ibn al-Beithar 2058; Tuhfa 267; Abd ar-Razzaq 529; Issa 68,
                5-6; Loew III, 409-411.

This article offers great difficulties because of the faulty transcription
of three names which lack diacritical points. One is dealing with the thymelea-
ceous plant Daphne Mezereum L., ("gentle wood, false garon; female mezereon, etc.)
and its relatives, many of which were described by Dioscorides under the name
thymelaia or khamelaia ("olive-tree of the earth", because of the resemblance
of its leaves to those of the olive-tree). The name māzariyūn is not Greek but
Persian (Vullers II,1117). The Greek name khamáileón of our manuscript and its
translation as "lion of the earth" are erroneous. It is a shrub with rose
flowers, rarely white, very fragrant, which grows in the mountains of nearly all
of Europe and North Africa. One employed the bark of its root and its trunk in

medicine. The corrupted Spanish name should read <u>lauro</u> (Simonet 300). Idrisi
(272) gives the Spanish <u>laureola</u> which in fact designates the spurge-laurel
(<u>Daphne Laureola</u> L.). At the same time he states that the name <u>al-hadrā'</u> is
very much in common use in Maghrib. As to the name <u>baftiraǧ</u>, - the reading is
uncertain -, it is perhaps the diminutive of the Persian word <u>baftarī</u> which
designates the comb or belch (?) of the weaving-loom. Steinschneider (<u>Die
Heilmittelnamen der Araber</u>, Frankfurt 1900,p. 319) reads <u>ba'tamraǧ</u>, but declares himself incapable of providing an explanation of this name.

238) <u>MUǴRA</u>   Rubric (Red chalk)

<u>MAIMONIDES</u>: It is <u>al-misǧ</u> and "the red earth" (<u>al-tīn al-ahmar</u>); and
it is also called (fol. 91^v) <u>urtukiz</u>.

<u>MEYERHOF</u>: [Dioscorides V, 96; Serapion 375; Ibn al-Beithar 2148; <u>Tuhfa</u> 196;
'Abd ar-Razzaq 579; Ducros 151.]

Dioscorides, already in his time, knew two types of rubric or Sinope earth
(<u>miltos</u>), a natural one, a clay impregnated with silicate and oxide of iron,
and an artificial one (<u>tektonike</u>) obtained by the calcination of yellow ochre.
The name <u>musǧ</u> or <u>musaqq</u> is lacking in the dictionaries, and the name <u>urtukiz</u>,
which simulates a Turkish form, defies all attempts for an explanation. It is a
mutilation of <u>psorikon</u>, of <u>tektcnikê</u> or of <u>syrikon</u> ("red lead") which is rendered into Arabic by <u>zarqūn</u> or <u>isriqūn</u>? Rubric once was used by surgeons for the
stanching of blood.

239) <u>MARTAK</u>   Litharge

<u>MAIMONIDES</u>: It is <u>al-mardāsang</u>.

<u>MEYERHOF</u>: [Dioscorides V, 87; Serapion 353; Ibn al-Beithar 2114; <u>Tuhfa</u> 256;
'Abd ar-Razzaq 523.]

<u>Mardāsang</u> is the Arabic form of the Persian <u>murdāsang</u> (originally <u>murdar-
sang</u> meaning "impure stone", Vullers II, 1157), and <u>martak</u> is the Arabic abbreviation of this name, from the Syriac <u>mardêkā</u> (see Brockelmann, Lex. 308a).
It designates the litharge ("silver stone") of the Greeks. It is the protoxide

of glazed lead, having a brilliant and silver appearance, by product of the ex-
traction of silver from galenas (composite sulfurs of lead). One used it primarily for the preparation of dry metallic collyria. The name martak is preserved in the Spanish language in the form almartaga meaning litharge.

240) MURŪRIYA   Escarole, etc.

MAIMONIDES: It is "wild lettuce" (al-hass al-barri).

MEYERHOF: [Theophrastus VII, 1-6 (thridakinê); Dioscorides II, 136 (agria

thridax); Ibn al-Beithar 2124; 'Abd ar-Razzaq 907; Issa: uncertain;

Loew I, 426-439.]

The name murūriyā is the Arabic form of the Aramaic mĕrāritā which designates a bitter herb (Assyrian: haššu and marāru). See the long exposition by
Loew on bitter herbs (mārŏr), the ingestion of which is part of the ceremonies
of the Jewish Passover. Ibn al-Beithar identifies it with the chondrilla
(see above number 110 and also number 114 Hindabā'). Loew argues in favor of
the sow thistle (sonchus oleraceus L., Compositae). However, there are so many
types of bitter chicory and lettuce, all designated in Arabic as murrār, muraïr,
murāra, marūr, etc. that the distinction is difficult. As to the designation
"wild lettuce", it is most in accord with the composite plant Lactuca Scariola L.,
(escarole) which has slightly bitter edible leaves and which is considered the
originator of our garden lettuce. Lactuca altissima BIEB. is considered as a
variety of escarole. Among the chicories, there are also many wild and very
bitter types which merit the designation murūriyā. In summary, it is impossible
to arrive at an absolute conclusion concerning the nature of this "bitter herb".

241) MĀMĪRĀN   Celandine

MAIMONIDES: It is "the plant of swallows" (baqlat al-hatātif)and one type

of "yellow roots" (al-'uruq as-sufr). Its name in ancient

Greek is khelidonion, and in Spanish ǧalidūniya (celidonia).

By contrast, the remedy which the Berbers call argis and

the Egyptians "fragrant wood" ('ūd ar-rīh) is the

bark of the wild pomegranate tree (ar-rummān al-barrī). Its
(medicinal) properties approach those of the celandine.

MEYERHOF: [Theophrastus VII, 15, 1; Dioscorides II, 180-181; Serapion 501-502;
Ibn al-Beithar 1525 and 2080; Tuhfa 252; 'Abd ar-Razzaq 144 and
503; Issa 47, 1; Loew II, 371-373; Dymock 31 and 248.]

The dictionaries are in agreement and identify the Persian name māmīrān
with khelidonion of the Greeks (e.g. Vullers II, 1124). The Arabic names are
in part translations of this Greek name "plant of swallows", and one has related
them to the papaveraceous plant Chelidonium majus L. Nevertheless, Renaud-Colin
have justly remarked that the Arabs probably confused the celandine that has
juice and a yellow root with an oriental drug that has yellow roots, the ranunculous plant Coptis Teeta WALL. This plant, as well as other species of Coptis,
originated in China. Their roots are imported to India and to Persia. They
are described by Mir Muhammad Husain in his large Persian pharmacopoeia (Mahzan
al-Adwiya). According to Sir George Watt (The Commercial Products of India,
London 1908, p. 130 and 405), the population of India used, apart from Coptis
Teeta, the juice of Corydalis Goraniana WALL, of Geranium Wallichianum SWEET,
and of Thalictrum foliolosum as astringents against eye illnesses, all under
the name mamiran.

As to the note of Maimonides at the end of his article, the names argis in
Berber and 'ūd ar-rih in Egyptian-Arabic (see Ducros no. 164) do not designate
the root of the wild pomegranate tree, but that of the barberry (Berberis
vulgaris L.). Therefore, it is interesting to note that several types of ranunculous
plants (Coptis and Thalictrum) contain, as the barberry, a large quantity of
berbenine (Dymock I, 35), and that their tonic properties are comparable, as
the ancient Arabic physicians have observed.

242) MISKITRĀ MASĪR   Dittany

MAIMONIDES: One also says miskitrā masī', as well as misk al-barr
("earth musk"); it is one of the species of mint (fūdanaġūt).

Its name in Spanish is <u>bulāyu g̊arbiyūnu</u> and in ancient

Greek <u>diktamnon</u>.

MEYERHOF: [Theophrastus IX, 16, 1-3; Dioscorides III, 32; Serapion 367;

Ibn al-Beithar 2138; 'Abd ar-Razzaq 553 and 694; Issa 129, 15;

Loew II, 83ff.]

These names are the Arabic forms of the Persian <u>musk-tiramsir</u> ("musked

pennycress", which derive from the Syriac language. It is the equivalent of

<u>diktamnon</u> of the Greeks. It is the dittany of Crete (<u>Origanum Dictamnus</u> L.

or <u>Amaracus Dictamnus</u> BENTH., Labiates), which was considered an excellent

remedy for the treatment of wounds during antiquity and the Middle Ages. It

is a Mediterranean plant which is sometimes cultivated in gardens. The Spanish

name, derived from the Latin <u>pulegium cervinum</u> ("cervine pennyroyal"), is in

modern Castilian <u>poleo cervuno</u> (Simonet 452). See below at number 309, the

species <u>fūdanag̊</u> or <u>fawdanag̊</u> (mint).

243) <u>MUZZ</u>   ? wild pomegranate-tree

MAIMONIDES: It is a wild pomegranate-tree (<u>rummān barri</u>), which is found

in aš-Šurāy, and has no fruits.

MEYERHOF: [Dioscorides I, 111; Serapion 293; Ibn al-Beithar 2144; <u>Tuhfa</u> 94,

180 and 287; 'Abd ar-Razzaq 205; Issa 151, 3; Loew III, 95; Ducros 65.]

See our articles 75 and 250. The name <u>muzz</u>, as we have mentioned, is also

vocalized <u>mazz</u> and <u>mizz</u>. The article is taken from the <u>Book of Plants</u> of

Abu Hanifa ad-Dinawari (see Ibn al-Beithar 2144). It is for this reason that

one should not read <u>Sarā</u> (meaning <u>Sierra</u>), but <u>Šuray</u> which is, according to

Yāqut (III, 286) a route in Arabia, between Tihama and Yemen. One is probably

dealing with the same wild pomegranate-tree (<u>Punica Granatum</u> L.) which grows

in the Mediterranean regions. See the name <u>muzz</u> in usage for an Indian herb

(at number 250 <u>nārmušk</u>).

244) MŪM   Wax

MAIMONIDES: It is the yellow wax (aš-šam' al-asfar).

MEYERHOF: [Dioscorides II, 83; Serapion 228 and 381; Ibn al-Beithar 1340 and 2193; Tuhfa 260; 'Abd ar-Razzaq 547 and 950.]

Mum is the Persian name for "wax", "candle". Here it is the technical term of physicians, such as the cera of pharmacists. The translation propolis given by Guigues (Serapion 381) is erroneous. See our number 122 (wasah al-kūr).

245) MŪRDĀŠURAĞ   Myrtle confection

MAIMONIDES: It is the confection of myrtle (rubb al-ās) in Persian.

MEYERHOF: This name is the transformation of the Persian mūrd-afsurağ meaning "confection of myrtle". The fruits of the myrtle preserved in honey constituted an astringent remedy greatly in vogue.

246) MĀST   Curdled milk

MAIMONIDES: It is skimmed curdled milk.

MEYERHOF: [Dioscorides II, 70; Ibn al-Beithar 2007 and 2076; 'Abd ar Razzaq 578.]

Māst is also a Persian name (Vullers II, 1118) in usage by physicians to designate curdled milk (coagulum lactis). Ibn al-Beithar states that it is a curdled milk whose acidity is not complete.

247) MĀISŪSAN   Wine of the lily

MAIMONIDES: A composite wine (šarāb) which is mentioned in the book of Aharun.

MEYERHOF: The name is Persian (mai meaning "wine" and sawsan or sūsan meaning "lily") and designates a composite potion whose complicated preparation is described in detail by Ibn Gazla (Minhāğ, under šarāb-as-sawsan): 400 flowers of white lily cleaned and dried with an Arabic costus, sweet rush, salt and balm, are macerated in cooked wine; then one adds musk, storax and balm-oil. One filters and then lets this wine mature in a jar placed in the cold. Aharūn (Ahron "the Priest") was a Syrian archiater who lived in the seventh

century and who wrote the <u>Medical Pandects</u> in thirty books which were translated from the Syriac into Arabic by the Jewish-Persian physician Masargawaih.

248) <u>MIDĀD</u>   Black ink from fumes

    <u>MAIMONIDES</u>: That which is mentioned in the medical books is composed of
                the fumes of the wood of the pine-tree (<u>sanawbar</u>), gum arabic
                and a little oil.

    <u>MEYERHOF</u>: [Dioscorides V, 162; Ibn al-Beithar 2098; 'Abd ar-Razzaq 561.]

    <u>Midād</u> is the Arabic term which corresponds to <u>melan</u> of Dioscorides and
is sufficiently explained in the article by Maimonides. Calcinated soot
(<u>asbolê</u> of Dioscorides I, 161) was the indelible material used in writing and
which permits us to decifer the Egyptian and Greek papyruses after thousands
of years. One used it in medicine against burns and gangrene and to accelerate
the cicatrization of sores. This ink was thus considered in some way as a
disinfectant.

CHAPTER NŪN

249) NĪLĀǦ   Pastel and indigo.

> MAIMONIDES: It is that which the people call an-nīl; mention thereof is
> found in preceding (paragraphs. see number 126 and 159). It
> is also called the "green earth" (at-tīn al-aḫḍar) and the
> "green fountain" (al-'aïn al-ḫaḍrā').

> MEYERHOF: [Dioscorides V,92; Serapion 157; Ibn al-Beithar 2244; Tuhfa 292;
> 'Abd ar-Razzaq 267 and 588; Issa 98,14 and 101,1; Loew I, 493-505.]

Nīlāǧ or naïlāǧ is the Arabic term (derived from the Sanskrit nīla through
the intermediary of Persian, Laufer 370) for indigo. However, we have expounded
(see number 126 and 159) that the Arabs always confused pastel (Isatis Tinctoria L.)
with indigo (Indigofera tinctoria L.). The term 'aïn ḫaḍrā' ("green fountain" or
"green eye") is found only in Maimonides; it is undoubtedly a popular designation.

250) NĀRAMUŠK   Rose chestnut-tree.

> MAIMONIDES: It is an-nāǧabašk and it is also called al-muzz as well as
> mušk (fol.92ᵃ) ar-rumman ("pomegranate musk"); it is an
> Indian herb.

> MEYERHOF: [Serapion 391; Ibn al-Beithar 2205; Tuhfa 287; 'Abd ar-Razzaq
> 603; Issa 118,14; Dymock I,170-172.]

Nār-mušk is Persian and signifies "pomegranate musk". We have already
mentioned in number 243 that muzz or mizz is an Arabic name of the wild pomegranate tree. One is here dealing with another confusion caused by the similarity of names which has disconcerted commentators to this very day. The drug
is certainly Indian, as Maimonides states. It is not a herb but a large and
beautiful tree with large white flowers, the gultiferous plant Mesua ferrea L.
("iron wood tree"). One of its names in Sanskrit is nagkesara from which is
probably derived nāgabašk (in Steingass 1375b, nāǧist). It is the bark of the
root which is utilized as an aromatic astringent, because of its strong grade
of resin (Dymock).

251) NAĞM   Couch-grass

MAIMONIDES: It is at-tīl, al-'ikriš and an-nagīl.

MEYERHOF: [Theophrastus IV, 6-11; Dioscorides IV, 29; Serapion 396 and 519;
          Ibn al-Beithar 458 and 2214; Tuhfa 409; 'Abd ar-Razzaq 101, 595
          and 900; Issa 7, 14 and 65, 4; Ibn 'Awwam II, 376; Ducros 156.]

The four Arabic names designate a creeping gramineous plant corresponding
to the agrôstis of the Greeks. One thought that it is primarily the small
couch-grass (Agrapyrum repens BEAUV.), but this plant is rare in the Near-East.
Today the name nagīl, in Syria and in Palestine, designates Aeluropus littoralis
GON. and the creeping dactyl Aeluropus repens DESF. (Post II, 756) which is
called 'ekriš in Egypt (Schweinfurth 52). In Egypt and in North Africa, the name
nagîl or nagīl is used for the large couch-grass of Italy (Cynodon Dactylon PERS.),
which also has the names nagm, nagîr and tīl. The rhizome thereof is sold in the
bazaars of Cairo as a diuretic (Ducros).

252) NAĪLUFAR   Nenuphar (water-lily)

MAIMONIDES: The "tomb of bees" (qabr an-nahl) and the "young bride" (al-'arus);
           it is also called bašnīn and in ancient Greek lôtos.

MEYERHOF: [Theophrastus IV, 8, 9-11; Dioscorides IV, 113; Serapion 400; Ibn al-
          Beithar 292 and 2243; Tuhfa 288; 'Abd ar-Razzaq 605; Issa 125, 15;
          Loew II, 280ff; Ibn 'Awwam II, 263ff; Ducros 38.]

Nīlūfar or naīlufar is the Arabic form of the Persian nilūpar, derived from
the Sanskrit nilotpala meaning "blue lotus". This name nīlūfar (transformed
into "nenuphar" in French and English) today designates both the white nenuphar
(Nymphae Lotus L. var. alba) and the blue one (Nymphae caerulea L.). The latter,
in particular, in Egypt, has the Arabic names indicated above. In addition,
one finds the popular names linufar and nufar. The dried flowers of the white
nenuphar are sold in the bazaars under the name bašnīn (Ducros). (See also
Ghafiqi number 129 and Schweinfurth in Bull. de l'Inst. d'Egypte, 1882, p. 62-67).
One administers them in compresses as a refreshing and calming agent. (The title

of this and the next three paragraphs in the Arabic text is found at the
beginning of each of the following paragraphs. The text here is placed in
proper order.)

253) <u>NISRĪN</u>   Musked rose and dogrose.

  <u>MAIMONIDES</u>: (It is) the wild rose (<u>al-ward al-barrī</u>) and it is the Chinese
               rose (<u>al-ward as-sīnī</u>).

  <u>MEYERHOF</u>: [Theophrastus IV,4,8,etc.; Dioscorides I,94; Serapion 392; Ibn al-
               Beithar 2222; <u>Tuhfa</u> 278; 'Abd ar-Razzaq 590; Issa 157 and 10;
               Loew III,194,211; Ibn 'Awwam I,377 and II,269ff.]

  The name <u>nisrīn</u> is Persian (Vullers II,1312) and designates both the musked
rose (<u>Rosa moschata</u> HERM., <u>gul-miškin</u>) and the dogrose (<u>Rosa canina</u> L., <u>gul-
nisrīn</u>). The latter furnishes the kitchen and the pharmacy with the fruits
(<u>cynorrhodous</u>) from which one prepares an astringent sugared preserve. Until
recently, the galls (<u>bédégars</u>, derived from the Arabic-Persian <u>badaward</u>. See
number 44) which are produced on these rose bushes by the prick of the hymen-
opter <u>Cyrups rosae</u>, were sold as an astringent remedy.

254) <u>NARĞIS</u>   Narcissus.

  <u>MAIMONIDES</u>: It is <u>al-'arār</u> and <u>al-'abhar</u>.

  <u>MEYERHOF</u>: [Theophrastus VII,6-8; Dioscorides IV,158; Serapion 392; Ibn al-
               Beithar 2221; 'Abd ar-Razzaq 135 and 598; Issa 123,3; Loew II,
               203-205; Ibn 'Awwam II,265ff.]

  The name <u>narğis</u> is the Arabic form of the Persian term <u>nargi</u> or <u>nargis</u>
(Laufer 427) which designates different species of narcissus (<u>Narcissus poeticus</u>
L., <u>Narcissus Tazzetta</u> L., etc.; Amarylidaceae). Loew claims there is no Arabic
name for this plant; the present article proves the contrary. '<u>Abhar</u> is given
by several authors as the name of the white narcissus, '<u>arār</u> (Lane 1990) as that
of the "wild narcissus" and fragrant plants in general. In Issa (25,23), '<u>arar</u>
is the composite plant <u>Asteriscus graveolens</u> L., also called <u>narğis barrī</u>. (The
title of this paragraph is lacking in the Arabic text).

255) <u>NAMMĀM</u>   Serpolet (wild thyme).

    <u>MAIMONIDES</u>: It is the <u>sisymbrium</u> (<u>as-sisanbar</u>) and in Spanish <u>qālamān-</u>
          <u>ta</u> (<u>calamento</u>).

    <u>MEYERHOF</u>: Theophrastus VI,6-7; Dioscorides II,128; Serapion 397; Ibn al-
          Beithar 2233; <u>Tuhfa</u> 282 and 378; 'Abd ar-Razzaq 600; Issa 181,2;
          Loew II,71.

The Arabic name <u>nammām</u> designates numerous labiates, notably the serpolet
(<u>Thymus glaber</u> MILL., <u>Thymus Serpyllum</u> FRIES.), but also water-mint, peppermint,
<u>Mentha sativa</u> L., etc., the same plants to which the Arabs gave the name <u>sīsanbar</u>
(<u>Sisymbrium</u>) which designates a cruciferous plant. See the commentaries of
Renaud-Colin (<u>Tuhfa</u>). The Spanish name <u>calamento</u> (Simonet 73) designates yet
another labiate, <u>Melissa Calamintha</u> L., which formerly was part of the famous
"melissa water of the Carmelites". There is thus confusion in this article of
Maimonides, just as in the remainder of all the Arabic pharmacological treatises.

256) <u>NA'NA'</u>   Mint.

    <u>MAIMONIDES</u>: It is that which one calls the "cultivated basilic" (<u>al-habaq</u>
          <u>al-bustānī</u>), and its name is also <u>manta</u> (<u>menta</u>) and <u>harma</u>; it
          is <u>hedyosmon</u>.

    <u>MEYERHOF</u>: Theophrastus VII,7,1; Dioscorides III,34; Serapion 388; Ibn al-
          Beithar 2227; <u>Tuhfa</u> 283; Issa 117,12 and 14; 'Abd ar-Razzaq 394,
          597 and 694; Loew II,75-77; Ducros 233; Ibn 'Awwam II,275-277.

<u>Na'na'</u> is the generic name of different species of mint (<u>Mentha piperita</u>
SMITH., <u>Mentha sativa</u> L., <u>Mentha aquatica</u> L.), as <u>habaq</u> is (the generic name) of
basilics or neighboring fragrant labiates. The name <u>harma</u> is only known as óne
of numerous Arabic names for purslain (Issa 147,10). Perhaps it is a faulty
reading for <u>hartā</u> (Suwaidi 1886). The Greek name <u>hêdyosmon</u> ("having an agreable
odor") is mutilated in the Arabic text and is nearly read as <u>androsaimon</u>.

In Cairo the druggists sell the leaves of <u>na'nā' filfilī</u> ("peppermint") in
the bazaars (Ducros).

257) NĀRIǦĪL   Coconut.

MAIMONIDES: It is "the Indian nut" (ǧawz al-Hind) that we have mentioned
             in letter ǧim. It is an-nāranǧ and ar-rānaǧ.

MEYERHOF: [Serapion 398; Ibn al-Beithar 2203; Tuhfa 286; 'Abd ar-Razzaq 601;
           Issa 53,17; Loew II,303-305; Dymock III,511-519; Ducros 229.]

See above our article number 82. Nāriǧil is the Arabic form of the Persian
nāriǧil which is derived from the Sanskrit nārikeli ("the juicy one") or narikera.
Nāranǧ and rānaǧ are Arabic mutilations; one also finds the form bāranǧ which
is even more corrupted. It is the coconut, fruit of the palm-tree Cocos nucifera
L. In Cairo, travelling salesmen market slices and preserves of coconut.

258) NAHŠAK   Wild carrot.

MAIMONIDES: It is the wild carrot (al-ǧazar al-barrī).

MEYERHOF: [Dioscorides II,139;III,73; Ibn al-Beithar 481 and 2240; Tuhfa
           353 and 445; 'Abd ar-Razzaq 202; Issa 69,5; Loew III,448-452.]

The name of the wild carrot is sometimes written nahšal and sometimes
nahšak (Dozy II,729). Vullers thinks that it is a Persian name which he writes
nahšal. This name is no longer in usage in Persia, Syria or Egypt. It probably
designated Daucus Carota L. var. Boissieri WITTM. or a related carrot among the
umbelliferaceae. We have seen above (article number 94) that the seed of this
plant, to the Arabs, had the Greek name in genitive, dūqū.

259) NĀNAHWĀH   Bishopswort.

MAIMONIDES: It is that which the people of Maghrib know under the name
             of al-fulaǧfala. It is the "Ethiopian cumin" (al-kammun al-
             habaši) and the "royal cumin" (kummun al-malik). Its name in
             ancient Greek is ammi.

MEYERHOF: [Dioscorides III,62; Serapion 33 and 390; Ibn al-Beithar 2202;
           Tuhfa 229 and 284; 'Abd ar-Razzaq 586; Issa 41,3; Loew III, 421
           and 423; Dymock II,116-119; Ducros 230.]

The name n̄anahwāh is Persian and signifies "bread spice". One can retrace this name to the Assyrian nīnu (Syriac ninyā) and n̄anhu (Loew III, 422). The Greek name ammi is also of Semitic origin: hamitā. These names designate numerous umbelliferous plants of the group Ammi, but here it refers to ammi itself or stonewort (Carum copticum BENTH). It is an African plant (from whence the name "Ethiopian cumin") whose fruits are sold in the bazaars of the Orient all the way to India. As the other cumins, they serve as carminatives and stomachics. The name fulaifila is given to many drugs that have a sour taste.

260) NŪRA   Quicklime

MAIMONIDES: It is that which the people call al-ǧir; it is al-kils before
water touches the calcinated stones.

MEYERHOF: [Dioscorides V, 115; Serapion 269; Ibn al-Beithar 1960 and 2242;
Tuhfa 290; 'Abd ar-Razzaq 475 and 589.]

The name nūra (in the text kura, error of the copyist) is derived from n̄ar meaning fire, and designates a caustic substance. It is quicklime and does not correspond to asbestos of Dioscorides. Today in Egypt, in Syria, in Morocco, etc. one still sells quicklime or slaked lime ǧir, whereas the term nūra, for many centuries already (see Dawud II, 159), signifies a mixture of lime and arsenic employed by the Musulmans as a depilatory. Kils is the Arabic form of the ancient Castilian word calza which originates from the Latin calx (Simonet 78).

261) NAŠĀSTIǦ   Starch

MAIMONIDES: It is that which the public calls an-naša' and in Greek
amylon and amtulun.

MEYERHOF: [Dioscorides II, 101; Serapion 401; Ibn al-Beithar 2224; Tuhfa
289; 'Abd ar-Razzaq 593.]

Našāstaǧ is the Arabic form of the Persian name našāsta meaning "starch". The popular name is today pronounced niša in Egypt. Amtūlūn is a mutilation of amilun or amylon. See also Simonet 16. Starch serves in medicine for the preparation of certain remedies; in the popular medicine of the Musulmans, for example, for making dry collyria.

262) NĀ'IMA   Sage

MAIMONIDES: It is aš-šalbiya (salvia).

MEYERHOF: [Theophrastus VI, 1-2; Dioscorides III, 33; Ibn al-Beithar 140, 1274
             and 1387; Tuhfa 30 and 394; 'Abd ar-Razzaq 42, 83 and 872; Issa
             162, 1; Loew II, 102ff and Ducros 219.]

The Arabic name nā'ima signifies "tender, delicate", and is one of the
Arabic terms for sage (above all Salvia officinalis L., Labiates). Another
name, as-sālima ("the salutary one") is an equivalent of the Latin name salvia
which passed into the Arabic vernacular in different forms (sālbiya, šālbiya,
Simonet 581). In the bazaars of Cairo, the druggists sell sage under the name
of maryamiyya ("the herb of Mary"), in small packages whose leaves are used as
a tonic, astringent and emmenagogue (Ducros).

263) NABTĀBILŪN   Cinquefoil

MAIMONIDES: One also says bantāfilūn, which means "having five leaves".

MEYERHOF: [Theophrastus IX, 13, 5; Dioscorides IV, 42; Ibn al-Beithar 355;
             Tuhfa 62; 'Abd ar-Razzaq 731; Issa 147, 17; Loew III, 190ff.]

Nabtāfilūn is a popular transformation of the Greek pentaphyllon which
designates the herb with five leaves or creeping potentilla (Potentilla reptans
L., Rosaceae). The rhizome and the leaves of this plant are sometimes employed
as astringents. I have not seen them in the bazaars of Cairo where, according to Schweinfurth, they were still sold around 1890.

CHAPTER SĪN

(fol. 92ᵛ)

264) SABASTĀN (SIC)   Sebesten.

> MAIMONIDES: It is al-muhaïtā, and the people of Maghrib know it under
>
>   the name az-zūfā; it is atbā' al-kalba ("dog's nipples").
>
> MEYERHOF: [Serapion 457; Ibn al-Beithar 1157; Tuhfa 254; 'Abd ar-Razzaq
>
>   576; Issa 57,20; Loew I,296ff; Ducros 59; Ibn 'Awwam II,317-318.]

The name sabistān or sibistān, as the dictionaries write it, is the Arabic
form of the Persian sag-pistān ("dog's nipples"; see the Arabic translation at
the end of the article by Maimonides). Muhaïtā is a Syriac form which is related
to the root m.h.t., "to be snivelly" (Dozy II,572), because the fruit in question,
the sebesten, is a mucilaginous drupe. It is the product of the sebesten-tree
(Cordia Myxa L., Boraginaceae). This Egyptian and Syrian tree has oval fruits
with the volume of a cherry. Within a viscous pulp they enclose a triangular
stone. This pulp serves as glue, and its viscosity gives rise to the comparison
with mucous (myxa in Greek) and snivel. The fruit is sold in the bazaars of
Cairo under the name tamr el-muhēt or nabq el-muhēt as a mild laxative and as
an antitussive. (Kohen p. 134 line 25 condemns the reading muhaït or muhēt and
sanctions the form muhāta as the only correct reading). The latter name gave
rise to confusion with nabq, fruit of the jujube-tree (Zizyphus Spina Christi W.,
sidr Rhamnaceae) which is totally different. (See below our number 269, and also
qarāsiyā at number 330). One has tried to see the sebesten in persea of Theophrastus and Dioscorides. De Sacy (Abdallatif 69-72) has for a long time refuted
this opinion which however keeps popping up anew. I adhere to the opinion that
persea was Mimusops Schimperi HOCHST., African and Asiatic tree which was cultivated in ancient Egypt (and whose leaves and fruits were found in Egyptian tombs).
Its Arabic name is labah. See the remarks of Issa (119,27) who states that this
tree is rare in Egypt; in fact it has already disappeared for several centuries.

265) SUNBUL   Nard.

MAIMONIDES: The Greek nard (as-sunbul ar-rūmī) is an-nārdin and the
"nard of sparrows" (sunbul al-'asāfīr) and 'utārid
("Mercury"). The Celtic nard (sunbul iglīti) is al-
mantaġūša.

MEYERHOF: [Theophrastus IX,7; Dioscorides I,7-8; Serapion 483; Ibn al-
Beithar 1237; 'Abd ar-Razzaq 813-814; Issa 186,20 and 123,9;
Loew III,483-488; Ducros 130; Dymock II,233-238.]

Sunbul "spike" is the Arabic name of all sorts of nard. Nārdin is the
Syro-Arabic transformation from the Greek nardinon. The "Greek nard" and 'utārid
designated Celtic nard (Valeriana celtica L.). The name nard originates from
the Sanskrit nalada meaning "fragrant". In Hebrew, the name is found in Song of
Songs (I,12;IV,13-14) in the form nērd, plural nērādin. In Egypt, the ear of the
true Celtic nard is rarely sold in the bazaars; it is known under the name sunbul
(or sinbil) galabi. One more frequently sells the rhizome of the Indian nard
(sunbul hindi or sunbul al-'asāfīr) which is the Valerianaceous plant Nardostachys
Jatamansi D.C., Indian drug originating in the mountains of Nepal. As to the
name mantaġūša, Dozy (II,627) has proven that it is a transformation of the
Persian ma'ibahūša meaning "dry wine of nard", translation from the Greek dia
nardou oínos (Dioscorides V,59). This name is applied by error to Celtic nard.

266) SARHAS   Fern.

MAIMONIDES: Its name in Persian is kīl-dārū and in Spanish falaġa (filiche,
helecho).

MEYERHOF: [Theophrastus IX,13-20; Dioscorides IV,184; Serapion 442; Ibn al-
Beithar 1167; Tuhfa 366; 'Abd ar-Razzaq 330; Issa 72,16; Loew I,
10-13.]

Sarhas is the Arabic form of the Persian sarahs; gil-dārū is a Persian synonym for the male fern (Dryopteris or Aspidium Filicismas S.W.), well-known fern
in temperate zones of the whole world. The dry rhizome is a known antihelminthic
and much used against ascarides and tenias. Today one uses the oily extract. In

Cairo, the druggists rarely sell the rhizome of <u>Filix mas</u> (<u>sarhas dakar</u>), but
rather the fronds of another fern, the "durable herb" (<u>sarhas dahabi</u>, <u>Ceterach
officinarum</u> BAUH.), which is considered as a specific remedy for illnesses of
the spleen and urinary passages (Ducros 86).

267) <u>SANĀ</u>   Senna.

> MAIMONIDES: There is one (type) from Mecca (<u>makki</u>) and another from Spain
> (<u>andalusī</u>). The Spanish one is the one called <u>šurbāns</u>; it is
> "the Greek myrtle" (<u>al-ās ar-rūmī</u>) and <u>al-qatwānita</u> which
> means "the green leaf". The one from Mecca is the one called
> "the senna of Holy Places" (<u>as-sanā al-haramī</u>).

> MEYERHOF: [Serapion 467; Ibn al-Beithar 1236; <u>Tuhfa</u> 373; 'Abd ar-Razzaq 823;
> Issa 42,9; Loew II,407-409.]

The senna of Mecca or "of Holy Places" (of Arabia) is the fruit of numer-
ous species of cassia of senna (<u>Cassia acutifolia</u> DEL., <u>Cassia angustifolia</u> VAHL,
<u>Cassia obovata</u> COLL., Leguminous plants), plants originating primarily in tropical
Africa. Their main country of export was and still is Egyptian Sudan. One finds
the flat kidney-shaped shells at the druggists in the Orient, and one also uses
the folioles (<u>senna Alexandrina</u>) as a purgative, primarily in Europe.

The Spanish senna (<u>sanā andalusī</u>) seems to have been incorrectly identified
with the fruit of the ash-tree (see Issa 84,20). These are probably the folioles
of the bladder-nut tree (<u>Colutea arborescens</u> L., the "bastard senna") which are
also laxative, and which were used to falsify the senna. As to the Spanish names
of this leguminous plant: <u>qatwānita</u> is probably a faulty reading for <u>qantawāša</u>
(in modern Castillian <u>cantueso</u>), name of the lavender Stoechas (Simonet 91),
whereas <u>šurbāns</u> is found in Simonet (589) in the form <u>šilbāša</u>, and probably corresponds to <u>silvanus</u>. It designates the "white turpeth" or "wild senna",
"Provencal senna" (<u>Globularia Alypum</u> L.), Spanish and Provençal plant which does
not belong to the leguminous plants.

268) <u>SIMSIM</u>   Sesame.

MAIMONIDES: It is al-ğulğulan.

MEYERHOF: [Theophrastus VIII,1-9; Dioscorides II,99; Serapion 466; Ibn al-Beithar 1218; Tuhfa 267; 'Abd ar-Razzaq 818; Issa 168,1; Loew III,1-11; Ducros 129; Dymock III,26-33.]

Simsim is a Semitic name (Assyrian šamaššammu; Hebrew šumšum; Aramaic sumsēnā, etc.) which designates the seed of Sesamum orientale L. (Pedaliaceae) and its varieties. The plant probably originated in Central Asia (Laufer 291) and reached Babylonia and Syria and later Egypt prior to the Christian era. In the word ğulğulan (the following names are derived therefrom: English gingelly; French jugeoline and zinzolin, Italian zuzzolino and Spanish aljonjoli), people have tried to see a word of Indian or Abyssinian origin; this is erroneous. I think this word is Arabic and is related to the word ğulğul meaning "small bell" because of the shape of the capsular fruit which encloses numerous seeds. In Egypt, where sesame seed is sold in all the bazaars, one calls nenuphar seed gulgulān masrī that of the black poppy gulgulān habašī (Ducros).

269) SIDR   Christ's-thorn.

MAIMONIDES: It is a thorny tree whose fruit is called an-nabq and which people eat. It is also called ad-dāl.

MEYERHOF: [Serapion 10,386 and 427; Ibn al-Beithar 1165; Tuhfa 293; 'Abd ar-Razzaq 594 and 731; Issa 192,5-8; Loew III,134-141.]

Sidr in Egypt is the Arabic name of the tree "Christ's thorn" (Zizyphus Spina Christi WILLD.,Rhamnaceae) which furnishes an edible fruit called nabq in Arabic. One has found this fruit in ancient Egyptian tombs. In Palestine one calls the fruit and the tree dōm or dūm, which has caused confusion with the palm-tree doum (see above our number 230). One has also confused sidr with the jujube ('unnāb or zufaizaf; Zizyphus sativas GAERTN., infra no 291). See also the discussion by Renaud-Colin in the Tuhfa. Dal is the Arabic name of the wild jujube (Zizyphus Lotus LAM.); this name exists in Hebrew: sāl.

270) SULT   Naked barley or spelt.

MAIMONIDES: It is an inferior species of wheat which greatly resembles
barley.

MEYERHOF: [Serapion 481; Ibn al-Beithar 1209; _Tuhfa_ 386; 'Abd ar-Razzaq
340; Issa 183, 18; Loew I, 789tf; Ibn 'Awwam II, 25.]

Ibn al-Beither identified _sult_ with _tragos_ of Dioscorides (II, 93) which,
however, was rather an alimentary preparation as pearl barley. _Tuhfa_ identifies
it with the "barley of the Prophet" (_sa'ir an-nabī_) which in Morocco, Algeria
and Egypt is _Hordeum tetrastichum_ KCKE. and its varieties. Clément-Mullet
(Ibn 'Awwam and _Journal asiatique_, March-April 1865) translates _sult_ as "naked
barley" (_Hordeum distichum_ var. _nudum_), Issa as spelt (_Triticum Spelta_ L.) and
finally Dozy (I, 671), translates _sult_ according to the dictionary of Alcala
(Grenada 1506) as "rye". M. Ch. Kuentz called my attention to the fact that
sult is an old Semitic word: Assyrian _siltu_: Hebrew _solet_ (meaning fine flour).
Spelt and rye are unknown in Egypt. In Upper-Egypt one calls _silt_ (in Palestine
sill) a wild graminaceous plant, _Imperata cylindrica_ P.B. The question of its
identification is thus far from settled. See also below at number 389.

271) SŪS   Licorice

MAIMONIDES: The roots of this plant are known; they are those which one
calls '_irq sus_ and '_urūq dar Hurmaz_. (_sic_). One cooks its
roots to extract the juice therefrom which is the juice of
licorice (_rubb sūs_). It is also '_asīr al-mahk_ ("juice of
mahk" meaning "licorice").

MEYERHOF: [Theophrastus IX, 13,2; Dioscorides III, 5; Serapion 485; Ibn al-
Beithar 1250; _Tuhfa_ 375; 'Abd ar-Razzaq 825; Issa 88, 6;
Loew II, 435-437.]

Sus is the Arabic name of licorice (_Glycyrrhiza glabra_ L., Leguminaceae)
'_Irq sūs_ is the name of the licorice root. The name seems to be Semitic (Assyrian
šūšu; Syriac and Babylonian Hebrew _šūšā_). The name _dār Hurmuz_ is lacking in the
dictionaries (in Ibn al-Beithar and Dozy _dār harm_). In Persian, it perhaps

signifies "wood of Hormouz" because licorice grows abundantly in Mesopotamia and its root was exported in part by way of Syria and Asia-Minor, and in part by way of the Persian gulf where is found an island and port of Hormouz. <u>Munk</u> is a faulty reading for the Persian <u>mahk</u> and <u>matk</u> (Vullers II, 1234) meaning licorice. The Arabic names are preserved in Spanish in the form <u>absus,</u> <u>orozuz</u>, etc. (Botica 976).

272) <u>SŪSAN</u>   Lily and iris

   <u>MAIMONIDES</u>: Its name in Berber is <u>lullūyu</u>; there is a white type (fol.
                  93^r) and a blue type (<u>asmāngŭnī</u>). The name of the white
                  lily in ancient Greek is <u>Irasā</u>, and the azure lily (<u>lazawardī</u>)*
                  is the blue one. In Spanish it is <u>luluyu</u> (<u>lilio</u>, <u>lirio</u>).

   <u>MEYERHOF</u>: [Theophrastus III, 13-18 and VI-IX; Dioscorides III, 102 and I, 1;
                 Serapion 486-487; Ibn al-Beithar 1253 and 216; <u>Tuhfa</u> 28 and 129;
                 'Abd ar-Razzaq 17; Issa 100, 12-14 and 109, 2; Loew II, 1-4 and
                 160-184; Ducros 182; Ibn 'Awwam II, 260 and 306.]

      <u>Sūsan</u> or <u>sawsan</u> is the Arabic form of a Semitic word (Hebrew <u>sosanna</u>; Aramaic <u>sosanta</u>, etc. borrowed into Egyptian <u>sšśn,</u> which designates the blue <u>nenuphar</u> (Coptic <u>sošen</u>) and several species of liliaceae and iridaceae. In this para- graph there is a mild confusion: the Greek <u>iris</u> (Arabo-Syriac form <u>irisa</u>) is the "blue lil   the iris of Florence (<u>Iris Florentina</u> L.) also called <u>asmāngŭnī</u> (Arabic form of the Persian: <u>asumān</u> meaning heaven, <u>gūn</u> meaning color), whereas the white lily (<u>Lilium candidum</u> L.) is called <u>krinon</u> and <u>leirion</u> in Greek, and <u>sawsan abyad</u> in Arabic. <u>Lillūyu</u> and <u>luluyu</u> are incontestably transformations of the Spanish <u>lilio</u> (modern Castilian <u>lirio</u>). The root of the iris is sold in the bazaars of Cairo under the name <u>qurmet el-banafsig</u> ("violet root", Ducros). See above article 34.

273) <u>SILGAM</u> (<u>sic</u>)   Long radish and turnip

   <u>MAIMONIDES</u>: One also calls it <u>šilgam</u>. It is <u>al-laft</u> and its name is also <u>kusad</u>.

---

* mutilated word in the text

MEYERHOF: [Theophrastus VII, 1-9; Dioscorides II, 110; Serapion 131 and 463;

Ibn al-Beithar 1338; Tuhfa 376; 'Abd ar-Razzaq 166, 831 and 952;

Issa 33, 1-9; Loew I, 487-489; Ducros 27; Ibn 'Awwam II, 171-176.]

Salǧam is the Arabic form of the Persian name šalǧam (Kohen p. 134 line 9; Vullers II, 457) which designates the cabbage-turnip (Brassica Napus L., Cruciferaceae). The Arabic name laft or lift is old-Semitic (Assyrian laptu; Hebrew lefet; Aramaic laftā or laptā) for the same plant, but also for the long radish (Brassica Rapus L., var. esculenta). Kuśād is a Persian name designating the root of gentian. There is here confusion with būśād, a Persian term for the long radish (Vullers I, 278). The two plants of the same genus correspond to gongylis of Theophrastus, gongyle of Dioscorides and bounias of the Greeks, in general. Ibn 'Awwam has detailed the different species of turnips that one cultivated in Spain in the twelfth century. The druggists of Cairo sell the oily seed of colza (Brassica Napus L., var. oleifera) (Ducros).

274) SU'D   Galingale

MAIMONIDES: It is that which one calls yunǧa (juncia) in Spanish; it is qurtuyūn (? qūtinūn).

MEYERHOF: [Theophrastus IV, 8-11; Dioscorides I, 4: Serapion 201 and 433;

Ibn al-Beithar 1186; Tuhfa 189; 'Abd ar-Razzaq 319 and 811;

Loew I, 558ff; Ducros 125.]

Su'd is the Arabic name of the long galingale (Cyperus longus L.), in Syriac se'dē. The Spanish name originates from junci radix ("seed of rush") (Simonet 618). The other name is mutilated; it is probably qūtinūn (from the Greek kotinon, "wild olive-tree", Dozy II, 419; Simonet 140) or ?kypeiros. The fragrant rhizome of Cyperus longus and of Cyperus rotundus L. (su'd al-himār) is sold in the bazaars of Cairo as a stomachic and emmenagogue (Ducros). See above our number 161 (habb al-azīz, edible galingale). In modern Castilian, the long galingale is called juncia larga or juncia olorosa (Botica p. 691).

275) SAQŪLŪFUNDŪRIYŪN   Hart's tongue

MAIMONIDES: It is al-uqrubān ("scorpioid") and "the herb of worms"
(al-hašīša ad-dūdiyya) and in Spanish al-ǧanǧabānsa
(cientopies) and in Arabic also al-'awt.

MEYERHOF: [Theophrastus IX, 18, 7; Dioscorides III, 134; Ibn al-Beithar 1194;
Tuhfa 399; 'Abd ar-Razzaq 360 and 809; Issa 164, 23-24; Loew I, 6-8.]

    This Arabic name is the transformation of the Greek skolopendrion, it is a
fern, the polypodiaceae Scolopendrium vulgare S.W., "hart's tongue" or "rat's
herb"; in Castilian lengua cervina; Professor J.M.Millas i Vallicrosa found
the same name in old Catalonian in a Hebrew manuscript in the Vatican Library
(Manucsrits hebraics d'origen catala a la Biblioteca Vaticana, in Homenatge a
Antoni Rubio i Lluch - Barcelona 1936, extract p. 4). The Arabic name al-'awt
is found in none of the dictionaries. The Spanish name is a faulty reading for
ǧantabāsa (see Dozy I, 223 and Simonet 159), which corresponds to centumpedes
(in Castilian cientopies) meaning "millipeds, scolopendria". "Herb of worms",
in modern Arabic, is also the name of two other vermifuges, tansy (Tanacetum
vulgare L., Composite plants) and golden herb (Ducros 85, 86; see our number 266,
sarhas). Hart's tongue is a drug not used today; it was prescribed in the past
against certain visceral obstructions.

276) SŪRUNǦĀN   Colchicum

MAIMONIDES: It is qalb al-ard ("heart of the earth") and hāfir al-muhr
("sabot of colt") as well as asābi' Harmas ("fingers of
Hermes"). Its name in Spanish is qaštaniyula (castanuela)
which means "small chestnut". Its name is also larahiyāra
(?) (? for modern Castilian merendera).

MEYERHOF: [Theophrastus IX, 16,6; Dioscorides IV, 83; Serapion 484; Ibn al-
Beithar 1249 and 1575; Tuhfa 365; 'Abd ar-Razzaq 816; Issa
54, 3; Loew II, 156-160; Ducros 175 and 209.]

    Sūrinǧān is certainly a Persian name, and this is erroneously contested by
Vullers (II,347), because one already encounters it in the earliest Arabic-Persian

physicians (Masargawaih, Rhazes, Avicenna, Abu Mansur Muwaffaq, etc.). Like its
Arabic equivalents, it designates different species of colchicum (Colchicum
autumnale L., Liliaceae, etc.) whose bulb is poisonous. Maimonides does not
mention the Arabic-Egyptian name 'ukna (for Colchicum Ritchii R. Br.). We also
find the Spanish name castañuela for the tubercle of the edible galingale
(Simonet 114). The other name (lārahiyāra ?) might be a mutilation of the
Spanish meriendas (Botica 463) or of its ancient form merenderas (Clusius 266).
In the dictionaries of the Castilian language of the nineteenth century, one
finds the following names for colchicum (Herbstzeitlose):colchico, colquico,
merendera, quita merienda and villarita. The term in our manuscript should
probably read marandara. Instead of hāfir al-muhr, I found hafir an-nahr in
Suwaidi (193b). Asābi' Harmas is the Arabic translation of the Greek hermo-
daktylos. The Egyptian druggists sell the bulb of Autumn colchicum under the
name la'ba barbariyya and the young bulb of Colchicum variegatum L. under the
improper name fuqqāh as-sūringān ("flower of colchicum"), the latter name as a
fattening remedy for women (Ducros). Kohen (p. 137, line 1) has the Arabic name
ša'līl for the flower of colchicum.

277) SUMMĀQ   Sumac

MAIMONIDES: It is al-tamtam.

MEYERHOF: Theophrastus III, 18; Dioscorides I, 108; Serapion 482; Ibn al-
           Beithar 1218; Tuhfa 368; 'Abd ar-Razzaq 413 and 815; Issa 156, 3;
           Loew I, 200-202; Ducros 128.

The name summāq originates from the Aramaic summāqā meaning "red", because
the fruits of this tree (the English oak, Rhus coriaria L., Anacardiaceae) are
a beautiful red or brown-purple. The name tamtam is also found vocalized timtim,
tumtum etc. The nearly oval small berries of the Mediterranean and Asiatic
plant served in medicine as an astringent, and are still used by oriental curriers
for making hides into leather (an art which originated in Cordova, in Andalusia).

278) <u>SANT</u>   Acacia gum-tree

    <u>MAIMONIDES</u>: It is a well-known tree in Egypt with a wide circumference;

               one heats with its wood. It is the "Egyptian thorn" (<u>aš-šawka</u>

               <u>al-misriyya</u>) and the "Arabic thorn" (<u>aš-šawka al-'arabiyya</u>),

               as well as <u>umm gaïlān</u>. One also says <u>agaïlan</u>. The fruit of this

               tree is called <u>al-qarad</u>; one extracts acacia juice (<u>aqāqiyā</u>)

               from <u>al-qarad</u>, as we have mentioned in chapter <u>alif</u>.* Its resin

               is gum arabic (<u>as-samg al-'arabī</u>).

    <u>MEYERHOF</u>: Theophrastus IV, 2, 8; Dioscorides III, 13; Serapion 6; Ibn al-

               Beithar 1758; <u>Tuhfa</u> 46; 'Abd ar-Razzaq 19, 740 and 967; Issa

               II, 2; Loew II, 377-391; Ducros 29 and 143.

    The plant in question is, in effect, an Egyptian tree, the "Egyptian gum-
tree" (<u>Acacia arabica</u> W. var. <u>nilotica</u> D., Leguminous plants). One sees it
everywhere in the Nile valley. Its Egyptian name <u>sndt</u> (Coptic <u>sonte</u>) passed
into Hebrew (<u>šitta</u>) and Arabic (<u>sant</u>). The facts of Maimonides are exact; the
fruit, still called <u>qarad</u> today, is sold in dried shells in the bazaars of
Cairo as an astringent. One also finds the seeds (<u>bizr es-sant en-nīlī</u>) and the
gum, but the latter is replaced more and more by gum arabic of superior quality,
imported from Egyptian Sudan, produced primarily by <u>Acacia Seyal</u> D., <u>Acacia
tortilis</u> HNE. and <u>Acacia Senegal</u> W.

279) <u>SADĀB</u>   Rue

    <u>MAIMONIDES</u>: There are many types thereof, for example, a wild type, a mountain

               type and a cultivated type (fol. 93^v). The cultivated type is the

               one which the Spaniards call <u>rūta</u>. The wild one is <u>al-faïgan</u> and

               <u>tāfisyā</u>; and one claims that <u>al-hazā'</u> and <u>az-zawfarā</u> are among

               its species.

    <u>MEYERHOF</u>: Theophrastus I, 3, 9 and 10; Dioscorides III, 45 and IV, 153: Serapion

               428; Ibn al-Beithar 1166; <u>Tuhfa</u> 364, 404 and 176; 'Abd ar-Razzaq

               712 and 819; Issa 159, 9; Loew III, 317-321; Ducros 14; Ibn 'Awwam

* see our number 12

II,293-295.]

Sadāb is the Arabic name of numerous species of rue, primarily Ruta
graveolens L. The name faiğan is the Arabic form of the Greek pêganon passed
through the Syriac peggānā. Tāfisyā originates from the Greek thapsia also
passed through the Syriac, but it is an Arabic name of the false fennel (Thapsia
garganica L., Umbelliferae). Hazā' is one of the names of anet (Anethum graveolens L.), and zawfarā is the Arabic-Syriac name of panace (Echinophora tenu-
ifolia L.), both of which are Umbelliferae. There is thus a certain confusion
among the Arabs in the classification of Rutacea. The druggists of Cairo sell
the small kidney-shaped seed of rue (bizr es-sadāb, Ducros) that one incorporates
into the preparation of collyria. The leaves of rue enter into tonic and stomachic preparations and are important as a preservative against a bad eye. On
this subject, see the thorough study of B.A. Donaldson, The Wild Rue. A Study
of Muhammadan Magic and Folklore in Iran. London 1939.

280) SAKABĪNAǦ   Sagapenum.

   MAIMONIDES: It is known. Its name in Spanish is sāka-bīnu (sagapeno).

   MEYERHOF: [Dioscorides III,81; Serapion 425; Ibn al-Beithar 1200; Tuhfa 372;

            'Abd ar-Razzaq 841 and 860; Issa 82,16; Loew III,459ff; Ducros

            126; Dymock II,160-162.]

   Sakbīnağ is the Arabic form of the Persian name sakbina (Vullers I,309)
from which is derived the Greek sagapenon. It is the root of certain Umbelliferae
(Ferula persica WILLD.?, Ferula scowitziana D.C.?) which is imported from the
Persian mountains to Indian ports and to western Asia. In the bazaars of Cairo,
one can see "sakbang" in shapeless granular masses, easily softened, and whose
odor reminds one a little of that of asa foetida (Ducros). Renaud-Colin think
that the product sold in Morocco should be a succedaneum.

281) SAQAMŪNIYĀ   Scammony.

   MAIMONIDES: It is al-mahmūda.

   MEYERHOF: [Theophrastus IX,1-20; Dioscorides IV,170; Ibn al-Beithar 1193;

'Abd ar-Razzaq 827; Issa 56, 21; Loew I, 451-452; Ducros 213.⌉

Saqamūniyā is the Syriac-Arabic transcription of the Greek skammônia,
name whose origin is unknown and which designates a convolvulus (Convolvulus
Scammonia L. Convolvulaceae) that grows on the oriental coasts of the Mediterranean, in Asia Minor and in Persia. The root is today imported into Egypt from
Greece and Syria, and it is sold in the bazaars of Cairo as a drastic purgative
(Ducros). The name mahmuda ("the commendable") is still in usage in Egypt; it
is probably related to the salutary effect of the drug.

282) SAQARDIYŪN   Water-germander

MAIMONIDES: One also says asqūdūriyūn. It is al-atariyūn (see the commentary) and the "wild garlic" (at-tūm al-barrī); one also calls
it "serpent garlic" (tūm al-hayya).

MEYERHOF: ⌈Theophrastus VII, 4, 1; Dioscorides III, 111; Serapion 111; Ibn al-
Beithar 1331; Tuhfa 395; 'Abd ar-Razzaq 897; Issa 179, 13; Loew
II, 104; Ducros 60.⌉

The first two names are Arabic transcriptions of the Greek name skordion
which one gave to the labiate Teucrium Scordium L. Nevertheless, in our days,
in the bazaars of Cairo, under the name tōm barri ("wild garlic") or tōm ta'bāni
("serpent garlic", corresponding to ophioskordon, Dioscorides II, 152), they sell
the white and ovoid bulb of "false spikenard" (Allium Victoriale L.liliaceae), a
sour and corrosive remedy (Ducros). This explains the "Spanish" name al-atariyūn:
its form in Ibn al-Beithar is matarqal, which Simonet (347) renders matricalis
herba. I think that the most exact denomination should be batarqāl or aqturiyāl
meaning victorial, Spanish name of the plant.

283) SASĀLIYŪS   Seseli and types

MAIMONIDES: It is that which the physicians in Maghrib claim to be the
seed of a type of kalh (Ferula). It is al-harrā ar-rūmi
('Greek mustard"). One also says taqāra, as-sasāliyūs, at-
tarādaliyūn and al-kāsim ar-rūmī ("Greek lovage"). More recent

authors state that it is the seed of mountain celery (al-karafs al-ǧabalī), and that sāsāliyūs and sāsālī are the same thing.

MEYERHOF: [Theophrastus IX,15,5; Dioscorides III,53-54; Ibn al-Beithar 1178; Issa 168,10 and 181,19; Loew III,470-472.]

Sāsālī is the transcription of the Greek name seseli, sāsāliyūs that of the genitive seselios. This name designated and still designates, to modern botanists, different Umbelliferae. This name was given to the "seseli of Marseille" (Seseli tortuosum L.). Tarādaliyūn is an Arabic form of the Greek tordylion or tordilon which designates the "seseli of Crete" (Tordylium offic-inale L.) whose fruits were utilized in medicine. Taqāra may by Spanish, or better yet a faulty reading for taffara. See above our number 203 (kašim: taqlīra). Kašim rūmi is one of the names of lovage of the "common seseli" (Levisticum officinale KOCH.); karafs ǧabalī is the name of the "mountain celery" (Petroselinum Oreoselinum MONCH.). Finally harra, Arabic-Syriac name, designates cruciferous plants of the species Diplotaxis; it is impossible to determine more accurately the significance of harrā rūmi. One no longer encounters any species of seseli in the bazaars of Cairo.

284) SAWĪQ   Semolina.

MAIMONIDES: It is wheat, barley and other similar roasted cereals, agi-tated with butter and then ground.

MEYERHOF: [Serapion 147 and 446 bis; Ibn al-Beithar 1255; 'Abd ar-Razzaq 855 (samīd).]

Semolina was not yet known to the Greeks who only had pearl barley (ptisane or ptisma) and barley-water made with pearl barley. The word sawīq in Arabic also signifies "fine flour, wheaten flour", corresponding to the Greek alphiton.

285) SARĪS   Chicory.

MAIMONIDES: Its foreign name is šariš with two punctuated šins. It is

Arabicized and pronounced <u>sarīs</u>. There are two species, a wild
type and a cultivated type.

The wild one is very bitter. It is the one with which the
physicians of Maghrib prepare the well-known potion. *

The cultivated type resembles lettuce (fol. 94^r) and the
people of Maghrib eat it as lettuce. It is the cultivated species
whose leaves are gathered before their maturity by the Egyptians,
and that their physicians call endive (<u>al-hundabā'</u>) and the
people call "the vegetable" (<u>al-baql</u>).

As-sarīs is also called <u>arhal</u> and <u>sakūtā</u> and <u>baltāmūn</u> (?).

<u>MEYERHOF</u>: [Dioscorides II, 132; 'Abd ar-Razzaq 846; Issa 48, 11 and 177, 15;
Loew I, 415-421.]

<u>Saris</u>, <u>sāris</u>, <u>šarīš</u>, etc. are the Arabic transcriptions of the Greek <u>seris</u>
which designates chicory or endive. It is the equivalent of the Arabic name
<u>hundabā'</u> or <u>hindabā'</u> that we have encountered above in article 114. Ibn al-
Beithar and the author of the <u>Tuhfa</u> had reason not to write a special article
on <u>saris</u>. <u>Baql</u> is still in Egypt a popular name for endive (<u>Cichorium Endivia</u> L.),
whereas the name <u>seris</u> is preserved in lower Egypt for wild chicory (<u>Cichorium</u>
<u>divaricatum</u> SCHOUSB.). (Schweinfurth 13). The same plant in Syria is called
<u>arhlilu</u> (Loew, according to Foureau); it is perhaps the <u>arhal</u> of Maimonides.
The following name, <u>sakūtā</u>, is undoubtedly a faulty reading for <u>šikūriyā</u> meaning
"chicory". The name <u>baltamūn</u> or <u>yaltamūn</u> may be a mutilation of <u>intybus</u> or of
<u>troximon</u> (?). See also Simonet 514.

* I do not know which potion Maimonides refers to. Ishaq ibn Salaiman, in
Ibn al-Beithar 2263, mentions one composed of juice expressed from chicory
cooked with oil. Ibn Sina, <u>ibidem</u>, makes a decoction thereof with cassia. He
wrote a treatise on the virtues of chicory which was printed in Istanbul:
<u>Hindiba risalesi Buharali Ibni Sina.</u> Ed. Suheyl. Univers. Istanbul 1937.

286) SARATĀN HINDĪ   Indian crab

MAIMONIDES: It is a stone that one imports from India and upon which one sees black striations and which resembles a crab.

MEYERHOF: In Ibn al-Beithar (1172), this chapter has the title "sea crab" (saratān bahrī), and copies in part Ibn Sina (I, 381) who states: "when one speaks of 'sea crab', one does not mean all the types of marine crabs, but one particular species with petrified limbs. A completely reliable person told me that this crab lives in the China sea, emerges from the sea water, enters into non-marine water near the sea, and dries in this water or emerges therefrom; it then becomes hard as a stone. This was told to me by some- one who witnessed this event many times in China". Suwaidi (207a) adds that one also finds this crab in the Indian ocean. Damiri (II, 44) is more succinct: "It is said that in the China sea there are crabs which, on ground, become hard as stones, and physicians prepare a collyrium therefrom which makes (corneal) opacities (of the eye) disappear". One finds the same account in (the book of) the traveler Sulaiman (Voyage du marchand arabe Sulayman en Inde et en Chine, rédigé en 851, etc. Translated from the Arabic...by Gabriel Ferrand. Paris 1922, p. 44).

The druggists of Cairo even today, sell the "eyes of cray- fish" ('ayūn es-saratān), a drug which is also known in Europe (Ducros 169). But in Maimonides it probably refers to a calcareous petrification imported from the Far-East.

287) SINGĀR   Gladiolus

MAIMONIDES: It is saïf al-ġurāb (the "sword of the raven"), and the Spaniards call it durhūnī. Its Arabic name is aš-šabibaīt; it is ad-dalbūt.

MEYERHOF: Theophrastus VII, 12-13; Dioscorides IV, 20 and 136; Ibn al-Beithar

875 <u>bis</u> and 984; Issa 87,11; Loew II,6-7.

The plant in question is the common gladiolus (<u>Gladiolus communis</u> L.,
Iridaceae). The name <u>singār</u> seems to be Persian, but is lacking in the dictionaries. Saïf al-ġurāb and <u>dalbūt</u> are known Arabic names. <u>Durhūni</u> is found in
Ibn al-Beithar (984) in the form <u>dūrhūli</u>; it is perhaps a mutilation of
<u>dragontea</u> (Simonet 531). The Persian dictionaries designate the name <u>dūr-hūli</u>
as Persian, but Vullers (I,893) states that the Persians took it for Greek. The
name <u>šabibaït</u> seems to be Berber rather than Arabic. The <u>Gladiolus communis</u> L.,
and <u>Gladiolus segetum</u> KER. pass for being poisonous; their bulbs were employed
against scrofula. One no longer finds this drug in the shop windows of the
Egyptian druggists.

288) <u>SULTĀN AL-ĠABAL</u>   Honeysuckle.

    MAIMONIDES: It is a known remedy in Maghrib. One calls it <u>sarimat al-ġadi</u>
          (the "bridle of a kid") and <u>umm aš-šu'ara'</u> (the "mother of
          poets") and <u>šaġarat at-tuhāl</u> (the "herb of the rat") and in
          Spanish <u>mātrašālba</u> (<u>madreselva</u>). One has said that it is
          the remedy called <u>qaqlamīnus</u> by Dioscorides.

    MEYERHOF: [Theophrastus IX,8-18; Dioscorides IV,14; Ibn al-Beithar 1395,etc;
          'Abd ar-Razzaq 48; Issa 111,7; Loew I,332ff.]

This plant is the garden honeysuckle (<u>Lonicera Caprifolium</u> L., Caprifoliaceae).
The Arabic names and the Spanish name are known and are also found in Ibn al-
Beithar. 'Abd ar-Razzaq gives the additional name <u>sultān al-ġāba</u> ("king of the
bush"). The Greek name, greatly mutilated in our text, is <u>periklymenon</u>. The
honeysuckle today only serves as an adornment in gardens. Only a century ago,
its stems were still used as an anticatarrhal and diuretic, and its flowers
as an ocular remedy. Fly honeysuckles (<u>Lonicera Periclymenum</u> L.) were employed
as succedaneum.

289) <u>SUKKAR</u>   Sugar.

MAIMONIDES: When physicians speak of <u>sukkar tabarzad</u>, it signifies solid
and hard sugar. It is said that it is the same that the
Egyptians call "vegetable sugar" (<u>as-sukkar an-nabāt</u>, sugar
candy), and this viewpoint is the most probable.

MEYERHOF: [Dioscorides II,82; Serapion 541; Ibn al-Beithar 1198ff; 'Abd
ar-Razzaq 829; Issa 159,6; Loew I,746-765.]

The art of extracting sugar from sugar cane (<u>Saccharum officinarum</u> L.,
Graminaceae) seems to have been invented in the Indies towards the beginning
of the Christian era. The name sugar in Sanskrit is <u>sarkarā</u>. Several centuries
later, this art was improved in Persia (Persian names for sugar: <u>šakar</u> and
<u>šakkar</u>) and brought to perfection by the Arabs who introduced the cultivation
of sugar cane into Syria, Palestine, Egypt, North Africa, Spain and Sicily. See
the history of sugar by E.O. von Lippmann (<u>Geschichte des Zuckers</u>, Leipzig 1890;
summary in <u>Abhandl.d.deutschen Zuckerindustrie</u> 6. XI,1916). See also E. Weide-
man, <u>Beitrage</u> XLI and LII, Erlangen 1915-1916.

<u>Sukkar tabarzad</u> is a Persian name (<u>tabar-zad</u> "pounded with the help of a
hatchet") which designates hardened white sugar. <u>Sukkar nabāt</u> today is still
the name for **candied sugar in Egypt.** Maimonides does not mention the Persian
designations <u>sukkar fānīd</u> (from the Persian <u>panid</u>; Vullers I,324) which is the
concentrated juice of the cane, and <u>sukkar qand</u> (from the Sanskrit <u>khanda</u>,
origin of the Arabic-Persian <u>qand</u>, French <u>candi</u>, English <u>candy</u>, German <u>kandis</u>,
etc. See G. Watt. <u>The Commercial Products of India</u>, London 1908, p.930), which
is the refined sugar.

290) SUKK   Confection.

MAIMONIDES: It is a remedy composed of date juice (<u>mā' al-balah</u>), from
gall-nuts ('<u>afs</u>) and Indian astringent and aromatic drugs.
If one adds some musk one calls it "muscated <u>sukk</u>" (<u>sukk</u>
<u>mumassak</u>).

MEYERHOF: [Serapion 479; Ibn al-Beithar 1201; <u>Tuhfa</u> 379; 'Abd ar-Razzaq

824; Laufer 551.

The preparation of this oriental aromatic remedy was indicated by Ibn al-Beithar according to Ishaq ibn 'Imran, Tunisian physician of the ninth century. See also E. Wiedemann, Aus Nuwairi's Enzyklopadie: Ueber Parfums, in Arch. f.d. Gesch.d.Naturwiss.u.d.Technik, IV, 1913, 418-426; and Seidel, Mechitar, p.217ff.

The Indian drugs mentioned by Maimonides include nard, the muscat nut, mace, clove, cardamomum, agalwood, sandalwood,etc. The origin of the name sukk has not yet been elucidated.

CHAPTER 'AĪN

291) 'UNNĀB   Jujube

MAIMONIDES: It is az-zufaĭzaf.

MEYERHOF: [Serapion 271 and 542; Ibn al-Beithar 1594; Tuhfa 293 and 302;

'Abd ar-Razzaq 665; Issa 192, 7; Loew III, 138-140.]

The name 'unnāb designates the fruit of several species of jujube (Zizyphus,
Rhamnaceae), above all that of Zizyphus sativa GÄRTN. (meaning Zizyphus vulgaris
LAM.). This name is related to the Arabic 'inab meaning "grape", because the
fruit of this bush is a globulous drupe which reminds one a little of the grape
because of its sweet and acid taste.

The jujube-tree was first cultivated in Syria. It was described in the
first century of the Christian era by Pliny (XV, 47 Zizipha) and mentioned by
Rabbi Eleazar ben Zadok in Jerusalem (sezafin) in the same epoch. The Arabic
name zafzūf (Tuhfa), diminutive zufaĭzaf, probably originates from the Greek.
It is preserved in jujube (French) and azufaifa (Spanish).

292) 'ALQAM   Wild cucumber (elaterium)

MAIMONIDES: It is "the donkey's cucumber" (qittā' al-himār) and one also
says "the wild cucumber" (al-qittā al-barrī); it is bābalūn
(boubalion), and the Arabs call it (fol. 94^v) as-sāb and its
juice is called ūmāzī.

MEYERHOF: [Theophrastus IX, 4-5; Dioscorides IV, 150; Serapion 312-315; Ibn
al-Beithar 1740 and 1584; Issa 73, 6; 'Abd ar-Razzaq 109, 688 and
738; Loew I, 549 ff; Ducros 176.]

The plant is the "trapped cucumber, wild cucumber" (Ecballium Elaterium
RICH., Cucurbitaceae), characteristic plant of the Mediterranean regions. It
was known to the Greeks (sikys agrios) and the Hebrews (Mishnaic name yerōqat
hamōr). The name 'alqam in Arabic designates bitter Cucurbitaceae (for example
the coloquinth), and is not characteristic of Ecballium except in Spain. As to
the Semitic name qittā', we will speak thereof below in number 343. Bābalūn is

very probably a mutilation of the Greek <u>boubalion</u>. <u>Sāb</u> is an Arabic name which is also discussed by Ibn al-Beithar (1385). Finally, the name <u>ūmāzī</u> (In Ibn al-Beithar 202 <u>umāda</u> and <u>ufādiyā</u>; in 'Abd ar-Razzaq <u>ūfādā</u>; in Ghafiqi ms. fol. 65b <u>ūmādā</u>) must be a mutilation of the Greek <u>omphakion</u> meaning "juice of green grapes", whereas <u>elaterion</u> was the name of the juice expressed from the wild cucumber or its seeds, according to Theophrastus, Dioscorides and Pline. One could also consider a mutilation of the Castilian name <u>zumo</u> meaning "juice, essence". In the bazaars of Cairo, under the name <u>gedūr faqqūs el-homār</u>)"roots of the donkey gourd"), one sells fragments of the roots of Elaterium as a drastic, a vomitive and for compresses (Ducros).

293) <u>'ULLAĪQ</u>   Bramble

<u>MAIMONIDES</u>: It is <u>al-bātūs</u> (<u>batos</u>). The Berbers call its fruit <u>nābiq</u> and
              the Spaniards call it in their idiom <u>arǧa</u> (<u>zarza</u>); its fruit
              is called <u>al-wahšī</u> (the "wild one").

<u>MEYERHOF</u>: [Theophrastus I, 3-10 and III, 18, etc; Dioscorides IV, 37; Serapion
            87; Ibn al-Beithar 2140; <u>Tuhfa</u> 311 and 388; 'Abd ar-Razzaq 657;
            Issa 158, 1; Loew III, 175-188.]

The plant <u>'ullaīq</u> ("that which hooks itself") corresponds to <u>batos</u> of the Greeks which is the common bramble (<u>Rubus fruticosus</u> L., blackberry, Rosaceae). However, the blackberry is unknown in the lands of the Arabic language. In Egypt and in Syria one calls <u>'ullēq</u> the <u>Rubus sanctus</u> SCHREB. and others. The name <u>nabiq</u> or <u>nabq</u> for the fruit is questionable. The Arabs and the Berbers often confused thorny trees and their fruits. The Arabic name of the fruit is <u>at-tūt</u> <u>al-wahšī</u> ("wild mulberry"). See the discussion of the name <u>'ullaīq</u> by Renaud-Colin in number 274 and 211 of <u>Tuhfa</u>. Suwaidi (212a-b) distinguishes two species of <u>'ullaīq</u>. The ancient Castilian name <u>arǧa</u> was explained by Simonet (21); the modern Castilian name for bramble is <u>zarzamora</u>.

294) <u>'AWSIǦ</u> (SIC)   Lycium

<u>MAIMONIDES</u>: It is also one of the species of thorny trees. It is the one

called al-ğulhum and al-ğarqad as well as rhamnos. It is

ašiyābardin and in Spanish it is called espina alba.

MEYERHOF: ⌈Theophrastus III, 18, 2; Dioscorides I, 90; Serapion 205 and 256;

Ibn al-Beither 1602; Tuhfa 312; 'Abd ar-Razzaq 314; 532 and 661;

Issa 112, 15; Loew III, 361-363; Ducros 168.⌋

'Awsağ is the Arabic name of lycium or African jasmine (Lycium afrum L.,
Solanaceae) and other plants of this same family. (In Biblical Hebrew ātād)
the names ğulhum or ğalham and ğarqad are also found in Ibn al-Beithar (506 and
1632). The latter name is preserved in Algeria and in Morocco in the form
ğerdeğ (Renaud-Colin). Rhamnos is the Greek name for Lycium; lykion is the name
of the expressed juice (see above our number 148 hudad). Ašiyābardin seems to
be a mutilated Syriac name; or Persian (ašk meaning drop, tear; bardin meaning
deposit, residue?). Simonet (p. 191), according to Ibn Gulgul reads asku-bardin
(exco-bardin) which is explained as a mutilation of the Latin spina ursina.
Alternatively, for example, one should read ašiyāf barf (Syro-Persian: "fresh
collyrium, refrigerant"). Espina alba (Simonet 195) is the Latin-Spanish translation from the Greek leukakantha which designates numerous thorny plants as well
as thistles. Ducros mentions that in Cairo one sells the branches of Lycium europaeum L. ("small purgative buckthorn") - I would add, those of Lycium afrum L. -
(are also sold) for the practice of witchcraft; for example, one burns them with
incense during the ceremony of zār (expulsion of bad spirits which cause illness).

95) 'AFS   Gall-nut

MAIMONIDES: It is al-qaşaf and al-bahaš.

MEYERHOF: ⌈Dioscorides I, 107; Serapion 210; Ibn al-Beithar 1564; Tuhfa 309;

'Abd ar-Razzaq 655; Issa 152, 10; Loew I, 631-634; Ducros 162.⌋

'Afs (in Syriac 'afsā) corresponds to kekis of Dioscorides and designates the
gall-nut, the excrescence of which forms on the buds of certain oaks (Cupuliferaceae)
following the puncture of a hymenopterum, the Cynips gallae tinctoriae. The name
qaşaf is lacking in the treatises and in the dictionaries. Bahas, according to

Ibn al-Beithar (273 and 371), is the name of the cork-oak (Quercus Ilex var.

Suber L.) or the gall-oak (Quercus lusitanica LAM. var. infectoria A.D.C.), which

is called 'afs like its gall-nuts. One sells the gall-nuts of this latter bush

in the bazaars of Cairo; they are the nuts of the Aleppo gall, originating in

Asia-Minor (gallae halepenses). They serve in medicine as a febrifuge and

intestinal astringent, but above all in dyeing for dyeing into black. The

gall-nuts of Quercus infectoria contain up to sixty per-cent tannic acid.

296) 'ŪD   Wood of agalloch (agalwood)

MAIMONIDES: That which has been confirmed is that it is the "Indian wood"

(al-'ūd al-hindī); it is the one physicians call "fragrant

wood" ('ūd at-tīb). It is the wood of well known fumigations;

it is the same one that one also calls "wood of nadd" ('ūd-

an-nadd) and "raw wood" (al-'ud al-hāmm), as well as the "dry

wood" (al-'ūd al-ǧaff)and the "wood from Tchampa" (al-'ūd

as-sanfī). Its Arabic name is al-anǧūǧ and in ancient Greek

agallokhe.

MEYERHOF: [Dioscorides I, 22; Serapion 266; Ibn al-Beithar 1603; Tuhfa 308;

'Abd ar-Razzaq 648; Issa 10, 10; Loew III, 411-414; Dymock III, 217-

223; Ducros 167.]

The Arabic word 'ūd signifies "wood"; but in pharmacology it is always

used for "fragrant wood", etc. which is the product of species of Aquilaria

(Thymeleaceae), above all Aquilaria malaccensis LAMK. and Aquilaria Agallocha

ROXB. These Indian trees develop resin in the sick parts of their wood. This

"raw wood" containing oleaginous substances has always been appreciated in the

Orient, and burned as perfume instead of incense. Its Sanskrit name was agaru

from which are derived the following names: Greek agalokhon, Biblical Hebrew

ahalim and ahalot, and Arabic anǧūǧ and alanǧūǧ. The variants of this name are

found in Muhassas (XI, 198). Nadd was an Arabic perfume whose principal ingredient

was agalwood. See E. Wiedemann, Arch. f. Gesch. d. Naturwiss. u. d. Technik VI,

1913, p.423-423. One should note that Wiedemann always incorrectly translates
'ud as aloe; it is the "wood of aloe" or better "wood of agalloch". The druggists in Cairo sell agalwood under the name 'ūd qaqullī or 'ud el-bahūr ("fumigations wood"), in flat fragments approximately 0.08 meters long; they have a
very aromatic odor.

297) 'INAB AT-TA'LAB   Black Nightshade.

> MAIMONIDES: It is the "wolf's grape" ('inab ad-di'b) and in Berber
>   yarbaquīna (yerba canina). It is 'inabā ahlā and al-'ubab and
>   al-fana' ("destruction"). One also calls it tulutān and in
>   Persian rūzbārağ. One of its species is called al-kākang as
>   well as ranūq.
>
> MEYERHOF: [Theophrastus VII,15 and IX,11; Dioscorides IV,71-75; Serapion
>   232; Ibn al-Beithar 1589; Tuhfa 219 and 310; 'Abd ar-Razzaq 651;
>   Issa 171,17; Loew III,379ff; Ducros 163.]

'Inab at-ta'lab ("fox's grape") is the most well-known Arabic name of black
nightshade (Solanum nigrum L.), a poisonous plant. The Syriac name 'enabē děta'lā
has the same meaning; it is thus that Hunain translated the Greek name strykhnos.
The other Arabic names are all known and mentioned in pharmacological treatises.
The Spanish name yerva, or better uva canina ("dog's grape", Simonet 557) is
preserved in the Arabic-Moroccan dialect in the form būquīna (Tuhfa 310), in
Algerian buqninu, muqnina, muqnin, etc. ('Abd ar-Razzaq). The Persian name
(rūzbārağ) is mutilated in all the texts; the proper reading is rūbāh-turlak
meaning "fox's grape".

The names of the alkekenge (winter-cherry) were discussed above in number
201 (al-kākang). Here Maimonides adds the name ranūq which is evidently a
faulty reading for rabraq. This name, according to Abu Hanifa ad-Dinawari
(Ibn al-Beithar 1027), was in usage by the inhabitants of Maghrib and Yemen.

The druggists of the bazaars of Cairo sell the dried plant of the black
nightshade under the name 'inab ez-zīb ("wolf's grape") for external usage.

One makes compresses and washings with a decoction of the plant on traumatic and cutaneous lesions.

298) <u>'ASĀ AR-RĀ'Ī</u>   Polygonum

<u>MAIMONIDES</u>: It is <u>al-batbāt</u> and one also says <u>šabatbāt</u>. It is the com-
bustible material well known in Egypt which is burned in fur-
naces. Its Persian name is <u>barsiyandaru</u>.

<u>MEYERHOF</u>: [Dioscorides IV, 4; Serapion 54; Ibn al-Beithar 1281 and 1547;
<u>Tuhfa</u> 305; 'Abd ar-Razzaq 670; Issa 145, 6: Loew I, 4ff and 343;
Ducros 160.]

The Arabic name <u>'asā ar-rā'Ī</u> signifies "shepherds stick" or "pastors rod".
Maimonides himself identified it (according to Tankhoum of Jerusalem, Loew I, 4)
with the <u>awōw rō'ēh</u> of the Mishnah which has the same sense. It is the equivalent
of <u>polygonon arrhen</u> ("male polygonum") of Dioscorides. One has identified it
with centinode and knot-grass (<u>Polygonum aviculare</u> L.); however, the remark of
Maimonides that it is a combustible material suggests another polygonum, <u>quddāb</u>
or <u>qurdāb</u> (<u>Polyganum equisetiforme</u> SIBTH. and SM.)which grows in the Egyptian
deserts and furnishes dry stems similar to those of the horsetail (<u>Equisetum</u>).
One has moreover identified the "female" polygenum of Dioscorides (IV, 5) with
the horsetail. <u>Šabatbātā</u> is a Syriac name which signifies "little stick".
<u>Barsiyān-dārū</u> or <u>barsiyān-dārū</u> is the Persian name for the polygonum. Ducros
has stated that the roots sold in the Cairo bazaars under the name <u>'asā er-rā'Ī</u>
are those of the snakeweed (<u>Polygonum bistorta</u> L.). They are used as astringent
and antidiarrheal.

299) <u>'ĀQIR QARHĀ</u>   Feverfew

<u>MAIMONIDES</u>: It is <u>al-karkarhān</u> and one also says <u>al-qarqarhān</u>. It is that
which the Berbers call <u>tāġandast</u> (fol. 95^r); its Greek name
is <u>taldarīm</u> and <u>bartilūn</u>.

<u>MEYERHOF</u>: [Dioscorides III, 73; Serapion 348; Ibn al-Beithar 1507; <u>Tuhfa</u> 301;
'Abd ar-Razzaq 652 and 886; Issa 14, 11; Loew I, 374ff; Ducros 166.]

'Aqir qarhā is a Syriac name which signifies "naked root". Kurkurhān is also a Syriac word and both are equivalents of the Greek pyrethron, which today designates the top-root of the Compositae Anacyclus Pyrethrum DC. The most well-known Syriac name passed into other oriental languages; for example, Sanskrit akarakarahka, and Armenian akrkarka. The Berberic name is encountered in different forms: tāgandast, tīgantast (Dozy I, 139), tīgandast (Ibn al-Beithar), etc. The last two names taldarim and bartilūn are undoubtedly mutilations of the Greek pyrethron.

Fragments of the root of feverfew are sold in the bazaars of Cairo under the name 'ud al-qarh ("ulcerated wood"; but in qarh there is a residue from the Syriac qarhā meaning "denuded"!). The drug comes from Maghrib and from Syria and serves as an aphrodisiac, a tonic and specific or remedy against gum ailments.

300) 'ASFUR   Safflower

MAIMONIDES: It is al-marīq and al-ihrīd; it is also called bahrām and
             bahraman. It is as-sukarī; the name of its seed is al-qirtim.

MEYERHOF: [Theophrastus VI, 1-6; Dioscorides IV, 188; Serapion 309; Ibn al-
           Beithar 1548 and 1761; Tuhfa 306 and 348; 'Abd ar-Razzaq 116,
           324 and 663; Issa 40, 16; Loew I, 394 and 404; Dymock II, 308-311;
           Ducros 161 and 180.]

'Asfur and 'usfur are Arabic names of the safflower blossom or bastard saffron (Carthamus tinctorius L., Compositae). This name passed through several European languages (English safflower; German saflor; Spanish alazor, etc.). The other known name of safflower is qirtim or qurtum which designates its plant and its seed. It is of Aramaic origin, qurtema, which Loew explains in a very plausible manner, i.e., from the fact that one tears or peels (Hebrew: qartem) the florets of the capitula in order to use them as coloring material. It gives a beautiful red-orange tint. It serves primarily to dye silk, but also to replace or falsify the styles of the true saffron (see above number 135). The name mariq or mirriq is also borrowed into Aramaic moriqā, from yāroq meaning "yellow"

(Fraenkel 150, according to Noeldeke). Bahram and bahramān are names which
resemble the Persian, but are given by Freytag (I, 166) as Arabic names, as well
as ihrīd. The name sukarī (sikri ?) is lacking in all the dictionaries.

Remnants of safflower have been found in Egyptian tombs of the eighteenth
dynasty. Schweinfurth thinks that the land of origin of safflower is not India
but anterior Asia. See the discussion of this question in Loew (I, 403ff) and
Laufer (324-328).

Ducros found red, dried safflower florets under the name 'usfur at the
druggists of Cairo. They are employed as coloring added to henna, and as rouge
(recently replaced by rouge imported from Europe). Besides, under the name
qurtum gabalī ("mountain safflower", that is, from Syria) one sells the seed of
Carthamus tinctorius L. var. inermis Schweinfurth, which dyes yellow. It is also
used to prepare an oil against scabies, and as a carminative and laxative remedy.

301) 'ILK AL-ANBĀT   Gum-resin of the pistachio or terebinth tree

MAIMONIDES: It is the resin of the pistachio tree (šaǧarat al-fustuq) and
some say that it is the resin of the terebinth tree (al-butm). Its
name in ancient Greek is ārā. It is the gum well-known in Egypt
which is sold by the druggists.

MEYERHOF: [Serapion 407; Ibn al-Beithar 1581; Tuhfa 317; 'Abd ar-Razzaq 671;
Issa 142, 1; Loew I, 198-200.]

'Ilk al-Anbāt ("gum of the Nabatheans"), according to several Arabic authors
(Ibn 'Imran, Ibn al-Gazzar, Ibn Gulgul, Ibn as-Suwaidi, 211b), designates the
resin of the pistachio plant (Pistacia vera L., Anacardiaceae). Others (Razi, Abu
Hanifa, Tuhfa) declare that it is the resin of the terebinth tree, an obvious
error. The "Greek" name ārā is probably Latin. I found it in Laguna (55) as an
equivalent of lentiscus. If Maimonides declares that 'ilk al-anbāt is the well-
known gum for sale from Egyptian druggists, he is probably confusing the resin of
the pistachio tree with that of the lentisk (Pistacia Lentiscus L.), which is none
other than the mastic-tree (see above at number 232). It is the latter alone that

is sold in the bazaars of Cairo, and it is unlikely that it was otherwise in
previous centuries.

302) 'ARTANĪTĀ   Root of the motherwort and cyclamen

MAIMONIDES: We have explained that it is the root of one of the two species
of Arum (luf). It is the "bread of monkeys" (hubz al-qurud).

MEYERHOF: [Serapion 85; Ibn al-Beithar 1524; Tuhfa 304; 'Abd ar-Razzaq 115,
159, 677 and 933; Issa 63, 12 and 107, 5; Loew I, 288f and III, 77-79;
Ducros 153.]

The name 'artanītā is purely Aramaic and formerly designated the root of
cyclamen (Cyclamen europaeum L., Primulaceae), which also has the name bahūr
Maryam (see supra number 55). The name of this drug which is a soapy tubercle,
was given by the Arabs to another root, that of the motherwort or "soapwort
from Levant" (Leontice Leontopetalum L. Berberidaceae) (Loew I, 188). In Cairo,
one recognizes the tubercles the size of a fist under the name raqaf (which is
however also used for cyclamen); they are used for cleaning woolen and carpet
fabrics. Ducros only saw tubercles of Cyclamen and never heard of the name raqaf.

We saw earlier (at number 209) that the Arabs also gave the name 'artanita
to the root of a species of Arum, hubz al-qurūd; which is serpentaria (Dracunculus
vulgaris SCHOTT., Araceae). I think that there is here a confusion of names
caused by copyists in the past. An Arabic-Spanish name of serpentaria is
garguntiya which is the Arabic form of the Spanish dragontia verva (Dozy II, 207).
The similarity of the writing of the two names is, I believe, the cause of the
confusion with the name cyclamen 'artanītā.

CHAPTER FĀ'

303) **FIDDIYYA**   Gnaphalium (cudweed) of Dioscorides.

    MAIMONIDES: A herb well-known to the public in Maghrib. It is the one which
                the Spaniards call tumantīl (tomiento, tomentello).

    MEYERHOF: [Dioscorides III,117; Ibn al-Beithar 1686 and 1813; Issa 137,12-14
                and 88,8; Loew I,371.]

    This Arabic name has the meaning silvered, and designates a Composita which
has a silvery-white down which is called gnaphallion by Dioscorides. Modern
botanists gave this name Gnaphalium to a species of composita which is distinguished by a cross blossom. It is the Gnaphalium dioicum L. (cat's foot; ground-
ivy) which corresponds to the ancient Castilian name tomiento.(Simonet 542) and
which has the sense of "oakum herb" (tomento meaning oakum). The Arabic name
tumantil originates from the Latin diminutive tomentellum which is preserved in
modern Portuguese (tomentello). The Gnaphaliums are praised as pectorals, sudorifics and diuretics. However, the botanist Fraas thought he was able to identify
the gnaphallion of Dioscorides with another Mediterranean Composita, the santolina
maritima SMITH., whose stems are covered with a very white down. Concerning
other identifications, see Leclerc in Ibn al-Beithar. Today the name fiddiyya is
applied primarily to the species Phagnalon, another Compositae with down but which
is not, however, employed in medicine.

304) **FAWĀNIYĀ**   Peony.

    MAIMONIDES: It is that which one calls "the one with five seeds" (dū al-
                hams habbāt). One also says that it is the root of the "donkey
                rose" (ward al-hamir).

    MEYERHOF: [Theophrastus IX,8,6; Dioscorides III,140; Serapion 182; Ibn al-
                Beithar 1648; Tuhfa 318; 'Abd ar-Razzaq 36,692 and 708; Issa
                132,7; Loew III,124; Ducros 165.]

    Fawāniyā is the Syriac-Arabic name of the Greek name paionia which designates
the "female" peony (Paeonia officinalis RETZ., Ranunculacea). The Arabic name

"one with five seeds" is the translation from the Greek pentorobon of Dioscorides, and the name "donkey rose" is in usage in Maghrib. However, the most well-known name in Egypt and in Syria is 'ūd as-salīb ("wood of the cross"). Under this denomination, in the bazaars of Cairo, one sells the roots of peony in the form of thick fusiform fragments. One adds them to beverages as an antispasmodic; one formerly used them against epilepsy, by promenading fragments of the root attached in the form of a cross over the chest of the patient (from whence the name 'ūd as-salib). This remedy is still in usage by certain superstitious Christians in the Near-East. (The title of this article is lacking in the original manuscript, an omission on the part of the copyist).

305) FŪ   Valerian

MAIMONIDES: It is the wild nard (an-nāridin al-barri), and in Spanish

              sastara. One has established that this plant is the one which

              the druggists in Maghrib sell to the inhabitants of the desert

              as a perfume. The Berbers call it aisimamun, and it is by this

              name that it is known throughout Morocco.

MEYERHOF: [Dioscorides I, II; Serapion 186; Ibn al-Beithar 1709 and 1318;

              Tuhfa 322; 'Abd ar-Razzaq 606, 701 and 813; Issa 137, 1; Loew III,

              482.]

    Fu is the Arabic transcription of the Greek phou which designates either the large valerian (Valeriana Phu L.) or Valeriana Dioscoridis SIBTH., both species being less efficacious than Valeriana officinalis L. (the "small valerian"). According to Renaud, the Berber name is pronounced asmāmen. The Spanish name is found in Ibn al-Beithar in the form šištra and is explained by Dozy (I, 755) and Simonet (600) as an equivalent of wild anet (Meum athamanticum JACQ., see above our number 231). The name of this latter plant in Arabic is mu, and it is therefore possible that there is confusion with fu. For the moment, we think Maimonides and Ibn al-Beithar who identify šištra with the large valerian should be followed, because the Spanish name of wild anet is yendro.

306) <u>FARĀSIYŪN</u>   Horehound

<u>MAIMONIDES</u>: It is <u>sandān</u> and the "herb of dogs" (<u>hašīšat al-kilāb</u>), so

called because dogs (fol. 95ᵛ) are in the habit of urinating

upon it. Its name is also <u>aš-šanār</u>, and it is one of the

species of horehound (<u>al-marrūya</u>) that was discussed above in

chapter <u>mīm</u> (see number 235).

<u>MEYERHOF</u>: ⌈Theophrastus VI, 2, 5; Dioscorides III, 105; Serapion 177; Ibn al-

Beithar 1674; <u>Tuhfa</u> 324; 'Abd ar-Razzaq 697; Issa 115, 7; Loew

II, 74ff; Ducros 172.⌉

<u>Farāsiyūn</u> is the Arabic transcription of the Greek <u>prasion</u>. <u>Sandān</u> is

probably an Arabic form of the Syriac <u>saddan ar'a</u> (Loew). In Kohen (p. 134, line 14)

one finds the faulty reading <u>saïdānū 'ā</u> and several lines later (line 27)

<u>sindibāz al-ard</u> (read <u>sindiyān al-ard</u> meaning <u>chamaedrys</u>); it is perhaps another

faulty reading of the Syriac name. The aforementioned two names designate the

horehound (<u>Marrubium vulgare</u> L., Labiates) that we have encountered above under

the name <u>marrūya</u> (number 235). <u>Šanār</u> is a Persian name of the white horehound

(Issa). The white and hairy stems of the horehound are still sold by the druggists

of Cairo under the Greek name <u>frāsiyūn</u>. The leaves are added into powders and

infusions against catarrhs of the respiratory passages (Ducros).

307) <u>FĀGIR (SIC)</u>   Xanthoxylum

<u>MAIMONIDES</u>: One says that it is the root of the Indian nenuphar (<u>an-</u>

<u>nilufar al-hindi</u>).

<u>MEYERHOF</u>: ⌈Serapion 172; Ibn al-Beithar 1650; Issa 191, 4; Loew II, 28;

Dymock I, 255-260.⌉

The Arabic name of this plant is generally written in the feminine <u>al-fāgira</u>

("the one with the open mouth"), and I think that in our manuscript there is a

copyist's error. It was first described by the Persian Ibn Sina (<u>Qānūn</u> I, 406),

who stated that one imported its pisiform seeds from Sofala (maritime port of

Oriental Africa, Mozambique, and, in the Middle Ages, an important port of call

for Indian navigation). It is for this reason that European botanists of the
sixteenth century gave this plant the name Fagara Avicennae. The Arabs did not
know the origin of this plant. In reality, it is an aromatic Rutacea from the
Indies and other tropical regions which is today called Xanthoxylum. In many
botanical treatises one finds the faulty spelling Zanthoxylum. The fāg̱ira of
Ibn Sina is probably Xanthoxylum Rhetsa DC., and is in usage as a condiment because of its peppery taste. The fruit is formed by several independent pistils,
dehiscent in two valves. The fragrant seeds contain an oil, a resin and a bitter
substance, the xanthopicrite.

In India, one still uses several species of indigenous Xanthoxylum:
Xanthoxylum alatum ROXB., Xanthoxylum acanthopodium DC., Xanthoxylum oxyphyllum
EDGW., and Xanthoxylum Budrunga WALL. They are all bitter aromatics which serve
as tonics, febrifuges, etc. (Dymock).

308) FANG̱AKUS̱T   Agnus-castus, chaste-tree

MAIMONIDES: One also says fang̱ankas̱t and bang̱anku̱s̱t. It is "the leprous
hand" (al-kaff al-g̱admā') and the "herb of Abraham" (s̱ag̱arat
Ibrāhīm) as well as the "Slavonian pepper" (fulful as-saqāliba).
One also calls it al-falaífula ("small pepper") and s̱atnā. Its
fruit is habb al-faqd. Its Spanish name is (?) faqra and its
Greek name agnos. One also says that it is the pentaphyllon,
which means "having five leaves".

MEYERHOF: [Theophrastus I, 3, 2 and III, 12, 2; Dioscorides I, 103; Serapion 174;
Ibn al-Beithar 354, 1700 and 1706; Tuhfa 62, 81 and 191; 'Abd ar-
Razzaq 325; Issa 190, 1; Loew III, 491-494; Ducros 44.]

The Arabic names of the first line are all transcriptions of the Persian name
pang̱-angus̱t ("which has five fingers", allusion to the shape of the leaves), which
designates the chaste-tree (Vitex agnus castus L., Verbenaceae). This Mediterranean bush has many different names in Arabic (see Issa). In Maghrib, however,
one gives it the same Spanish (rig̱ino) and Arabic (hirwa') name as the castor-oil

plant, but a separate Berber name (angarf, Renaud-Colin). The name šatnā, which
is lacking in the dictionaries, seems to me to be a faulty spelling of šunyā, from
the Syriac šūnāyā (Loew). The spelling of the Spanish name is uncertain: Latin
ficaria, Castilian figuera? (Simonet 213).

The Egyptian druggists sell the fruits of the chaste-tree (habb el-faqd), in
the bazaars. They are black seeds resembling a little black pepper, from which
are derived the Arabic names "small pepper","Slavonian pepper", etc. The former
druggists of Europe called it "monk's pepper" because, since antiquity, one attributed to the fruit an antiaphrodisiac and antihysteric action (Ducros).

309) FAWDANAǦ   Mint

MAIMONIDES: There exist numerous species:

a) The fluviatic type (nahrī) is called habaq al-mā' ("aquatic mint") and
al-habaq an-nahrī ("fluvial mint"). It is ad-dawmarān and in Egypt one says
habaq at-timsāh ("crocodile mint") and in Spanish muštaraštara (mentastro or
mastranzo). However, the Maghribians have corrupted the name and read mašištrū.

b-c) The mountain type is the one which is called an-nābuta, and the wild
type is that which is called bulāyu (poleo) in Spanish. It is the one which in
all of Maghrib one puts into aliments, and which one calls bulāy. One also calls
it al-gubaïrā. One says fawdanaǧ and fantanaǧ, and in Arabic it is al-'irmid.

d) One of its types (fol. 96^r) is the one which the Arabs call at-tarnīq,
in ancient Greek flīsun and in Persian ǧālīǧun.

e) Al-faïtal and as-sufaïra are species of al-fawdanaǧ and al-kartabāš
as well as al-miskitrāmašir; we have discussed it earlier (see numbers 242, 247,
255).

MEYERHOF: [Theophrastus VI, 1-7 and IX, 16; Dioscorides II, 128 and III, 31-35;
Serapion 175-367; Ibn al-Beithar 1712 and 2138; Tuhfa 325, 330 and
378; 'Abd ar-Razzaq 317, 363, 597 and 694; Issa 117, 10-15 and 129,
13-15; Loew II, 75-84.]

This chapter offers considerable difficulties because of the confusion that existed among the Greeks and the Arabs on the subject of mints and related species, and, in our case in particular, because of the mutilation of several names in the text. Fawdanaǧ, etc. is the Arabic form of the Persian pūdana (Vullers I,380), synonym of the Arabic habaq which designates fragrant plants of the labiate type, above all the mints and thymes.

a) Fawdanaǧ al-mā' is the aquatic mint (Mentha aquatica L.) which corresponds to sisymbrion of the Greeks. However, the Spanish mentastro or mastranzo (Simonet 359) signifies Mentha rotundifolia L., another variety of mint.

b) Nābuta is the transcription of the Latin nepeta (Spanish nebeda) (Dozy II, 636 and Simonet 397) which designates wild pennyroyal. According to Dioscorides (III,35), it is a mountain species of kalaminthê which modern botanists have identified as Mentha tomentella LINK.

c) The "Wild mint" of Maimonides corresponds to pennyroyal mint (Mentha Pulegium L.) which is proved by the Spanish designation bulāyu, equivalent to the Latin pulegium and Spanish poleo. This name is preserved in popular Moroccan (flēyyu) and Egyptian (flēya, Schweinfurth 30) dialects. Nevertheless, ǧubaïrā'— name given to more than ten plants, above all the sorb-tree— is not found except in Ibn al-Beithar (2138) in the form ǧubaïrat al-aíyil, referring mainly to poleo cervuno, meaning dittany, which we will discuss below in e). The name 'irmid does not designate mint to any Arabic author; it is perhaps an error of the copyist.

d) The name tarnīq is lacking in all the (botanical) dictionaries and treatises. One might think of tiryāq ("theriac"), a name sometimes applied to aromatic plants. The two other names are mutilations, the first probably of blêkhôn, the second of glêkhôn, both from Dioscorides III,31; the last name is thus not Persian but Greek. These two names are also equivalents for pennyroyal (Mentha Pulegium L.), but the author here wished to speak of another species of mint whose identity we cannot establish because of the mutilation of the Arabic name.

e) According to Ibn-al-Beithar 1717, Dozy II,73 and 294, and Simonet 548, the name faital designates a species of cow-parsnip (spondylium) which is an umbellif-

erous plant and thus has nothing in common with mints. Sufairā' is,
in general, a name for buckthorn (Rhamnus) and has as little in common
with mints as faltal. Al-kartabāš is also a name that we have not been
able to locate in (botanical) treatises. It is probably a faulty spelling for karkabāš (Dozy II, 458), Persian term which designates the nettle-
tree (Celtis australis L.), or for karkāš (Vuller II, 820) which is applied to the seeds of darnel. Finally, miskitrāmašir is known; it is
the dittany that we have discussed above at number 242 (Origanum
Dictamnus L.).

310) FALFAMŪNIYA   Root of the long pepper-plant

MAIMONIDES: One also says falfalmūniya. It is the root of the pepper
plant.

MEYERHOF: [Theophrastus II, 20, 1; Dioscorides II, 159; Serapion 173;
Ibn al-Beithar 1696 and 1699; 'Abd ar-Razzaq 715; Issa 140,
20 and 141,3; Loew II, 61; Dymock III, 177-180]

The Arabic name in its different forms - the most used is fil-
filmūja - originates from the Sanskrit pippalī-mūl (meaning "pepper
root"); in Persian pilpilmūwa, Vullers I, 370; in Syriac falfalmūr,
Brockelmann Lex. 576. This name still exists in hindi dialect and de-
signates the root of the long pepper (piper longum L., or Chavica
Roxburghii MIQ.) and several other Piperaceae. Chavica officinarum
MIQ. furnishes an even longer fruit. These climbing plants grow in
Oriental India and in the Sunda Islands. They were known to the
Greeks but their fruits were confused with those of other pepper plants.
The Arabs knew the fruit by the Arabic-Persian name dār-filfil
("long pepper"). The root, which in India (Dymock) and in China
(Laufer 375) is still in the commerce, was first described by Al-Beruni

in his <u>Book of Drugs</u> (<u>Kitāb as-Saïdana</u>, unique Arabic manuscript in
Brusa, Turkey), where he correctly transcribes the Indian name <u>bibal-mūl</u>,
and states, according to Ibn Masa and others, that it was the root of the
long pepper-plant. This root serves as a warming remedy in the Orient.

311) <u>FAWFAL</u>   Areca-nut

<u>MAIMONIDES</u>:

It is the "Indian Hazel-nut" (<u>al-bunduq al-hindī</u>) and <u>al-atmūt.</u>

<u>MEYERHOF</u>:

[Serapion 178; Ibn al-Beithar 1711; Issa 20, 4; Loew II, 302; Dymock
522-532; Ducros 192.]

<u>Fawfal</u> is the Arabic form of the Persian <u>pūpal</u> (Vullers I, 379) which
is derived from the Sanskrit <u>pūgaphala</u> (Laufer 548) and designates the
"areca-nut", fruit (seed) of the Indian palm-tree <u>Areca Catechu</u> L. This
fruit, mixed with the leaves of betal (<u>Piper Betle</u> L.) and a bit of pulverized lime, forms a masticatory much in use in India. The areca-nut, in
addition, is praised as an antihelminthic remedy.

By contrast, <u>atmāt</u> or <u>atmūt</u> is the Arabic name of another Indian seed,
the "bonduc nut", derived from an Indian Caesalpinia, <u>Caesalpinia Bonducella</u>
ROXB. This "nut" also has the names <u>bunduq hindi</u> and <u>ratta</u>. See Meyerhof
& Sobhy, commentary on number 102 of Ghafiqi (<u>atmūt</u>). There is thus confusion between two different Indian drugs in this paragraph of Maimonides.

In Egypt, one sells the areca-nut (<u>kad-hindī</u>) in the bazaars as a
constituent of dry collyria (Ducros).

312) <u>FĀSRĀ</u>   Bryony

<u>MAIMONIDES</u>:

One also says <u>basrā</u>. It is the herb one calls the "white vine"
(<u>al-karma al-baïdā'</u>), and one also says <u>al-karm al-abyad</u>, the "serpent

grape" ('inab al-hayya) and "hair shearer" (haliq aš-ša'ar); in Spanish
abrāla and in Persian hazār ğušān.

MEYERHOF:

[Theophrastus IX, 14-25; Dioscorides IV, 182; Serapion 183; Ibn al-
Beithar 1654; Tuhfa 328; 'Abd ar-Razzaq 450, 694 and 722; Issa 34, 2;
Loew I, 553 ff; Ibn 'Awwam II, 371.]

Fāšīrā is a Syriac name, bāšrā one of its Arabic forms, hazār ğušān
("one thousand ells")* its Persian synonym (Vullers II, 632). These names
and the Arabic names of this article designate the white bryony (Bryonia
alba L., Cucurbitaceae,equivalent to the Greek ampelos leukê). The branch-
ing, fleshy, white root ("devil's turnip"), having a sour and burning flavor,
is employed against hydrops and ailments of the skin. The Spanish name
abrala or abobrilla, also bobrinella, is explained by Simonet (1 ff) as a
transformation from the Greek name bryônia.

313) FĀŠRAŠĪN   Black-vine

MAIMONIDES:

It is the herb called the "black-vine" (al-karma as-sawdā', al-karm
al-aswad). Its name in Spanish is būtāniya. The roots of this plant are
a drug which dyes red; it is that which the women of Maghrib employ to
rouge their cheeks. Its well-known name among the people is al-maïmūn
("the happy").

MEYERHOF:

[Dioscorides IV, 183; Serapion 184; Ibn al-Beithar 1655; 'Abd ar-Razzaq
451 and 723; Issa 177, 9; Loew I, 585.]

Fāšrašīn and fašaršīn are both Arabic transcriptions of a Syriac name
faser astin (Brockelmann Lex. 614b; Vullers II, 632) which was the equivalent
of ampelos melaïna ("black-vine") of Dioscorides. One has identified this latter
plant with the dioic bryony (Bryonia dioica LACQ. Cucurbitaceae, see Issa 34,3).

* an ell or aune is an old French measure, about 1.88 meters

However, the majority of modern botanists argue in favor of the black-vine (black-bryony, soft bryony with black fruits, "herb with beaten women") which is not a Cucurbitacea, but the Dioscoreacea   *Tamus communis* L. The large tubercles of this plant are still in use against contusions and burns.

The Spanish name *butaniya* is explained by Vullers (I, 278) as a transformation of the Greek *batanouta* of Dioscorides. However, this word is not found in the editions of Dioscorides nor in the Greek (botanical) dictionaries! By contrast, the proposition of Simonet (64) that the name is derived from the Latin *vitinea* (meaning *vitis nigra*) seems more acceptable.

314) FARSAH   Peach

MAIMONIDES:

It is a red species of peach (hawh); it is known by the name "flowery one" (az-zahrī).

MEYERHOF:

[Dioscorides I, 115; Serapion 471; Ibn al-Beithar 830; Issa 149, 5; Loew III, 159; Ibn 'Awwam I, 315.]

Farsah is the Arabic form of the Persian *farsank* which signifies the parasang, itinerary measure of the Persians. I believe that there is an error of the copyist here for *firsik*, Arabic, Persian and Hebrew name derived from the Greek *Persikon mêlon* ("Persian apple"). For example, this name is found in the Arabic (botanical) dictionary *Muhassas* (XI, 138) and in Vullers (II, 657). It is a type of peach (*Prunus Persica* SIEB. & ZUCC., Rosaceae) which was known in Spain. Today in Egypt, one cultivates a type of peach which is also called el-hōh ez-zahrī. The synonym hawh zahrī ("flowery peach") is also found in Ibn 'Awwam. See below number 397 (hawh).

315) FĪL (read: FĪLZAHRA or FĪLZAHRAǦ)

MAIMONIDES:

It is the flower of the Persian lycium (al-hudad al-fārisi).

MEYERHOF:

[Theophrastus III, 18; Dioscorides I, 90 and I, 100; Serapion 180 and 205; Ibn al-Beithar 1720; Tuhfa 166; 'Abd ar-Razzaq 314; Issa 112, 15; Loew III, 133ff; Ducros 168.]

There is here also a copyists's error. One should read "fīlzahra; it is Persian lycium". We have seen above (at number 148) that hudad was considered as the Arabic name of the plant fīlzahraǧ (fīl-zahra meaning Persian "elephant bile", because of its color and the bitter taste of the juice). However, there existed a certain confusion regarding the identification of these names. See also 'awsiǧ (at number 294). In general, one can state that to the Arabs, hudad (Arabic) and fīlzahra (Persian) were the equivalents of the Greek lykion, and that 'awsiǧ was the equivalent of the Greek rhamnos. Ghafiqi (ms. fol. 60b-61a) states among the synonyms: "Aqsiāqus (read oxyakanthos), this is šaǧarat al-fīl ("the elephant tree") and by this name one also designates 'ullaiq al-kalb (the "dog bramble" meaning eglantine)....The significance of this name is "the pointed thorn". One also says that it is the tree which has berries called zirisk and which is al-ambarbāris ("barberry"); one brings them from Khorassan.

316) FĀZAHRAǦ (read: FĪLZAHRAǦ)   Elephant bile

MAIMONIDES:

This name to the Persians designates the bile (fol. 96^v) of the elephant.

MEYERHOF:

The confusion caused by the copyist continues in this article which is probably part of the preceding one. It should be read fīl-zahraǧ; then the explanation of the name is exact.

Fāzahr or fādzahr and bāzahr are Arabic forms of pādzahr, pāzahr, etc,
Persian names of bezoar. The latter is a stony concretion which forms in
the intestines of certain animals, particularly the wild goat of Persia
(Capra Aegagrus), and to which one formerly attributed curative and prophy-
lactic properties against poisons. See Anastase p. 75 ff (chapter al-fādzahr
in al-Akfani and commentary.)

CHAPTER SĀD

317) SANAWBAR   Pine

MAIMONIDES:

According to the first subdivision, there are two types, one male and
one female. The male is the one which has no fruits. The female is of
two types; one produces large seeds, the other small seeds. The small
seeds are those which are called qadm Qurais and al-kirkir and bītus (pitys).

MEYERHOF:

[Theophrastus III, 9,2-5; Dioscorides I, 69; Serapion 438; Ibn al-Beithar
1417; Tuhfa 298, 'Abd-ar-Razzaq 320 and 620; Issa 139, 15 and 140, 15-17;
Loew III, 40-47.]

Loew (III,41ff) proposes that the Syriac-Arabic name sanaw-bar is derived from the Syriac astrubila, transcription of the Greek strobilos
meaning "fruit or cone of the pine". To the Arabs, the name sanawbar
next took on the meaning of "pine" and was employed as the translation
from the Greek penke and pitys. The distinction between "male" pine and
"female" pine is already found in Theophrastus. Modern botanists have not
yet been able to identify the names of all the different species of Conifers
of the Greeks and Arabs. One has considered the sanawbar dakar ("male pine")
to be the false-fur-tree (also called pine or spruce, Picea
excelsa LINK.) which, however, does not grow spontaneously in the Mediterranean
region. One should rather consider Pinus orientalis LINK. These trees are,
of course, not "male" (this word here means akarpos or without fruits);
their cones are small. The "female" pines probably represent the parasol
pine (Pinus Pinea L.) which has large cones, and the Aleppo pine (Pinus
halepensis MILL) which has slightly smaller cones. The Arabic names for
the small cones are also found in Ibn al-Beithar and in the (botanical)
dictionaries.

318) <u>SABIR</u>   Aloe

<u>MAIMONIDES</u>:

It is the juice of the plant which the people with us know by the name <u>as-sabbāra</u>. The name of this plant in Arabic is <u>al-muqr</u> and in ancient Greek <u>aloê</u>.

<u>MEYERHOF</u>:

Dioscorides III, 22; Serapion 422; Ibn al-Beithar 1388; <u>Tuhfa</u> 294; 'Abd-ar-Razzaq 619; Issa 10,9; Loew II, 149-152; Ducros 141; Laufer 480.

For the most part, the Greek name <u>aloê</u> passed through oriental languages until Chinese (<u>lu-wei</u>, Laufer 480). Its Arabic equivalent <u>sabir</u> or <u>sabr</u> designates the juice of every bitter plant, and in particular the <u>aloes</u>. This Arabic name is preserved in Spanish as <u>acibar</u> and in Portuguese as <u>azebre</u> or <u>azevre</u> meaning "aloes". See M. Meyerhof, <u>Essay on the Portuguese</u> <u>names of drugs derived from the Arabic</u>, in <u>Petrus Nonius</u>, vol. 11, Lisbon 1938, p.1-8. Among the numerous kinds and varieties of this Liliaceae, it was above all the <u>Aloe vera</u> L. and <u>Aloe Perry's</u> BAK. which gave the resinous juice so appreciated in medicine. This latter plant inhabits the Island of Socotora and furnishes the drug called <u>Aloe socotrina</u> or <u>succotrina</u>; one has erroneously given this name to another species which grows in southern Africa and which was probably unknown to the Arabs. In Syriac, aloes were called <u>sĕbārā.</u> The Arabic name <u>Sabbara</u> is today in usage to designate the American aloe (Amaryllidaceae) because of its external resemblance to the aloes. The concentrated juice of aloes is sold by the druggists of Cairo under the name <u>sabr suqutrī</u> ("socotrin aloes"). It is employed as a gastric and emmenagogue (Ducros). The name <u>muqr</u> or <u>maqr</u> is today unknown.

319) <u>SA'TAR</u>   Savery, thyme, origan

<u>MAIMONIDES</u>:

There are many types:

(a) The wild thyme (<u>as-sa'tar al-barrī</u>) is called <u>an-nadg</u> in Arabic.

(b) The Persian thyme (<u>as-sa'tar al-fārisī</u>) is the one which is called "Slavonian pepper" (<u>fulful as-Saqāliba</u>); it is savory (<u>aš-šatiriyya</u>, Satureia).

(c) As to the "donkey thyme" (<u>sa 'tar al-hamīr</u>), it is a species of Southern-wood (<u>al-qaisūm</u>) that one calls <u>tummālu</u> (tomillo) in the foreign language (Spanish).

(d) When physicians speak of "substantial thyme" (<u>sa'tar ǧawharī</u>) or of "roast thyme" (<u>sa-tar aš-šiwā'</u>), they mean the known thyme that people use as a condiment for (cooked)dishes.

<u>MEYERHOF</u>:

⌈Theophrastus VI, 2-7; Dioscorides III, 36-41; Serapion 432; Ibn al-Beithar 1398; <u>Tuhfa</u> 299 and 163; 'Abd ar-Razzaq, 626-629 and 771; Issa 129,13; 163,9-10; 180, 23 etc; Loew II, 103-106; Ibn 'Awwam II, 298-301.⌉

I share with Renaud-Colin the opinion of Fraenkel (143) that the Aramean name <u>satrā</u> is the equivalent of the Latin satureia and, in Arabic, adopted the interpellation of the letter <u>'ain</u>. One finds the forms sa'tar, vulgar <u>sa'tar</u> and <u>za'tar</u>. This name designates numerous species of Labiates of the origan, thyme and savory types.

(a) "Wild thyme" or <u>an-nadg</u> is the savory (<u>Satureia hortensis</u> L.)

(b) The name "Persian thyme" is perhaps an equivalent of <u>sa'tar al-furs</u> of Issa (117,13), which is, however, a name of the pennyroyal (<u>Mentha Pulegium</u> L., see above number 309). But here we are undoubtedly dealing with the "savory of Crete" (<u>Satureia Thymbra</u> L.).

It is the one which is designated by the "Spanish" name šātiriyya
(Simonet 586, in modern Castilian ajedrea). In Syria and in Palestine,
the name za-tar farisi today designates thymus capitatus (Post II, 337).
By contrast, the name "Slavonian pepper" does not designate a Labiate but
(see our numbers 308 and 163) the chaste-tree (Vitex Agnus Castus L.)
and the water-cress (Nasturtium officinale R. Br.)

(c) "Donkey thyme" is in Arabic also the name for southern-wood (Artemisia
     Abrotanum L., see below number 337), and for the thyme (thymus
     capitatus L.K. and HOFFM.) that Maimonides discussed under the name
     of hāšā (see above number 157). It is the one which, in effect, is
     called tomillo (Simonet 550) in Spanish.

(d) Finally sa'tar aš-šawwā' "the thyme of the roaster" - one can also
     read sa'tar aš-šiwā' meaning "roast thyme" - is probably identical
     to common thyme (Thymus vulgaris L.). Kohen (p. 137, line 7) has the
     spelling sa'tar gazarī instead of gawharī and states that it is the
     thyme one eats with a roast (ši'wā'). 'Abd ar-Razzaq (626 bis) has
     the form sa'tar gawzi.

320) SAMG AL-BUTM   Terebinth resin

MAIMONIDES:

     It is that which one calls tayābašt.

MEYERHOF:

     [Theophrastus IX, 1-2; Dioscorides 1-71; Serapion 59 and 84; Ibn al-
Beithar 1581; Tuhfa 317; Issa 141,14; Loew I, 191-195, Ducros 142]

     We are dealing with the resin of the Pistacia Terebinthus L.
(Anacardiaceae) with which we dealt above at number 66. It was the tur-
pentine of the ancients. See also the commentary of Renaud-Colin at
numbers 178 and 317 of Tuhfa. The Berberic name tayābašt is not cited by
other physicians, as much as I was able to verify. Perhaps it resembles
tadist or tidekšt of Trqbut (p. 204), meaning pistachio-tree?

321) <u>SAMĠ AL-BALAT</u>   Lithocolla

<u>MAIMONIDES</u>:

A remedy composed of white marble (<u>ruhām abyad</u>)and of beef paste
(<u>ġirā 'al-baqar</u>).*

<u>MEYERHOF</u>:

<u>Samġ al-balāt</u> signifies "paste of pavement" and it is the transla-
tion of the Greek <u>lithokolla</u> meaning "lithogenic cement". Maimonides gives
the composition according to the formula of Dioscorides. Dawud al-Antaki
(I, 437) gives another much longer and complicated formula: alum, sarcocolla,
Dragon's blood, terebinth, vitriol, coral, - all crushed and cooked together.
He also distinguishes another type of natural lithocolla, with a red color.
In medicine, one used both against ailments of the skin. Kohen (p. 137,
line 10-12) describes the composition of lithocolla as Maimonides, but
adds some resin (<u>rātīnaġ</u>). He contests the existence of <u>samġ al-balāt</u> which
was presumed to be a simple drug from India, and cites as evidence a book
of ar-Razi.

322) <u>SINĀB</u>   Mustard

<u>MAIMONIDES</u>:

It is the seed of mustard (<u>al-hardal</u>) whose active substance was extracted by means of vinegar.

<u>MEYERHOF</u>:

[Theophrastus VII, 1-3 (<u>napy</u>); Dioscorides II, 154 (<u>sinepis</u>); Ibn al-
Beithar 767-769; <u>Tuhfa</u> 417; Issa 169, 17-21; Loew I, 516-527; Ibn 'Awwam II,
252 ff.]

The name <u>sināb</u>, undoubtedly borrowed into Greek <u>sinêpi</u> or into Latin
<u>sinapis</u> (in modern Castilian <u>jenabe</u>, Simonet 152), is also found in Ibn
al-'Awwam and in Ibn al-Beithar, but as the name of the wild plant,

* extracted from the skin or tendons of cattle

the wild mustard (hardal barrī or Sinapis arvensis L.) The explanation

given here by Maimonides is unique in its kind. Here sinab corresponds

to our table-mustard. It is extracted from the seeds of several species

of Brassica and Sinapis (Cruciferaceae). The flour of mustard seeds

was always used in medicine as a rubefacient, irritant and stimulant.

See above number 218 (labsān) and below number 400 (hardal).

(fol. 97$^{\alpha}$)

323) SĀBŪN   Soap

MAIMONIDES:

The soap which is mentioned by physicians is the solid soap known by

the name "soap of Raqqa" (as-sābūn ar-raqqī).

MEYERHOF:

⌈Serapion 423; Ibn al-Beithar 1283, Tuhfa 295; 'Abd ar-Razzaq 622.⌉

One attributes the invention of soap to the Gauls (Pline XXVIII,51).

The Arabic name sābūn is the transcription of the Greek sapon or the Latin

sapo (Simonet 149), in Castilian jabon. Raqqa was a town in Mesopotamia

(Iraq) celebrated for its pottery. The geographer Yāqut does not mention

the fabrication of soap. In Egypt, one uses the soap of Nablus (Nabulus,

Palestine) as a medical soap (sābūn nābulsī). However, it is being more

and more replaced by soaps of European production.

CHAPTER QĀF

324)   QULQUL   Crotolaria?

MAIMONIDES:

One also says qilqil and qulqulān as well as qalaqil. The seed of
this plant is al-basam. It is that which the druggists call "balsam
seed" (habb al-balasān); one uses it in our times as a substitute for
the (true) balsam seed.

MEYERHOF:

[Serapion 198; Ibn al-Beithar 1822; Tuhfa 180 and 335; 'Abd ar-Razzaq
229; Issa 43,1 and 60,10; Loew II, 515 and III,90; Dymock I, 400 ff;
Muhassas XI, 150.]

The identification of this plant has been in doubt to this very
time. In Maghrib where one only knows the imported seeds, it was sometimes thought to be the wild pomegranate tree. According to Renaud-Colin,
in Morocco, the name qiqlān designates the cassia-tree (Acacia Farnesia-na
WILLD.). In Arabia, Forskal identified qilqil or qulqal with Cassia Tora L.
("wild senna"), the identification accepted by Leclerc (Ibn al-Beithar
1822) and Schlimmer (114).

However, I think it is probable to recognize qulqul, qalāqil, qulqulān
(see Freytag III, 492 and Dozy II, 399) as species of Crotolaria
(Leguminous plants). Their characteristics are well in accord with the
description given by Abu 'Amru and Abu'1 'Abbas an-Nabati (Rihla) in
Ibn al-Beithar: when the plant is dried, the seeds elicit a rattling sound
in the swollen and hollow shells, from which (are derived) the Arabic names
and the modern Latin botanical name Crotolaria. In Yemen, Crotolaria
retusa L., still today has the name qulqul (Shweinfurth 164). In

India , one sows this plant and related species whose leaves are eaten
as a vegetable; the seeds serve as an antibilious remedy and one ex-
tracts therefrom a type of hemp from the stems of Crotolaria juncea L.
(Dymock). See the article on Crotolaria juncea ("san-hemp") in Sir
George Watt's The Commercial Products of India (London 1908), p. 430-437.
Basam and habb al-balasān, by contrast, are the seeds of the balm-tree
(Commiphora Opobalsamum ENGL.) and has nothing to do with qulqul.

325) QĀQULLA   Sea rocket, water parsnip and varieties

MAIMONIDES:

    This herb is called al-qullām in Arabic. It is that which is called
al-mullāh and aš-šaraǧir and ar-rawāš and al-kāšir. Its Spanish name
is bilihta and mardanīla and aš-šartila. In Maghrib one also calls it
karyūniš; the root aqaryūniš of this name is foreign. One also calls it
badīlubā (ped de lobo).

MEYERHOF:

    [Theophrastus VII,1-5; Dioscorides II, 155; Serapion 109 and 134;
Ibn al-Beithar 1725; Tuhfa 337 and 342; 'Abd ar-Razzaq 739; Issa 27,13
and 35,7 and 77,13-15 and 170, 11; Loew I, 489 ff, I, 506-510.]

    The explanation of the names of this paragraph offers many difficul-
ties. Firstly, the Greek and Arabic names produce confusions: the Greek
name kardamon, which designates cruciferous plants (Lepidium or Erucaria)
is often confused with kardamomon, Greek name for the small cardamom, the
well-known Indian drug. Similarly the Syriac-Arabic name qāqullā (already Assyrian qāqullu) which designates species of Cruciferaceae (Cakile,
Lepidium, etc.),is confused with qāqula, Arabic name of the small cardamom.

    The synonyms of this paragraph also designate different plants.
The names qāqullā and qullām have been identified as the sea-rocket

(Cakile maritima SCOP.), annual plant of the sandy beaches of the North,
sometimes praised as a diuretic (see Muhassas XI, 172). Mullah is an
Arabic name which designates totally different salty plants, here perhaps
the purslain orach (Atriplex halimus L. Chenopodiaceae), which also has
the name qāqullā. However, Muhassas (XI, 175, line 13) states that the
plant has the name Mullāh because of its salt-like color, and not because of
its salty taste. The names šaršar, šarāšir, etc. are found in Freytag
(II, 411), but without identification, as well as kāšir (Freytag (IV, 38).
Rawās is, to Ibn al-Beithar (1070), a name of water parsnip (karafs al-ma'
Sium latifolium L., umbelliferaceae)that we discussed above at number 196.
We have also found the name karmūniš there, which is explained by Renaud-
Colin (Tuhfa 337) as being derived from a Roman plural acriones (which is
confirmed by our manuscript) and as an equivalent of water cress (Nasturtium
officinale L., Cruciferae). The spelling of Dozy (I, 30) and Simonet (3)
agriokardamon is not confirmed. Among the Spanish names, bilihta originates
from the low-Latin plecta, in modern Castilian pelosilla (Simonet 439).
Mardanila is perhaps related to murtilla (Simonet 366), and šartila to
šartil, in low Latin sertula, representing a garland (Simonet 585).

Ped de lobo is old Castilian for "wolf's foot". The spelling of this
name, which is mutilated and devoid of diacritical points in our manuscript,
would have been impossible without the benevolence of Misters Renaud and Colin
who were kind enough to communicate to me a passage relative to this, from
the manuscript by Umda belonging to Mr. Colin, where the anonymous author
cites the name badīlubā according to the celebrated Abu'l-Qasim az-Zahrawi.
In modern Castilian, pata de lobo ('wolf's foot') is one of the names of
Orchids (Botica 992).

326) <u>QULB</u>   Lithospermum

<u>MAIMONIDES</u>:

    These are white seeds, hard as rocks, and for that reason they are
called "seeds of rock" and it is <u>stomakhos</u>.

<u>MEYERHOF</u>:

    Dioscorides III, 141; Serapion 324; Ibn al-Beithar 1823; Issa 110,10;
Loew 297.

    <u>Qulb</u> or <u>habb al-qulb</u> is the Arabic name of hard and white seeds of
the "herb with pearls" (<u>Lithospermum officinale</u> L. Borraginaceae),
European mountain plant. These seeds were reputed to be able to dissolve
vesical calculi. It is for this reason that the plant also has the Arabic
name <u>kāsir al-haǧar</u> ("stone-breaker"; see Ibn al-Beithar 1873). The Greek
name of our text <u>istūmāhūs</u> - probably a mistake of the copyist for <u>istāhūs</u> -
(<u>stakhys</u>) - is an error of the author. The Greek name of the seeds is
<u>lithospermon</u>. In Simonet (393), we find two additional names for lithospermum
which passed into the Arabic language: <u>muštīya</u> (<u>mustela</u>?) and <u>saišafrāga</u>
(<u>saxifraga</u>).

327) <u>QANBĪL</u>   Kamala

<u>MAIMONIDES</u>:

    It is an earth that one finds in India where it exists below sand,
and from where it is imported. It is said that it is the earth with
which one prepares the artificial honey wine and which is called <u>ad-dādī</u>.

<u>MEYERHOF</u>:

    Serapion 303; Ibn al-Beithar 1842; Issa 114,2; Loew II, 26 ff; Dymock
III, 296-301.

The powder of kamala is a red dust which covers the fruits of the
tropical plant "rottlera of dyers" (<u>Rottlera tinctoria</u> ROXB. or <u>Mallotus
philippinensis</u> MÜLL. ARG., Euphorbiaceae), which one detaches from the
fruits when one mashes them in a basket and when one rubs them with the
hands. This powder is formed from projecting glands, capitate, nearly
sessile, and with starry hairs, which have a resinous content of red
yellowish color. The powder contains up to 80% earth and debris of
leaves and stems. For this reason it was considered by the Arabic authors
as earth or manna which falls in Yemen and in India. In reality, this
powder has been known for a long time in the Oriental India where it has
the name of <u>kampila</u> or <u>kampilla</u> (Dymock) from where are derived the Arabic
names <u>qanbīl</u> and the European <u>kamala</u>. <u>Kampila</u> is derived from the Sanskrit
<u>kapila</u> (Chopra 338). See also Sir George Watt's <u>The Commercial Products
of India</u>, London 1908, p. 755-757. One has confused <u>quanbīl</u> with <u>wars</u>
(tinctorial powders of <u>Flemmingia rhodocarpa</u> BAK., see above number 123)
and here Maimonides confuses it with <u>dadi'</u>, the edible lichen (<u>Lecanora
esculenta</u> EV; see above number 86 and 96). Another Arabic name for
<u>kamala</u> is <u>wars hindi'</u>. <u>Kamala</u> serves as a purgative and antihelminthic.

328) <u>QĀTIL ABĪHI</u>   Strawberry-tree

<u>MAIMONIDES</u>:

It is <u>al-qadlab</u> and in ancient Greek one calls it <u>qāmāriyūn</u>; it is
the same which one calls <u>abariqun</u> and it is <u>manaquli</u> (fol. 97^v). It is
well-known, among all the physicians of the Maghrib, that this remedy is
the edible fruit which the people call "juice for the bears" (<u>asīr ād-dubb</u>)
and which the Berbers call <u>asāsra</u>. It is a fruit which resembles the
mulberry in terms of its volume and size, but it is redder than the jujube
(<u>al-'unnāb</u>); the tenderness of its substance is as that of the plum; it
has no stones.

MEYERHOF:

[Theophrastus III, 16; Dioscorides I, 122; Serapion 252; Ibn al-Beithar 1553, 1729 and 1807; 'Abd ar-Razzaq 515 and 751; Issa 19, 14; Loew I, 591 ff.]

The plant in question is the strawberry-tree (Arbutus Unedo L. Ericaceae) or "tree with strawberries". The name of the tree in Greek was komaros, that of the fruit, a beautiful spherical berry, memaikylon. Abārīqūn is perhaps a mutilation of the name ağdarhān which in Syria designates Arbutus Andrachne L. The other Arabic name is nearly always written qutlub. One eats the fruit of this tree. Its root was employed as astringent and tonic. The Berber name is given by 'Abd ar Razzaq and Tuhfa (97) in the form asāsnū or sāsnū which Renaud and Colin still heard in our times in Morocco (in Rabat). The Arabic name qātil abīhu ("his father's murderer") originates from the fact that its fruits do not dry out before the emergence of a new shoot of the plant. (Ibn al-Beithar 1729).

329) QASAB AD-DARĪRA   False sweet-flag

MAIMONIDES:

It is al-qalamās (kalamos), al-qamha and the "Persian reed" (al-qasab al-fārisī). Recent authors have claimed that the sweet-flag comes from foreign countries, from Persia, and not from India. And because people demanded much of it from a place other that its land of origin, that is India, and did not demand it from the country of its production, it was lacking in this region, and it was thought that it was lacking in its land of origin.

MEYERHOF:

[Theophrastus IX,7; Dioscorides I,18; Serapion 248; Ibn al-Beithar
1779; Tuhfa 349; 'Abd ar-Razzaq 756; Issa 5,6 and 176,4; Loew I, 692-694;
Dymock III, 569-571; Ducros 189.]

The Arabic name qasab ad-darīra signifies a "perfumed reed" and
corresponds to kalamos enodes of Theophrastus and kalamos aromatikos of
Dioscorides. The identification of this drug gave rise to very great difficulties, and the European botanists have discussed this question since the
16th century (see the commentaries of Berendes 25f. and 44f.). In the
Near-East, the druggists always confuse qasab ad-darira with wagg, the true
sweet-flat (Acorus Calamus L. see number 125). Eminent botanists, such as
Acherson, have tried to see Swertia Chirata HAM,in kalamos and qasab ad-darīra,
identified with qěně bosem of the Bible, a Gentianaceae. It is only since
1906 that Stapf seems to have found the plant and the drug in the "oily herb
of Rusa" (Andropogon or Cymbopogon Martini ROXB., Graminaceae), from which one
extracts two types of essences of Rusa: the essence of Palmerose and the
essence of Sofia. Concerning this plant and its products, see Sir George
Watt's The Commercial Products of India London, 1908, p. 451.

We have mentioned above that the rhizome of true sweet-flag is sold in
the bazaars of Cairo, erroneously under the name qasab ad-darīra. One should
reserve for it the other name of 'irk ekar which is derived from akoron.
In medicine, the false sweet-flag was employed as a stimulant, carminative
and antispasmodic, and it is still in usage in British India against the
rheumatisms and neuralgias. Concerning the Arabic name qamha or better
qumha, see below number 336 (qummuhān).

330) QARĀSIYĀ   Cherry, here sorb-apple

MAIMONIDES:

It is a type (of fruit) that resembles the plum but is much smaller, has
an acid taste and is widespread in Egypt and in Syria. It is not habb al-mulūk
("berries of kings") nor one of its species, as numerous authors have thought.

MEYERHOF:

[Theophrastus III, 2-15; Dioscorides I, 120; Ibn al-Beithar 1749; Tuhfa
334 and 436; 'Abd ar-Razzaq 737; Issa 148, 18 and 151,18; Loew III, 169-175.]

Qarāsiyā is the Arabic form of the Greek name kerasia. It designates the
cherry, fruit of the cherry tree, but here the fruit of the domestic sorb-
apple tree or service-tree (Pirus sorbus GAERTN.) which is widely prevalent
in Syria. The cherry-tree does not grow today in Egypt where its fruit is
imported from Syria, from Cyprus, from Anatolia, etc. The name habb al-mulūk
in Maghrib is the name given both to the cherry as well as the fruit of the
sebesten-tree (Cordia myxa L.) which grows in Egypt, where it is often taken
to be a yellow cherry. See Tuhfa (254) and the commentary of Renaud-Colin;
compare also above number 264 (Sabastān). Furthermore, one should note, that
Ibn 'Awwam (I, 316), under the name "Egyptian cherry" (qarāsiyā misriyya),
designates a small species of plum. For the fruit of the service-tree, Dozy
gives the Arabic-Egyptian synonym hawh ad-dubb ("bear peach") and the Arabic
synonym mas'a. The former signifies the fruit of the mandragora to Issa
(114,13). See below number 372 (sarāsiyā).

331) QATAF   Orache

MAIMONIDES:

It is as-sarmaq and one also says as-sarmag. It is that which one calls

the "vegetable of the Greeks" (baqlat-ar-Rūm) and "the golden vegetable"
(al-baqla ad-dahabiyya) and in Latin būlaš.

As to the plant (fol. 98^{z}) that the Arabs call as-sa'dān, it is one
of its species.

MEYERHOF:

[Theophrastus VII, 1-5; Dioscorides II, 119; Serapion 105; Ibn al-Beithar
1810; Tuhfa 363; 'Abd ar-Razzaq 141, 761 and 820; Issa 27,14; Loew I, 344 ff;
Ibn 'Awwam II, 153 ff.]

Qataf is the Arabic name, sarmak the Persian name (Vullers I, 98 and II,
286) of the garden orach (Atriplex hortensis L., Chenopodiaceae), culinary
plant to whose fruits one attributes laxative qualities. One also calls it
isfānāh rūmī ("Greek spinach") in Arabic, etc. The Arabic name "golden
vegetable" is the translation of the Greek word khrysolakhanon (Pseudo-
Dioscorides II, 119). I believe I can explain the "Latin" name būlaš by the
Spanish pollo or polluelo (Botica 965) which designates a chenopodiaceae related to orache, the herbaceous saltwort (Salicornia herbacea L.),known in
Egypt by the name qures. As to the name sa'dān, according to Issa (124,12)
and Loew (III,190), it designates a plant totally different from the Chenopodiaceae, the Rosaceous plant Neurada procumbens L., thorny desert plant.
Maimonides perhaps compared it to the Chenopodiaceae because many of the
latter are salty desert plants. See also Muhassas XI (155 in the middle),
where one finds the description of sa'dān which is related to qutb (qataf?).

332) QAR'   Pumpkin, gourd

MAIMONIDES:

It is ad-dubbā', and the people of Egypt know it by the name al-yaqtīn;
al-yaqtīn is al-fasag. It is all that does not elevate itself upon a stem and which
is perfectly round or approximately round, such as the coloquinth (al-hanzal),

the melon (al-bittīh), the gourd (al-qar') and similar fruits; all this is
called al-yaqtīn.

MEYERHOF:

[Theophrastus VII, 1-5; Dioscorides II, 134; Serapion 58 and 239;
Ibn al-Beithar 1752; Tuhfa 116 and 347; 'Abd ar-Razzaq 242; Issa 62, 13-14
and 104,2; Loew I, 542-548; Ibn 'Awwam II 226-235.*]

Renaud-Colin have discussed the question of the identification of
the names garʿ, dubbāʾand yaqtin. Ibn'Awwam, distinguished four species
of round or long gourds under the name gar and yaqtin. Among them are the
pumpkin, the calabash, etc. He also describes the cultivation of these cucurbitaceae and finds support therefore in several ancient authors. Regarding
the generic name yaqtīn, as Maimonides expounds it in conformity with the
Arabic (botanical) dictionaries, it designates the cucurbitaceae and other
plants witn creeping stems. It is for this reason that I think that the
word yaqtīn, which is not Arabic, was borrowed into Hebrew or Aramaic,
because the root of the word qaton is found in several Semitic languages
(Assyrian:qatānu) and has the sense of "being small, insignificant".
(See also Gesenius, Hebräisches und aramäisches Handwörterbuch, Leipzig s.v.).
From the botanical point ot view, garʿand dubbāʾ may designate Cucurbita
maxima DUCH. (pumpkin), Cucurbita Pepo L. (small round pumpkin) and
Lagenaria vulgaris SER. (calabash). For the different species of garʿ, see
Issa. The name I have rendered fašaġ is of uncertain spelling, because it
is lacking diacritical points. Fašaġ is the Arabic name of a thorny, climbing plant (Similax bona nox L., Liliaceae), according to Ibn al-Beithar
(1683). See also numbers 54, 98, 292 and 388 in this glossary.

* One should add to the bibliography the detailed study ot Arabic Cucurbitaceae
  by J.J. Clement-Mullet, Etudes sur les noms arabes de diverses familles de
  végétaux; in Journal Asiatique, 6th series vol. 15, 1870 p. 90-122.

333) QANTŪRYŪN   Centaury

MAIMONIDES:

There are two types, a small one and a large one. The small one
is the one which the people in Maghrib call buqūl al-hayyāt ("vegetable
of serpents"as well as qussat al-hayya ("serpent's tassel"), and in
Spanish ǧantūriya (cintoria, Simonet 162). The Arabs called it al-'aǧūr
and the Greeks also call it ǎǧīliyu.[*] Its ancient Greek name is qanturiyun
(kentaureion).[**]

As to the large type, it is the one which the Maghribians call
mukainasat Quraiǧ ("the small broom of Qurais").

MEYERHOF:

[Theophrastus VII, 9,5 etc.; Dioscorides III, 6-7; Ibn al-Beithar
1839-1840; 'Abd ar-Razzaq 78, 735-736; Tuhfa 333; Issa 44,15 and 78,2;
Loew I, 405 ff and I, 652.]

The small centaury of the Greeks and Arabs was most probably
Erythraea Centaurium PERS. (Gentianaceae), the large one, or officinal
centaury, Centaurea Centaurium L. (Compositae). The Arabic names of these
plants are, for the most part, well-known and mentioned by the (botanical)
dictionaries, except 'asur whose spelling is uncertain. For mukainasat
Quraiǧ, one finds in Dozy (II, 493), according to Ibn Biklaris, the name
miknasa quraǧiyya which has the same meaning ("Quraisite broom"). To
explain the "Greek" name aǧilːya, I propose the spelling aǧiāna which
corresponds to the Spanish aciano, name of the bluet (Centaurea cyanus L.)
(Botica 224). Simonet (267) found the spelling hiliya in Ibn Biklaris

* One considered here rather a mutilation of the Berber name arǧīqna or
arǧāqnu, cited by Ibn al-Beithar 49 and 'Abd ar-Razzaq 78. See the commentary.

** In the text an error of the copyist has saturiyun instead of qantūriyūn.

which he explains as a derivative of the Latin _fellea_ ("bitter as gall")
because of the bitter taste of the juice of the centaurium. In modern
Castilian it is called _hiel de tierra_ ("earth gall"). The modern Greek
name _ges khole_ meaning "earth gall" (Langkavel, p. 47) is not excluded.

334) QARDAMĀNĀ   Bastard cumin.

MAIMONIDES:

One also says qartamānā. It is the Greek caraway (al-karāwiyyā ar-
rūmiyya); it is a wild type of this plant as we have mentioned at letter kāf.

MEYERHOF:

Dioscorides III, 61; Serapion 100; Ibn al-Beithar 1747; _Tuhfa_ 340;
'Abd ar-Razzaq 745; Issa 104,4; Loew III, 439 ff; Ibn 'Awwam II, 244;
Ducros 179.

Arabic herbalists, translating the Greek authors, confused kardamon,
kardamomon and kyminon agrion and gave to the wild or bastard cumin
(Lagoecia cuminoides L., Umbelliferaceae) the Greek-Syrianized name qardamana.
Ducros erroneously gives this latter name to the lady's smock (Cardamine
pratensis L., Cruciferaceae), whose fruit is sold in the bazaars of Cairo
by the name of hurf ez-zarif. According to Hooker and Field (p.97), the
drug sold in Persia by the name qardamana is the Chaerophyllum sp.(Umbelliferaceae). See above number 195 (karāwiyā).

335) QASTAL   Chestnut

MAIMONIDES:

It is qastāniya (castana) and aš-šāh-ballūt.

MEYERHOF:

Theophrastus III, 2 to IV, 8; Dioscorides I, 106; Serapion 474; Ibn
al-Beithar 339 and 1270; _Tuhfa_ 452; 'Abd ar-Razzaq 183 and 981; Issa 43,3;
Loew III, 612-615.

Qastal is an Arabic form of the Greek kastania. In Maghrib one
writes qustāl. The name šāh-ballūt is Persian-Arabic and has the significance "royal acorn" by analogy with the Greek Dios balanos meaning
"acorn of Jupiter". Castana is the Spanish name (from the Latin castanea)
whose Arabic forms are varied (Simonet 110ff). It is the fruit of the
chestnut-tree (Castanea vulgaris LAM. or Castanea vesca GAERTN., Fagaceae)
which only grows in the northern regions of the Arabic world. The popular
name of the chestnut (imported from Europe) in Egypt is abū farwa ("doubled
fur") because of the double lining of the down of the seminal tegument.

336) QUMMUHĀN   False sweet-flag and varieties

MAIMONIDES:

It is ad-darira.

MEYERHOF:

[See the bibliography at number 329 (qasab ad-darira).]

Qummuhān, qummahān and qumha are, according to Lisan (III,400), three
Arabic names which may designate false sweet-flag (qasab ad-darira), as
Maimonides indicates. In addition, (it may designate) saffron (za'faran),
the red of Andrinople (wars) and an aromatic (tīb). Among the European
(botanical) dictionaries, Freytag (III, 495) translates qummahān as
Crocus, and Dozy (II, 403) as "sweet-flag".

337) QAISŪM   Southern-wood

MAIMONIDES:

It is a species of artemisia (šīh) with an aromatic odor. It is the
one called the "shepherd's tooth healer" (miswāk ar-rā'ī), in ancient
Greek abrotonon and in Spanish šarrīn. The Arabs (fol. 98) call it
'ubaitarān.

MEYERHOF:

[Theophrastus VI, 1-7; Dioscorides III, 24; Serapion 107; Ibn al-Beithar 1861 and 1510; 'Abd ar-Razzaq 675 and 771; Issa 21,20; Loew I, 379-384; Ibn 'Awwam I, 46; Dozy I, 753; Simonet 585.]

Qaïsum is the Arabic name ofthe Greek abrotonon. Dioscorides distinguishes a male abrotonon and a female abrotonon, and the Arabs have imitated him in believing in a qaïsum dakar and a qaisum intā. One identifies the former with the "male Southern-wood" (royal herb, citronnelle, Artemisia Abrotanum L.) and the latter with the "female Southern-wood", (lavender-cotton, small citronnelle, Santolina Chamaecyparissus L.) both of the Compositae family. The name miswāk ar-rā'ī is found in Ibn al-Beithar (2131) for Levisticum or Lepidium. It seems to me that there is here a copyist's error and that one should read habaq ar-rā'ī ("Shepherd's basilic"), generic Arabic name for the genus Artemisia. The "Arabic" name 'ubaïtaran (to the Bedouins bu'aïtaran or ba'ēterān) is undoubtedly a transformation of the Greek abrotonon. The "Spanish name šarrīn is the transcription of the Castilian sarrilla, generic name of the thymes and mints (Dozy I, 753; Simonet 585).

In Syria, the names qaïsum ǧabalī and bu'aïtarān today designate Achillea fragrantissima SCH.BIP. (Post II, 48). In Egypt, ba'ēterān is Artemisia judaica L. (Schweinfurth 53).

338) QUST   Costus

MAIMONIDES:

It is al-bustaǧ.

MEYERHOF:

[Theophrastus IX, 7,3; Dioscorides I, 16; Ibn al-Beithar 1785; Tuhfa 350; 'Abd ar-Razzaq 484 and 757; Issa 58,15; Loew I, 391÷393;

Dymock II, 296-303; Ducros 135.]

Qust is the Arabic form of the Greek name kostos which originates
from the Sanskrit kustha (Laufer 584); in Aramaic kŭṣṭā. Dioscorides distinguishes three types: an Indian, an Arabic and a Syrian. The name Costus
was given by botanists of the 16th century to a species of Zingiberacea.
Today, one identifies the kostos of the Greeks and the qust of the Arabs
with an Indian composita, Aucklandia Costus FALC. (or Saussurea Lappa
CLARKE), whose root which grows in the mountains of Kashmir was imported
by the Arabs into mediterranean countries. According to Sir George Watt
(The Commercial Products of India, London 1908, p. 980), the harvesting
of the root of the Saussurea Lappa is a state monopoly in Kashmir; it is
the government which sells this product abroad or to private contractors.
The Indian and "Arabic" Costus are thus the same drug, whereas one identifies
the Syrian Costus with elecampane (Inula Helenicum L.)(Issa 99,4). The
druggists of Cairo, under the name of qust hindī, sell large fragments
of a white or grayish root which Ducros has identified as that of the
Saussurea hypolenca SPR. Its aromatic odor reminds one of the carnation.
One employs it in fumigations, as an expectorant and as an antiasthmatic.
As to the name bustaǧ, it is the Arabic form of the Persian name bustak
which means very simply "incense" (also "resin", etc., Vullers I, 239).

339) QINA   Galbanum

MAIMONIDES:

It is the resin of the herb which in Spain is called al-baštanāqa
(pastinaca). This resin is also called 'asal al-qina ("galbanum honey")
and al-barzad.[*]

* in the text al-bāzard, a copyist's error

MEYERHOF:

[Theophrastus IX, 7,3; Dioscorides III, 83; Serapion 120; Ibn al-
Beithar 1841; Tuhfa 353; Issa 82,12; Loew III, 455-457; Ducros 191.]

Qina or better qinna is the Arabic name of the gum-resin called khalbane
by the Greeks. The latter name is Semitic. Biblical-Hebrew helbēna; Syriac
halbēnītā, that is "milky". It is the resin of several species of Ferula
(Umbelliferaceae), particularly Ferula galbaniflua BOISS.and BUHSE, or
Ferula rubricaulis BOISS, Ferula Schair BARSZ, etc. The majority of these
plants grow in Central and Oriental Persia, in Afghanistan, etc., from
where they were imported into Syria and Palestine. Bārzad is the Persian
name of the resin which forms brownish or greenish masses that are sold in
the bazaars of Cairo under the name qanna-wašaq (not to be confused with
wašaq meaning gum-ammoniac. See No. 124 above) for antiasthmatic fumigations. Pistanaca of the Latins,pastenaga of the Spanish (Simonet 430) was
the generic name of several umbelliferacea (Daucus, Peucedanum etc.) which
only furnished latex, but not gum-resin resembling galbanum.

340) QURRAT AL-'AĪN   Water-parsnip

MAIMONIDES:

It is also ġirġir al-mā' ("water-cress"). It is karafs al-mā'
("water-celery") and in Spanish qunāla (cunilla).

MEYERHOF:

[Dioscorides II, 127: Ibn al-Beithar 1751; Tuhfa 337; 'Abd ar-Razzaq
433 and 752; Issa 170, 11; Loew I, 510,]

The Arabic name qurrat al-ʲaīn signifies "freshness of the eye" and
is the equivalent of sion of Dioscorides which has been identified with
the umbelliferous plant Sium latifolium L. (water-parsnip, water-celery).
According to Ibn al-Beithar (656), since the middle ages, this plant has

been confused with gernūneš (meaning water-cress, Nasturtium officinale L.,
Cruciferaceae) to which the other Arabic names were also applied. See
above Number 162 (hurf) and the discussion of Renaud-Colin in Tuhfa. As
to the Spanish name, it is disfigured in the editions of Ibn al-Beithar
(qatāla). In Maimonides, we find the exact term which, according to
Simonet (146) who follows Ibn Biklaris, corresponds to the Castilian
name cunilla. In effect, it designates our plant, the aquatic celery.
It was used as a resolutive but is no longer employed in medicine at the
present time.

341) QITRĀN   Tar

MAIMONIDES:

It is an oil that one extracts from the cedar-tree (aš-šarbīn)that one
calls šabīn (fir tree) in Maghrib.

MEYERHOF:

[Theophrastus XI, 1,2; Dioscorides I, 77; Serapion 25,321 and 470;
Ibn al-Beithar 1317; Tuhfa 352 and 458; 'Abd ar-Razzaq 954; Issa 43,14;
Loew III, 30 ff.]

Qitrān or qatrān (from the Arabic root q.t.r. meaning "to drip") is
the vegetable tar obtained by the distillation of the wood of different
Coniferaceae. Maimonides cites the cedar-tree (šarbīn), but it may also
refer to the juniper (Juniperus Oxycedrus L.) or the cyprus (for example
Cupressus horizontalis GORD.), which is still today called sarbin in
Syria. By contrast,the Arabic-Spanish name šabīn or šabbīn (sapino) designates firs and pines (Abies pectinata DEC. oxud Pinus Picea L.,
Simonet 571). One should not confuse this name with šabīna which designates Juniperus Sabina L. (Simonet 572). The thorny question of the
different species of oil of the cedar and the tar was discussed by Renaud-
Colin in Tuhfa 150 and in other places.

342) <u>QALĪMĪYĀ</u>   Cadmia

<u>MAIMONIDES</u>:

One also says <u>iqlĪmiyā</u> and <u>qadmiyā</u>. It is the slag (<u>al-habat</u>, the
impurity) of all melting bodies.

<u>MEYERHOF</u>:

⎡Dioscorides V, 74; Ibn al-Beithar 1826; Tuhfa 354; 'Abd ar-Razzaq 47.⎤

The Arabic name is the corruption of the Greek <u>kadmeia</u>, probably passed
through Syriac (see Brockelmann, <u>Lex</u>. 668b). Maimonides, as certain more
recent Arabic authors (Dawud and 'Abd ar-Razzaq), take the word <u>qalĪmiyā</u>
in a very broad sense, excluding the natural cadmia which contains zinc,
iron, arsenic, etc. The artificial cadmias are the oxides of zinc, of
arsenic, etc., sublimated in furnaces, or formed on the surface of melting
massess. They were in usage, in ancient medicine, above all as ingredients
in dry collyria.

343) <u>QITTĀ</u>   Cucumber, melon, gourd

<u>MAIMONIDES</u>:

It is <u>as-sawāf</u> in the language of the Arabs. Its round species is
called ....*; <u>al-faqqūs</u> is the long species.

<u>MEYERHOF</u>:

⎡Serapion 58 and 106; Ibn al-Beithar 1739; <u>Tuhfa</u> 347; 'Abd ar-Razzaq
741; Issa 61, 17 and 62,5; Loew I, 530-538; Ibn 'Awwam II, 205-221.⎤

<u>Qittā</u> is a Semitic name (Assyrian <u>quiššu</u>; Hebrew-Mishnaic <u>quiššut</u>)
which designates primarily the cucumber, but also other Cucurbitaceae.
As Renaud and Colin have remarked in <u>Tuhfa</u>, the synonymy of the Cucurbitaceae
to the Greeks and Arabs is complicated and not yet sufficiently clarified.

* name lacking due to a copyist's error. See the commentary

In Egypt, the names qittā and faqqūs today designate varieties of melon
(Cucumis Melo L. var. Chate NAUD.),and faqqūs in particular a long and
curved form with grooved skin. The Arabic name sawāf for "cucumber" is
attested to by the Qāmūs (according to Freytag II, 377). The name of the
round species may be 'aggūr or 'abdillāwi, but this is not certain, because
today 'aggūr is a pointy melon. Cucumis Melo var. Chate was cultivated in
ancient Egypt (Loew according to Schweinfurth). See above number 292
('alqam) and below number 388 (hiyār).

344) QUNĀBARĀ   Uncertain

MAIMONIDES:

It is the plant which in Persian is called bargast and in Arabic qumlūl;
one says that it is al-usturgāz.

MEYERHOF:

[Ibn al-Beithar 1838; Issa 144,1]

The name qunābarā is of Syriac origin and is undoubtedly derived from
the Greek (Brockelmann 675b). The Arabic equivalent qumlūl (in Ibn al-Beithar
qumlūl and tumlūl, ? corruptions) is certified by the Qāmus (Freytag III, 502).
The Persian name bargast (Vullers I, 222) designates a vegetable resembling
spinach. All this is uncertain, as well as the identification by Sontheimer
of qunābarā as the leadwort (Plumbago europaea L.). In Syria, the name
qunnābarā or qunaïbrā is given to Lepidium Draba L., Cruciferae (Post I, 106).
If it was so in the Middle-Ages, why did not the Arabs identify qunābarā as
drabê of Dioscorides (II, 157)? The identification with usturgāz is erroneous; it is the name of the root of Asafoetida. Ghafiqi (ms. fol. 62b), on
this subject, states: "Asqlīnās (read asklepias).It is a plant we have

mentioned and discussed above. Hunain called it qunābira in his translation of the book of Galen on simple remedies. But al-qunabira is
something different. I have seen qunabira in many books and I think there
is an error here, since the description of al-qunabira is far from that of
asklepias." Later (fol. 102a), Ghafiqi states: "Bargast in Persian; this
is al-qunabira in Latin, and al-gumlul in Persian". The "Latin" or Spanish
name remind one of the Castilian cambronera which, however, designates a
Rhamnaceae. The name gumlul is purely Arabic, and is also found both in
Lisan (XIV, 21 line 5; cited according to Abu Hanifa ad-Dinawari) and in
Tag (VIII, 51 line 1 ff).

345) QALĪ   Alkaline ashes

MAIMONIDES:

It is the "alum of safflower" (šabb as-'usfur) and the "alum of
shoemakers" (šabb al-asākifa); one also calls it as-šarbarār. We have
already mentioned that it is the residue of the combustion of the vegetable soda (al-gāsūl).

MEYERHOF:

[Dioscorides V, 119; Ghafiqi 76; Serapion 515; Ibn al-Beithar 87
and 1828; Tuhfa 341; 'Abd ar-Razzaq 35; Issa 161,6; Loew I, 645 ff.]

Qallī, qalī or qilī is an Arabic name which designates the cinders
of alkaline plants. The French word alcali and the German word kalium
come from qalī. The principal plants which the Bedouins still use today
to extract the qali are the salt-wort (Salicornia fruticosa L., "sea
coral"), Suoeda fruticosa FORSK, and kali (Salsola Kali L.). It is a
product which substituted for and still substitutes for soap to the inhabitants of the desert.

The name šarbarār (perhaps mutilated by the copyist?) seems to be the Spanish sabonera, name of a halophyte plant of Alicantia. See number 24 above (ušnān). See also the important article Soda by A. Steiger and J.J.Hess in Vox Romanica II, Zurich and Leipsig 1937, p. 53-76.

346) QATT   Lucern

MAIMONIDES:

It is that which is called as-safsaf and al-fasfasa and 'alaf ad-dawābb ("fodder for beasts of burden") and al-qadb. The one which remains green is called ar-ratba ("the fresh one") and its name in Spanish is yarba da-mūla (yerba de mula), which means "herb of the mule" ('ušbat al-baġla).

MEYERHOF:

Theophrastus VIII, 7,7; Dioscorides II, 147; Serapion 18; Ibn al-Beithar 1684 and 1738; Tuhfa 359; 'Abd ar-Razzaq 2 and 612; Issa 116,4; Loew II, 463-465; Ibn 'Awwam II, 126 ff.

It is the lucern (Medicago sativa L., Leguminous plants), well-known fodder plant. It is the equivalent of the Greek Mêdike, name given because the plant came to the Greeks from Persia (Hehn p. 306). The Arabic names safsaf and fasfasa (or fisfasa) are derived from the Persian aspa-astī ("horse fodder") through the intermediary Syriac fasfisĕtā (Geoponics). This name is also found in Assyrian as aspastu (see G. Contenau's Drogues de Canaan, d'Amorru et jardins botaniques in Mélanges syriens offerts a M.R. Dussaud, p. 14). The Spanish name yerba de mula is found in Simonet (614). The modern Spanish name of lucern is alfalfa, derived from the Arabic al-nafal (name of the wild lucern Medicago ciliaris HOOK.). See also the following chapter (number 347:qurt) which deals with another leguminous fodder plant

related to lucern. It also has the Arabic names qatt and 'alaf. The
seed of the lucern was an astringent remedy in ancient times.

347) QURT   Alexandrian trefoil

MAIMONIDES:

It is the well-known plant (fol. 99^{k}) in Egypt that one gives to
beasts of burden as fodder, and which is called aš-šabdar; it is also
called al-barsīm.

MEYERHOF:

Serapion 190; Ibn al-Beithar 1759; 'Abd ar-Razzaq 710 and 782;
Issa 182,15; Loew II, 474; Ibn 'Awwam II, 127 ff; Ducros 18.

This plant is the Alexandrian trefoil (Trifolium alexandrinum L.,
Leguminous plants) which furnishes the fodder for beasts of burden in
Egypt during the winter. The name used in Egypt is barsim or birsīm.
(This name is probably of Coptic origin. See G.P. Sobhy in Bull. de l'Inst.
d'Egypte, vol. XX, 1938, p. 12). Šabdār is the Arabic form of the Persian
name šabdar, genetic name of trefoils or Trifoliaceae (Steingass 731).
The round or kidney-bean shaped reddish seed of barsīm baladī ("indigenous barsim") is sold in the bazaars of Cairo as a fortifiant and
tonic (Ducros).

348) QINNAB   Hemp

MAIMONIDES:

It is aš-šahrānağ; one also says šahdānağ al-barr ("wild hemp");
it is habb as-samna ("fattening seed" or "seed of fat").

MEYERHOF:

Dioscorides III, 148; Ibn al-Beithar 1845; Tuhfa 444; Issa 38,6-7;
Loew I, 255-263; Ducros 71.

The name qinnab originates from the Greek kannabis and designates hemp (Cannabis sativa L., Ulmaceae-Cannabinaceae). The Persian name is šāh-dāna ("seed of the king"), and both names in effect designate the seed of the hemp enclosed in the fruit (hemp-seed). The Arabic physicians do not often speak of the intoxicating effect of the resin of the female Indian type of the variety of Cannabis sativa. On this subject see M. Meyerhof "Hashish" in the supplement of the Encyclopedia of Islam. In Egypt, cultivated hempseed is sold by the druggists under the name habb at-tīl, as a nourishing and fortifying agent. One extracts the oil from hemp. The resin (hašīš, "herb") is clandestinely introduced as a narcotic to be smoked with tobacco, or consumed in electuaries (manzūl). A fierce strife is always in progress between the authorities and the contrabanders who carry out the illicit commerce in this drug.

349) **QUTN**   Cotton

MAIMONIDES:

It is al'utb and al-kursuf.

MEYERHOF:

Serapion 269; Ibn al-Beithar 1808; Issa 89,4; Loew II, 235-242.

Qutn is the Arabic name which passed into the European languages in the forms coton, cotton, kattun, etc. It is the cotton-bush (Gossypium herbaceum L. Malvaceae) and its product, cotton. The Arabic name "utb designates something marrowy. As to the name kursuf, I am following the opinion of Loew (II,236); that is, in final analysis, it is derived from the Sanskrit karpasa which also passed in Biblical Hebrew (karpas meaning "coton material, cotton cloth"). Ibn al-Beithar provides an additional half dozen names for cotton, discussion of which is beyond the scope of this brief commentary. In medicine, cotton served the Arabs, as it does for us, as material for dressing (wounds). See also Laufer (p.490 ff and 574).

CHAPTER RĀ'

350) **RĪBĀS**   Rhubarb-Currant; currant

MAIMONIDES:

It is that which is called aǧtiyālla in Spanish.

MEYERHOF:

[Serapion 418; Ibn al-Beithar 1072; 'Abd ar-Razzaq 803; Issa 155,22 and 156,16; Loew I, 357 ff.]

Rībās is considered the Arabic form of a Persian name rēvās, rīwās, rīwīz, rīwīǧ, rīwāǧ, etc. (see Vullers II, 88, 99 and 100). This name designates primarily the rhubarb-currant (Rheum Ribes GRONOV., Polygonaceae) as well as currant and the currant bush (Ribes rubrum L., Saxifragaceae). Here, as in Ibn al-Beithar, one is probably dealing with rhubarb-currant, drug whose use has disappeared. As to the Spanish name, it is found in Simonet (4) in the form aǧtiyālla (achethiella), derived from the Latin acetosella (in Castilian acetosilla and acederilla), which designates the sorrels (Rumex and Oxalis). I voluntarily admit the suggestion of M. Renaud that here the sourish taste of currant should make one use the same adjective that one does to the sorrel.

351) **RĀZIYĀNAǦ**   Fennel

MAIMONIDES:

It is that which the Egyptians call aš-šamār; but the Maghrīb calls it al-bisbās. Its Greek name is marathon.

MEYERHOF:

[Theophrastus VI, 1-2 etc., Discorides III, 70; Serapion 408; Ibn al-Beithar 1019; Tuhfa 358; 'Abd ar-Razzaq 186 and 775; Issa 84, 11; Loew III, 460-465; Ibn 'Awwam II, 250 ff; Ducros 136.]

The name rāziyānag̃ is the Arabic form of the Persian rāziyāna or rāziyām (Vullers II, 5) which designates the fennel or sweet anet and its species (Foeniculum vulgare MILL., Foeniculum capillaceum GILL., Foeniculum dulce BAUH., etc., Umbelliferaceae). The name šamār is still un usage in Egypt. It is ancient Semitic: Assyrian: šamrānu, šimru; Hebrew šummār; Aramaic šummārā; Arabic-Syrian šamra, šōmar, etc. The name bisbās for fennel is conserved in Maghrib, whereas in the oriental Arabic world it designates mace. The Greek name marathon was corrupted in the Latin Middle Ages into marathron. The fruits of the fennel in all times had the reputation of being a powerful carminative.

352) RĀTINAG̃   Resin

MAIMONIDES:

One also says rātīnā (rhêtine). It is the resin that the Maghribians call ragīna (resina) and the Egyptians qulfūniyā (colophony). It is that which one(also) calls zaft al-ġadāwā. It is the resin of the male pine (as-sanawbar ad-dakar) or the dry terebinth (ad-darw al-yābis). By contrast, the resin which in ancient Greek is called kolophonia, is the resin of the small pine (tannūb), and it is not al-qulfūniyā.

MEYERHOF:

[Dioscorides I, 71; Ibn al-Beithar 1021,1417, 1581; Tuhfa 357; 'Abd ar-Razzaq 779 and 787; Loew III, 42; Ducros 190.]

Rātīnag̃ is the Arabic-Persian form of the Greek word rhêtine meaning "resin". By this name one has designated primarily the resins of pine. However, at all times, there has been a certain confusion among the Greeks as well as the Arabs, as to the application of the name rhêtine which was sometimes a generic name. Qalafūniyā to the Egyptians is still, in our times, the name of different types of resin, but above all that of the terebinth resin (Ducros). According to Renaud-Colin, this same name is applied in Morocco to the dry residue of the resin, after distillation. I cannot explain the name zaft (or zift) al-gadāwā (or 'adārā, "pitch of virgins or young lads" or qadārā, "of prostitutes") which one encounters in no other place.

Among the names of trees, sanawbar dakar probably designates Pinus orientalis LINK. (see above chapter 318, sanawbar). Darw yābis is a type of terebinth, and tannūb is the false-fir (Picea excelsa LINK) or another coniferacea with small cones. The name of the colophony of the Greeks is derived from the Ionian city Colophon on the coast of Asia-Minor, from where the resin was imported into Greece (Dioscorides). It is probable that this colophony was the residue of the distilled terebinth of Chio. In our days, one extracts the colophony from the terebinth, above all in the vicinity of Bordeaux, in the waste lands of Gascony, from oily-resinous drainage obtained from the incision of the trunks of Pinus Pineaster SOL.

353) RĀSIN (SIC)   Large Elecampane

MAIMONIDES:

It is the "ginger of Syria" (az-zangabīl aš-šāmī).

MEYERHOF:

[Theophrastus IX, 11,1; Dioscorides I, 28; Serapion 280; Ibn al-Beithar 1017; Tuhfa 356; 'Abd ar-Razzaq 230, 303, 470 and 802; Issa 99,4; Loew I, 421-424; Ducros 155; Ibn 'Awwam II, 303-305.]

The vocalization in usage of this name is rāsan. It is a Persian name which designates the large elecampane (Inula Helenium L., Compositae).

Its Greek name is <u>panakes cheironeion</u> in Theophrastus, and <u>Helenion</u> in Dioscorides. This drug is the thick and fleshy underground portion of the stem (not the root, as Ducros claims). It is aromatic, tonic and stimulant. The plant grows in all of central and southern Europe and in central and western Asia. In Egypt, the druggists sell the dried, brown and wrinkled stem under the name <u>'irq el ganāh</u>. It is recommended by Ibn 'Awwam as a remedy against strangury.

354) <u>RA''ĀD</u>   Electric Ray

<u>MAIMONIDES</u>:

It is the benumbing fish well-known in Egypt; it is the "aquatic scorpion" (<u>aqrab al-mā'</u>).

<u>MEYERHOF</u>:

[Dioscorides II, 15; Serapion 403; Ibn al-Beithar 1047; 'Abd ar-razzaq 804.]

Under the name <u>narkê</u>, Dioscorides described an electric marine fish which has the property of making (a person) numb. Pliny (IX) describes it by the name <u>torpedo</u> and enunciates its different usages in medicine (XXXII). It is the electric numb-fish of the Mediterranean (<u>Torpedo Narce</u> RISSO). The Egyptian fish of which Maimonides here speaks, is the electric silure of the Nile (<u>Malapterurus electricus</u> LACÉPÈDE). The Arabic name <u>ra''ād</u> ("the thundering one") is imprecisely applied to all electric fish. The electric catfish is also called <u>ra"āš</u> ("trembler") in Egypt, and in the Sudan <u>barrāda</u> (Malouf 156). The Egyptian ad-Damiri seems to have omitted this Egyptian fish in his big (book of)zoology. By contrast, Kohen mentions it twice: firstly (p. 129, line 14) under the names <u>ra''ād</u> or <u>hūt Mūsā</u> ("fish of Moses", name today reserved for Sole and other

- 250 -

Mediterranean Pleuronectides). A little further (p. 139, line 17) Kohen
states: "Aqrab al-mā' (the "water scorpion"). It is ar-ra''ād and hūt
Mūsā. If you take it in the hand, you tremble and become benumbed until
you throw the fish away, and then you will be healed. Exalted is the
Creator who did not create anything that is deprived of utility or
noxiousness. It was believed that the noxiousness was not indispensible,
but it is required for treatment." As a consequence, the "electric"
treatment of certain ailments by means of this fish was in vogue in
the 13th century. During antiquity (Galen, Dioscorides), and in Persia
(Ibn Sina I, 432), one applied the electric ray on the head to cure
cephalalgia and epilepsy, and the oil in which the electric ray was
boiled was employed against rheumatism. Today, one no longer makes use
of this animal in medicine.

355) RATA   Bonduc-nut

MAIMONIDES:

It is the "Indian hazel-nut" (al-bunduq al-hindī). It is that which
one calls atmat.

MEYERHOF:

[Ibn al-Beithar 358 and 1028; Ghafiqi 102; Issa 35,16; Dymock I,
496-499.]

Rata is the Arabic form of the Persian name rata or ritta (Vullers
II, 22) which designates the bonduc-nut, or the seed of Caesalpinia
(Guilandina) Bonducella FLEM. (Leguminous plants). I suppose the Persian
name is derived from the Indian. In Hindoustani it is rithā which designates another drug somewhat resembling the bonduc-nut, the fruit of the

soapberry-tree (<u>sapindus trifoliatus</u> L., Sapindaceae). The <u>Caesalpinia</u> <u>Bonducella</u> is an Indian tree known today on the coasts of all tropical countries. The seeds ("dunce's eyes") of the thorny plant are brown and contain a resin, tannin, and a bitter substance. They were much in use in   British India (Honigberg 285 ff) against ailments of the spleen, and are even included in the Anglo-Indian pharmacopoeia. The seeds of a related species <u>Caesalpinia Bonduc</u> ROXB. are gray (See G. Watt <u>The Commer-</u> <u>cial Products of India</u>, London 1908, p. 191). In the bazaars of Cairo, Ducros (p. 137) found hazel-nuts under the name <u>bunduq hindi</u>. I cannot explain the name <u>atmat</u> which is probably of Sanskrit origin. According to Laufer (581), it designates the seeds of the Indian Lotus (<u>Nelumbium</u> <u>speciosum</u>).

356) <u>RĀZĀQI</u>   Jasmine oil

MAIMONIDES:

It is the oil of jasmine (<u>al-yāsimin</u>); it is that which is called az-zanbaq in Maghrib.

MEYERHOF:

[Serapion 290 and 530; Ibn al-Beithar 895, 916, 1024 and 1129; <u>Tuhfa</u> 138; 'Abd ar-Razzaq 295 and 421; Issa 101, 11 and 109,2; Loew II, 160 ff.]

The Arabic name <u>rāzaqī</u> or <u>rāziqī</u> may designate a type of small grape, the white lily, the jasmine and the oil one extracts therefrom (see Ibn al-Beithar in four places and Dozy I, 524). <u>Zanbaq</u>, Arabic form of the Persian name <u>zanba</u>,also has the meaning "white lily" and "jasmin". Here Maimonides clearly states that he refers to the oil of jasmine (extracted from <u>Jasminum officinale</u> L. or from <u>Jasminum Sambac</u> ÁITCH., Oleaceae). Ibn al-Beithar (1129) states that it is the oil of sesame in which one preserved (the flowers) of the jasmine. The ancients did not know jasmine oil; the pertinent passages in the work of Dioscorides are apocryphal.

357) <u>RAWSAHTAĞ</u>   Burned copper

<u>MAIMONIDES</u>:

   It is burned copper (<u>an-nuhās al-muhraq</u>) which the people in
Maghrib call <u>hadīd al-harqūs.</u>

<u>MEYERHOF</u>:

   [Dioscorides V, 76; Ibn al-Beithar 1071 and 2217; 'Abd ar-Razzaq
383 and 778.]

   <u>Rawsahtağ</u> is the Arabic form of the Persian name <u>rō-suhta</u> or <u>rōy-suhta</u>
("calcinated or burned copper", Vullers II, 74) and the translation from
the Greek <u>khalkos kekaumenos</u>. <u>Harqūs</u> or <u>halqūs</u> which, according to Dozy
I, 317, was the name of calcinated copper in the Maghrib, is also de-
rived from the Greek <u>khalkos</u>. <u>Hadīd</u> here appears to mean the "causticity"
of burned copper. This substance, both to the Greeks and Arabs, played
a major role in the composition of certain dry collyria against trachoma
and corneal specks in the eyes. Leclerc ('Abd ar-Razzaq 778) observed
the medical use of this impure copper sulfide in Algeria.

- 253 -

CHAPTER ŠÍN

(fol. 99ᵛ)

358) SĀHTĪRAǦ   Fumitory

MAIMONIDES:

It is the "coriander of the fox" (kazburat at-ta'lab) and one
also says the "wild coriander" (al-kazbur al-barrī) and in Spanish
ǧinšīla (cenicilla). It is qulintruāla (culiantrolo). It's Greek name
is gingidion and kapnos.

MEYERHOF:

[Dioscorides IV, 109; Serapion 452; Ibn al-Beithar 1264; Tuhfa 440;
'Abd ar-Razzaq 942; Issa 85,7; Loew I, 651; Ibn 'Awwam II, 313.]

Šāhtīraǧ or šāhtaraǧ are Arabic forms of the Persian šāh-tara or
šāh-tarra (Vullers II, 394) which has the meaning "king of vegetables"
and designates fumitory ("earth gall, hen's leg", Fumaria officinalis L.,
Fumariaceae). The Spanish names are found explained in Simonet (158 and
146); cenicilla is the Castilian name for certain parasitic plants;
culantrillo is the modern Castilian diminutive of culantro (coriander).
Kapnos ("smoked") is, in effect, the Greek name of fumitory, but gingidion
is the name of the gummiferous carot (Daucus Gingidium L., Umbelliferaceae).
There is here an error on the part of the author, perhaps confusion with
šītaraǧ, name of the large pepperwort (Lepidium latifolium L. Cruciferaceae
see below number 347). Fumaria officinalis was used in the Middle-Ages
against maladies of the digestive tract. The plant and the fruits are
still in usage today in   India and in Afghanistan as a laxative and
diuretic (Hooper & Field, p. 121).

359) ŠAQĀYIQ   Anemone

MAIMONIDES:

It is šaqāyiq an-Nu'mān and aš-šaqir. It is that which the Berbers
call takard, and its Greek name is anemônê. There is a cultivated species

and one with white blossoms.

MEYERHOF:

[Theophrastus VI, 8 and VII, 7; Dioscorides II, 176; Serapion 277; Ibn al-Beithar 1329; Tuhfa 441; 'Abd ar-Razzaq 106 and 941; Issa 17,6; Loew III, 118 ff; Ducros 138.]

The orientalists are not in agreement on the Arabic designation of this plant which is, for the most part, the anemone with the color of blood (Anemone coronaria L., Ranunculaceae), abundant in Syria and in Palestine. Some derive the Arabic name Nu'man from the Greek anemône; others, on the contrary, attribute an Arabic origin to the Greek name. Some translate šaqāyiq (or šaqā'iq) an-Nu'man as "the sisters of King Nu'man"; others (Lagarde, Casanova) as "bloody wounds of Adonis" (see Renaud-Colin in Tuhfa). The Berberic name was corrupted by an error of a copyist; it should be tikūk (Tuhfa). Trabut (Répertoire des noms indigènes des plantes etc., Algier 1935, p. 105) applies the name tikoukt to the small centaury (Erythraea Centaurium PERS.). The juice of the plant and its decoction are still in usage as a collyrium against corneal specks and cataracts. The dried flower is sold by the druggists of Cairo (Ducros).

360) ŠĀH-ŠUBRUM   Small basilic

MAIMONIDES:

One also says šāh-šafram. It is a species of basilic (habaq) with small leaves, and it is the one known as "basilic of Kirman" (al-habaq al-kirmānī.

MEYERHOF:

[Serapion 454; Ibn al-Beithar 1268; Tuhfa 443; 'Abd ar-Razzaq

970; Issa 126,10; Loew II, 81 ff; Ducros 112.⌉

Šāh-šubrum, šāh-šafram, etc. are Arabic transformations of the
Persian name šāh-asparagm (itself transformed into neo-Persian as
šāh-isparam, šāh-isfaram, etc., Vullers II, 393) which has the meaning
"king of fragrant plants". Originally it designated the large basilic
(Ocimum Basilicum L., Labiates). The translation of this Persian name
into Greek furnished the name basilikon ("the royal"), which is only
found in (the writings of) Byzantine physicians (Aetius, 6th century,
and Simeon Seth, 11th century). To the Arabs, it designates a species
of basilic with small leaves, as Maimonides states, probably above all
Ocimum minimum L., which also has the name dawmarān or daïmarān. Kirman
is a vast province of southern Persia. I did not find the small basilic
at the druggists in Cairo.

361) SAQĀQIL   Sea holly, parsnip and others

MAIMONIDES:

It is that which is called qunīla in Spanish; one also says šaǧ-
mīla. In certain countries it is called the "wild carrot" (al-ǧazar al-barrī).

MEYERHOF:

⌈Serapion 449; Ibn al-Beithar 1330; Tuhfa 445; 'Abd ar-Razzaq 946;
Issa 135,47; Loew III, 450.⌉

The origin of the name saqāqil (or saqāqul) is not clear. The
ancient forms that one encounters in Syriac (hasqīqalā) and in Arabic
(hasqāqul and šašqāqul) speak in favor of a Persian origin. This name
designates umbelliferous plants with edible roots. The Arabic name was
given to Pastinaca Schekakul (synonym Pastinaca dissecta VENT.) and to

Malabaila Sekakul RUSS. Others argue in favor of Eryngium campestre L.
(panicaut) which still had the name seqaqul in Egypt in the 18th century (Forskal). The Arabic name ğazar-barrī ("wild carrot") designates
the beet (Beta vulgaris L.), species of carrot, and the wild anet (Meum),
as well as other umbelliferaceae.

As to the Spanish names, the first corresponds perhaps to the
Castilian cunilla (Simonet 146), from the Greek konilē; the second, according to a communication from M. Renaud, is a faulty spelling for
šahmālla (Simonet 575 xahamiella), name of obscure origin.

362) SUKĀ‘Ā   Cotton thistle and others

MAIMONIDES:

It is the "shepherd's needle" (ibrat ar-rā‘ī) and the "prickling
musk" (misk al-hidda), as well as the "monk's needle" (ibrat ar-rāhib),
the "foreign thorn" (aš-šawka al-barrāniyya), al-karī‘a and al-kunğur;
one also says al-kunkur. In Berber it is tāfrūt.

MEYERHOF:

[Theophrastus VI, 4,3; Dioscorides III, 12; Ghafiqi 26; Serapion
477; Ibn al-Beithar 1335; Tuhfa 457; 'Abd ar-Razzaq 104; Issa 128, 6;
Loew I, 445.]

The Arabic name šukā‘ā (or šukā‘ī) designates different species
of thistles. According to Issa, it is the wild prickly artichoke or
cotton thistle (Onopordum Acanthium L., Compositae). Kunkur and kunğur
are Arabicized Persian names which designate the artichoke (Cynara
Scolymus L., Compositae), whereas ibrat-ar-rā‘ī and ibrat ar-rāhib are
names of geranium. Tāfrūt, according to a personal communication from
M. Renaud, is a Berberic name which does not designate thistles but the
gladiolus. Nevertheless, Trabut (Répertoire des noms indigènes des plantes,

etc. Algiers 1935, p. 57) gives <u>tafront</u> as the name of a thistle,
<u>Carduncéllus pinnatus</u>.

363)   SABAT   Anet

<u>MAIMONIDES</u>:

    It is <u>as-sanūt</u> and <u>as-samāl</u>. It is that which is called <u>aslīlī</u>
in Berber.

<u>MEYERHOF</u>:

    [Theophrastus VII,1-6; Dioscorides III, 58; Serapion 523; Ibn al-
Beithar 1275; <u>Tuhfa</u> 453; 'Abd ar-Razzaq 949; Issa 17,10; Loew III,466 ff;
Ibn 'Awwam II, 312 ff.]

    <u>Šabat</u> is the vulgar form of the Arabic name <u>šibit</u> or <u>šibitt</u> which
designates anet ("stinking fennel"), <u>Anethnam graveolens</u> BENCH & HOOK.,
Umbelliferaceae. This name is ancient Semitic: Assyrian <u>šibittu</u>; Aramaic
<u>sibita</u>; Hebrew-Mišhnaic <u>šebēt</u>. The Arabic name <u>sanūt</u> or <u>sannūt</u> for anet
is confirmed by the <u>Qamus</u>, according to Freytag II, 362. It simultaneously
designates two other Umbelliferacea with edible seeds: fennel (Freytag, ibid,)
and cumin (Issa 62,18). <u>Samāl</u> is perhaps a corruption caused by a copyist.
Dr. Renaud proposes that <u>as-sasāl</u> means seseli,whereas I would rather think
of <u>bisbās</u>, name which in Maghrib designates numerous umbelliferous plants
related to fennel. The Berber name <u>aslīlī</u> is exactly rendered (Renaud).

364)   SAĞARAT MARYAM   Cyclamen (sow-bread)

<u>MAIMONIDES</u>:

    It is that which one calls <u>faqlāmīnus</u> (kyklaminos, cyclanen), and it
is <u>qālibsīt</u>. It is not <u>bahūr Maryam</u>, as (fol. 180^R) many physicians think.

<u>MEYERHOF</u>:

    [Theophrastus IX,9; Dioscorides II, 164-165; Serapion 520; Ibn al-Beithar
354; 1307, 2051; <u>Tuhfa</u> 1,25,62,89,233 and 304; 'Abd ar-Razzaq 5 and 53; Issa
63,12; 15, 6; 48, 6; 63,12 and 115,12; Loew I, 288 and III,77; Ducros 153.]

Šaǧarat Maryam ("tree of Mary ") is an Arabic name common to
several plants, Cyclamen, Parthenium, Vitex, Cachrys, etc., etc.
We have seen earlier (number 55) that the name buhūr (or bahūr) Maryam
("incense of Mary ") also designates numerous plants, particularly motherwort. By the name šaǧarat Maryam, Maimonides both here and in number 55,
designates the cyclamen (Cyclamen europaeum L., Primulaceae) which, however, is called bahūr Maryam by other Arabic authors. Its root has the
Syriac name ʿartanītā. The tubercle of motherwort (Leontice Leontopetalum L.
Berberidaceae) resembles the one of the cyclamen; it is for this reason
that the rhizomes and the plants were often confused by the druggists.
In the bazaars of Cairo, the two rhizomes are sold under the name raqaf
(Acherson, Zeitschr, des Deutsch.Palästinavereins XII, p. 155).

Qālibsīt is certainly a name mutilated by a copyist, perhaps
Galeopsis. However, the name Galeopsis is not in its place in this paragraph.

365) SŪNĪZ   Nigella

MAIMONIDES:

It is aš-šamīt, aš-šaibartar, aš-šašmar and the "black cumin"
(al-kammūn al-aswad); one also calls it the "black seed" (al-habba as-sawdā').

MEYERHOF:

[Dioscorides III,79; Serapion 521; Ibn al-Beithar 1351; Tuhfa 454;
'Abd ar-Razzaq 362 and 948; Issa 125,3; Loew III,120-123; Ducros 203]

Sūnīz is a Persian name (Vullers II, 482) sometimes transformed into
Arabic as siniz. In addition, one encounters the synonym sānuǧ in the
popular language of Maghrib. It designates cultivated nigella or black
seed (Nigella sativa L., Renonculaceae), plant cultivated in the Orient
for its seeds ("black cumin") which were known to the Greeks under the name
melanthion and to the Hebrews under the name

qesah. It is strange that Maimonides does not mention the name most used in
Egypt: habbat al-baraka, meaning "seed of benediction", because it is given
to women after parturition and as a tonic. The first three names of our
article were corrupted by the copyists. I recognize in aš-šamīt the ximente
of Simonet (596); in Castilian one should read simiente maura (=negra)
or"black seed". The mutilated word šaïbartar has perhaps the same significance. The third name probably reads šišm or šišmaq, popular Egyptian
name, derived from the Persian čašm ("eye") and common to (both) black seeds
of nigella and of Cassia Absus L. (Leguminous plants).

366)   SUBRUM   Euphorbia

MAIMONIDES:

We have already explained that it belongs to the plants with latex
(al-yuttū'āt) and its name in Spanish is lahtarwāla,* which signifies "the
milky one" (al-labaniyya). Its name in Berber is tānāgat and its Greek
name is qālīqūn.

MEYERHOF:

[Dioscorides IV, 165; Serapion 456; Ibn al-Beithar 1276; Tuhfa 449;
'Abd ar-Razzaq 951; Issa 80,6; Loew I, 605.]

Šubrum is the Arabic vocalization of the Persian name šibram which
designates Euphorbia Pithyusa L., euphorbia with an irritating, evacuant
and hydragogic latex,and related types. See above number 178. The
mutilated Hispanic name should be read lahtaïruwala, in Latin lactariola,
in modern Catalanian lleterola (Simonet 290) meaning "small milky one",
in Arabic lubanïna. The Berber name is rendered tānāgat by Ibn al-Gazzar
(Dozy I, 140). The Greek name is probably a mutilation of paralion,
another name for pityousa, or of fāfliyūn (peplion), name given by
Dioscorides (IV,168) for Euphorbia Peplis L. One also considered the Latin-

* in the text bahtarwala, mutilation of the name by the copyist

Hispanic name calcarium to be a euphorbe of the species šubrum (Simonet 74).

367) ŠĪTARAG̃   Leadwort and pepperwort

MAIMONIDES:

It is al-'ussāb and in Spanish balīsā. It is that which is called
a'ras and asrīs as well as lepidion.

MEYERHOF:

⌈Dioscorides II, 174; Serapion 460; Ibn al-Beithar 1369; Tuhfa 442;
'Abd ar-Razzaq 672-943; Issa 107,12 and 144,1; Loew I, 505 ff and III,68ff;
Dymock II, 329-340.⌉

The majority of authors identify the name šītarag̃ with the lepidion
of the Greeks, and modern botanists consider it the pepperwort (Lepidium
latifolium L. Cruciferaceae). Several (Vullers, Dozy, Loew) confuse this
name with šāhtirag̃ (fumitory; see above number 358). Nevertheless,
Freytag has already explained, following Qamus, that the name šītarag̃ is
derived from the Indian čītrag̃. In effect we find in Dymock that the
Sanskrit name čītraka designates different species of Indian leadwort
(Plumbago rosea L., Plumbago zeylanica L., etc.) This name must have
passed into Arabic through Persian. It was then transferred to pepperwort
which also shares several Arabic names ('ussāb, g̃awz̃ar-ru'yān,and hāmīsa)
with leadwort (Plumbago europaea L.) Finally, we should note that the
Spanish name balīsa (Simonet 29) is preserved in modern Castilian (velesa
and belesa; Botica 1111) as the name for leadwort. The two names without
Arabic prefixes, a'ras and asrīs, are also probably Hispanic, corresponding to iberis (Lepidium Iberis; Simonet 269) or perhaps hirsuta
(in Simonet 271). Kohen (p. 122 line 6) also has the spelling a'ras.

The roots of Plumbaginaceae are still used in   India   against all
sorts of maladies. Pepperwort has fallen into oblivion; it is no longer
sold in the bazaars of the Near-East.

368) ŠABB   Alum

MAIMONIDES:

One also calls it the "white vitriol" (az-zāǧ al-abyad) and the
"humid alum of Yemen" (aš-šabb ar-ratib al-yamānī). Aš-šabb ad-dawr
is the Egyptian alum.

MEYERHOF:

[Dioscorides, V, 106; Serapion 448; Ibn al-Beithar 1279; 'Abd ar-
Razzaq 962-964.]

The Arabic name šabb (from the root š.b.b."to light, to burn") designates alum (disulfate of alumina, potash, ammonia etc.). It was well
known to the Greeks by the name styptêria, and to the ancient Egyptians,
because it is found in abundance in the raw state in the deserts of
Egypt. The one in Yemen had the best reputation to the Arabs. The name
šabb dawr, in my opinion, perhaps designates a raw alum in the form of
round masses that one finds in Egypt. One uses it for the preparation of
dry collyria. Kohen (p. 135, line 5) has the spelling šabb mudawwar
("rounded alum") according to Ibn Gulgul who explains that it referred to
a white and round alum imported from Tripolitania into Spain.

369) ŠADANA   Hematite

MAIMONIDES:

One also says šādinaǧ. It is the "stone of Tor" (haǧar at-Tūr) and
the "stone of blood" (haǧar ad-dam).

MEYERHOF:

[Dioscorides V, 126; Serapion 450; Ibn al-Beithar 1267; 'Abd ar-Razzaq 356; Ducros 132.]

Šādana, šādina and šādinaǧ are the Arabic forms of the Persian name šādana (Vullers II, 384) which designates the hematite (haïmatitês lithos) of the Greeks. Ṭūr or Ṭūr Sīnā' is the Arabic name of Sinai from where, in effect, comes the hematite (a sesquioxide of iron) since antiquity. The ancient Egyptians manufactured beetles, styles for collyria and figurines with these minerals. In medicine, one still uses hematite in ocular ointments and interiorly as a styptic against hemorrhages.

370) ŠAǦARAT AL-KALAB   Madwort and diverse(plants)

MAIMONIDES:

It is the herb one calls ǧamliǧ in Spanish.

MEYERHOF:

[Dioscorides III, 91; Ghafiqi 38: Ibn al-Beithar 1 and 1295; Issa 11,10; Loew I, 468 ff and 473 ff.]

The Arabic name šaǧarat al-kalab has the meaning "herb against the rage; antirabies". It is the translation of the Greek alysson, plant described by Dioscorides, but until now not sufficiently identified. This name was given to the genus Alyssum (Cruciferaceae) and in particular to Alyssum saxatile L.(yellow allyssum). Others have thought it is Farsetia clypeata R. BR. (Cruciferaceae) or Marrubium Alysson L. (Labiates). Unfortunately the Hispanic name ǧamliǧ or ǧamlōǧ has not been well identified. In our text the word hamlīh is an error. The Arabic authors sometimes have ǧamlaǧ, ǧamlūǧ and ǧamlāǧ (Freytag). Simonet (154) derives the name ǧamlōǧ from khamailykos of Pseudo-Dioscorides (IV,60), name of a species of vervain. Freytag (I,308) and

Dozy (I,219) see, in the name gamlig, the hemp-nettle (Galeopsis L.,
Labiates), following Arabic physicians in this deduction. Simonet (153)
writes chamelocho, following Ibn Gulgul, who was the first to mention this
Spanish name.

The "antirabies herb" is no longer sold in the bazaars of the Orient;
its use has fallen into oblivion and one can no longer identify it.

371) SARĀSIYĀ   Cherry

MAIMONIDES:

One also says ǧarāsiyā. It is the fruit known in Maghrib by the name
of "seed of kings" (habb al-mulūk) and one also calls it šāh-dawrān.

MEYERHOF:

[Dioscorides I, 113; Serapion 441; Ibn al-Beithar 480 and 1749; Tuhfa
334; 'Abd ar-Razzaq 225 and 737; Issa 148, 18; Loew III, 169-175; Ibn 'Awwam
I, 248-250.]

The first names are transcribed from the Greek kerasia which passed
into Syriac and Arabic in the form qarāsiyā. According to Ibn al-Beithar,
garāsiyā is the Sicilian pronunciation. According to Simonet (160), šarāsiyā
is the ancient Hispanic form. In modern Castilian it is cereza. They designate the cherry, fruit of the Prunus Cerasia Br. (Rosaceae). Habb al-mulūk
in Maghrib is the name of the cherry, but also of the fruits of the plum
tree, the croton, the spurge and the curcas. Šāh-dawrān is a Persian name
which is lacking in the (botanical) dictionaries. Perhaps it should be
šāh-dāna ("seed of a king") or šāh-wār ("worthy of a king")? Šadurwān or
šadirwān is, according to Vullers (II, 383), the Persian name of a carpet
or curtain which covers the door of the royal palace. Šadurwān or

siāh-dawārān is, to Serapion (429) and 'Abd ar-Razzaq (838 and 862),

a gum   which furnished a black coloring material.See above number 330

(qarāsiyā).

372) SĬBRIQ   Rush, convolvulus, ononis

MAIMONIDES:

It is that which one calls yarba barnīya in Spanish. It is the rush

(al-asal).

MEYERHOF:

[Theophrastus IV,12; Dioscorides I,17; Ibn al-Beithar 1282; Tuhfa 22;
'Abd ar-Razzaq 85; Issa 56,16 and 102,9.]

The name šibriq is Arabic; its significance is uncertain. Maimonides

identifies it with asal,Arabic name of several rushes (Juncus acutus L.,

Juncus arabicus POST, etc.), but I believe this is an error because Abu

Hanifa ad-Dinawari, whose article is preserved in its entirety in Muhassas

(XI, 165), states that this plant resembles rush. He continues by stating

that šabāriq are slender plants having leaves harsh to the touch,and a hard

wood from which amulets are made for cattle. Issa gives the name šibriq

to a convolvulus (Convolvulus Hystrix V.). In effect, according to Fleischer

(Studies on the Supplement to the Arabic Dictionaries of Dozy, in Berichte der

phil.-histor. Klasse der Kgl. Saechs Gesellsch.der Wissensch III, Leipzig 1884,

p.2), Sweinfurth found the name šibriq in Palestine for Ononis antiquorum L.

(Papilionaceae), in Egypt for Convolvulus Hystrix. Also Post (I,305 and II,

203) marked the name šibriq or šibrug in Palestine for the two plants in

question. This name, therefore, in any event, designates a plant armed with

prickles. I propose to spell the Spanish name yerba barrina meaning "tendrilled

herb" (Simonet 38) which would mean that the plant in question has pointed

ends or (the form of) a corkscrew. The modern Castilian word for "tendril"

is barrena. In French the small field liseron (Convolvulus arvensis L.)
also has the name tendril.

373) SABAH   Brass

MAIMONIDES:

It is the yellow copper (an-nuhās al-asfar).It is so called because
of its resemblance to gold.

MEYERHOF:

⌈Dioscorides V, 75; Ibn al-Beithar 1283; 'Abd ar-Razzaq 965.⌉

Brass was described by Dioscorides under the generic name khalkos,
"bronze". It was very well-known during the Arabic era.Ibn al-Beithar
calls it šabahān, a name which, like šabah or šibh, signifies "resemblence".
Ibn al-Beithar cites Ibn Gulgul who states that natural brass was found in
Khorassan (Eastern Persia) and one uses its filings in the preparation of
certain collyria.

374) SĪR-AMLAǦ   Preserved emblic

MAIMONIDES:

It is emblic (fol. 100ᵛ)   preserved.

MEYERHOF:

⌈Serapion 71 and 171; Ibn al-Beithar 145 and 1379; Tuhfa 43 and 126;
'Abd ar-Razzaq 27; Issa 139,1; Loew I, 607; Ducros 6; Dymock III, 261-264.⌉

Šīr is the Persian name for milk. Amlaǧ is the Arabic form of the
Persian name āmala or āmula (Laufer 581) which is derived from the Sanskrit
āmālaka (Dymock) or amālaki (Chopra 590). It is the emblic myrobalan, fruit
of Phyllanthus Emblica L. (Euphorbiaceae). Ibn al-Beithar states that
šīr-amlaǧ was the emblic macerated in milk. But šīr can also be a wine

or syrup. The emblical myrobalans are always for sale in the bazaars of Cairo (Ducros) under the name of amleg. They are administered against intestinal ailments. They are fruits resembling small blackish plums. It is an oriental drug which was unknown to the Greeks.

375) ŠAHMĀNAǦ   Fleabane elecampane

MAIMONIDES:

It is that which one calls al-barnūf in Egypt.

MEYERHOF:

[Theophrastus VI,12; Dioscorides III,121; Ibn al-Beithar 264 and 1273; Issa 98,18; Loew I, 423; Ducros 16.]

The usual form of the name is šāhbānaǧ, from the Persian šāh-bānag meaning "fanfare of the king". It is the fleabane elecampane ("herb with bugs", Inula conyzoides D.C. Compositae) and related types. By the name konyza the Greeks designated various species of Erigeron (Compositae) and Inula britannica L. The plant which is called barnūf in Egypt was identified by Schweinfurth (54) as Inula Dioscoridis DESF. It is also mentioned by Ramis (p.190) as a plant which is widespread in Egypt in humid locations. In the bazaars of Cairo, under the name bernūf, the druggists sell the dried leaves which Ducros determined as from Conyza squarrosa L. (synonym is Inula Conyza D.C.). It is used as vulnerary and sudorific. The name bernuf appears to be Coptic in origin. See P.G.Sobhy, Remains of Ancient Egyptian Medicine in Modern Domestic Treatment in Bull. de l'Inst. d'Egypte. vol. 20 Cairo, 1938, p.12.

376) ŠANǦĀR   Alkanet

MAIMONIDES:

It is "donkey lettuce" (hass al-himār) and the "pigeon's foot"

(<u>riğl al-hamām</u>), a known plant.

<u>MEYERHOF</u>:

⌈Theophrastus VII, 809; Dioscorides IV,23; Serapion 234; Ibn al-Beithar 1344; <u>Tuhfa</u> 362; 'Abd ar-Razzaq 781; Issa 9,2; Loew I, 292-296; Ducros 109.⌉

<u>Šanğār</u> is the Arabic form of the Persian name <u>šangār</u> (or <u>šangāl</u>, Vullers II,471) which designates the alkanet (<u>Alkanna tinctoria</u> TAUSCH identical to <u>Anchusa tinctoria</u> L., Borraginaceae). Its Biblical name is probably <u>hallāmūt</u>, its Greek name is <u>ankhousa</u>. In addition to the two Arabic names indicated by Maimonides, there are many others to be found in Issa. In the bazaars of Cairo, one sells pieces of the bark of alkanet under the name <u>riğl el-hamām</u>. The people use it as a remedy against intestinal ulcers and as a tintorial material for dyeing into red (Ducros). In Syria, Guigues (Serapion 234) understood <u>hawā ğuwānī</u> ("interior air") as the vulgar name for alkanet because of its fistulous texture.

377) <u>SUKK</u>   Arsenic or vegetable rat poison

<u>MAIMONIDES</u>:

This name is in usage for the sawdust of a tree that is imported from India and which kills rats. Its well-known name is "rat poison" (<u>simm al-far</u>).

<u>MEYERHOF</u>:

⌈Ibn al-Beithar 1336; <u>Tuhfa</u> 460; 'Abd ar-Razzaq 863 and 959; Dymock III, 641; Ducros 84.⌉

The Arabic name <u>šukk</u> or <u>šakk</u> was translated by Leclerc and others as "arsenic" because the Arabic authors describe the drug in question as a powder which kills rats. Arabic synonyms are <u>at-turāb al-halik</u> (the "earth which kills") and <u>rahag al-far</u> (rat powder). But no Arabic author states that it is arsenic (zarnih). The Qamus (III,299) relates the following passage: "Šakk...is a remedy which kills rats, is imported from Khorassan, from silver mines; it is white and yellow." This speaks in favor of arsenic, all the more so since oriental Persia till this day furnishes orpiment (yellow sulfur of arsenic).

Kohen (p. 136,last lines)states: "....there are two types, one white and one yellow. The one of good quality is imported from Khorassan, according to ar-Razi." Dawud (I,423ff), among the names of this drug, uses the term al-muksamūh, probably a mutilation of the Persian margi-mūš ("rat poison"). In another place (II,160), Dawud writes the name harkasmuh and markasmuh. He further states that šukk is a product of mercury and of sulfur of poor quality, spoiled by the cold. It was prepared in the "island of Venice" and in Khorassan, and its white product, solid and brilliant, was the better one; the yellow was the poorer one. It was used against pruriginous afflictions of the skin. Maimonides is the only one to affirm the vegetable origin of šukk. However, Dymock furnishes a valuable piece of information: he says that the Indian medical books give the name šuka to a white powder which has irritating effects on the skin. I here see the origin of the name šukk which passed into Persian (Vullers II, 437). Nevertheless, Dymock identifies the substance suka with fossil dust (diatomaceous earth), which one knows in Egypt under the name husn Yūsuf ("beauty of Joseph"). It is a type of powder used by women, and not a poison. It may thus perhaps consist of a mixture of arsenic and diatomaceous earth.

378) SŪ   Ben (East Indian horseradish-tree)

MAIMONIDES:

It is the "ben-tree"(šaǧarat al-bān).

(In the text, the name su̅' is written s̆ada', an error of the copyist. In
Kohen, p. 136, line 20, one finds the faulty spelling s̆u̅h instead of su̅.
The latter name is the one given by Abu Hanifa ad-Dinawari. One also en-
counters it in ancient Arabic poetry.)

<u>MEYERHOF</u>:

[Dioscorides IV,157; Serapion 197; Ibn al-Beithar 226 and 1354; <u>Tuhfa</u>
382; 'Abd ar-Razzaq 165 and 327; Issa 120,20; Loew II, 124; Ducros 70.]

The tree of the ben belongs to the genus <u>Moringa</u>, in our case above
all <u>Moringa pterygosperma</u> GAERTN. ("oil-bearing ben, myrepsic ben") and
<u>Moringa aptera</u> GAERTN., the <u>balanos myrepsikê</u> (<u>glans unguentaria</u>) of the
ancients. The fruits of these trees are sold by the druggists of Cairo
under the names <u>habb el-ba̅n</u> or <u>habba ga̅liya</u> ("precious seed"). They contain a very oily white almond which is consumed by women who wish to ac-
quire plumpness (Ducros).

CHAPTER TĀ'

379) <u>TURMUS</u>   Lupine

<u>MAIMONIDES</u>:

   It is <u>al-basīla</u> and <u>al-ǧarǧar</u>.

<u>MEYERHOF</u>:

   [Theophrastus VIII,2-11; Dioscorides II,109; Serapion 494; Ibn
al-Beithar 406; 'Abd ar-Razzaq 881; Issa 112,13; Loew II, 453-463;
Ducros 51; Ibn 'Awwam 97-99.]

   The Greek name for lupine <u>thermos</u>, passed into Egyptian (Coptic),
into Hebrew and into Aramaic, and from there into Arabic, into Persian
and even into certain Indian dialects. The Greeks knew a wild species
(<u>Lupinus angustifolius</u> L., Leguminous plant) and a cultivated one
(<u>Lupinus hirsutus</u> L.). The seed is bitter and needs to be crushed in
water to become edible. That which one grows in the Near-East today is
the <u>Lupinus Termis</u> FORSK. In Egypt there are, in addition, two wild species,
<u>Lupinus digitatus</u> FORSKAL and <u>Lupinus angustifolius</u> variety <u>aegyptiacus</u>
SCHWEINF. On this subject and in general on the history of lupine see
Hugo Michaelis' <u>Zur Geschichte der Lupine</u>, in <u>Berichte der Deutschen
Pharmazentischen Gesellschaft</u> (29th year, Berlin 1919, p.518-530).
In the bazaars of Cairo, one sells the white lupine (<u>Lupinus albus</u> L.)
as a remedy, in Arabic <u>termis gabalī</u> (Ducros). The name ǧarǧar (or ǧirǧir,
Issa) is Arabic; the name <u>basīla</u> Hispanic, from the Latin <u>pisellum</u>
  (diminutive of the Latin <u>pisum</u> meaning "pea")(Simonet 444ff).

380) <u>TĀFISYĀ</u>   Thapsia (false fennel)

<u>MAIMONIDES</u>:

   It is <u>al-yantūn</u> and <u>al-matinān</u>. It is the wild rue itself (<u>as-sadāb</u>

al-barrī), or it is said that it is the resin of the wild rue. That
which I have seen at the physicians of Maghrib are white-reddish roots;
they are those which are called al-yantūn.

MEYERHOF:

Theophrastus IX,8-20; Dioscorides IV,153; Serapion 279 and 492;
Ibn al-Beithar 441 and 2321; Tuhfa 14 and 404; 'Abd ar-Razzaq 244,408
and 879; Issa 180,3; Loew III 473ff.

Tāfisyā or tāfsiyā is the Arabic transcription of the Greek name
thapsia for Thapsia garganica L.("false fennel, bastard turpeth",
Umbelliferaceae). This plant is abundant in the north of Africa where,
because of its sour, irritating and drastic juice, it is considered as
a sort of panacea. The name yantūn is also confirmed by Ibn al-Beithar,
but matnān, as we have seen in number 222, designates a different plant,
the mezereon (Daphne Guidium L.) The identification of tafsiyā with
wild rue or with its resin was refuted by Ibn al-Beithar. It is strange
that Maimonides fails to mention the name diryās, which was in usage for
Thapsia in the Maghrib (see Tuhfa), and also known in Cairo (Kohen p. 126,
line 6ff).

381) TAMR HINDĪ   Tamarind

MAIMONIDES:

It is the name of the tree al-humar. The Egyptians call the "date"
itself (i.e. the fruit) humar, and the Arabs call this "date" as-subār.

MEYERHOF:

Serapion 491; Ibn al-Beithar 426; Tuhfa 407; 'Abd ar-Razzaq 877;
Issa 176,16; Loew II, 409; Ducros 52.

The Arabic name tamr hindī has the meaning "Indian date" and designates the pulp of the pods of the tamarind tree (Tamarindus indica L.,
Leguminous plants), beautiful tree of the Sudan,   India and other
tropical lands. The name humar was given to it in western Arabia, subār
in Southern Arabia. One sells the pulp of tamarind, together with its
hard and irregular seeds, above all in the bazaars of Cairo. One uses it
as a laxative and for the preparation of refreshing beverages.

382) TŪTIYĀ   Tutty

MAIMONIDES:

It is that which is called "cadmia of brass" (iqlīmiyā as-sufr)
as well as qasqatūta; it is also called qadmiyā.

MEYERHOF:

[Dioscorides V, 75; Serapion 511; Ibn al-Beithar 473; Tuhfa 403 and
854; 'Abd ar-Razzaq 884.]

The name tūtiyā is Syriac and probably originates from tūtā meaning
"ripe", because of the "annoying and inflated aspects of the product"
(Renaud-Colin). See the discussion of the name tutiya in Laufer (512ff)
who doubts that the Sanskrit name tuttha (green vitriole) is of Syriac
origin. See also the commentary of Guigues at number 511 of Serapion.
It designates the impure oxides of zinc, of differing colors according
to the nature of their impurities (copper, etc.). White tutty was considered the best. The Syrians and the Arabs identified it with the pom-
pholyx of the Greeks ("metallic bubble"), natural or artificial product
of the condensation of the vapors of cadmia (see above number 342).
One often confused it with cadmia which it resembles from the chemical

standpoint. The name qasqatuta is undoubtedly Spanish, cascatutia,
from cascar "to break" (Simonet 144) and tutia. Tutty was an important
ingredient of dry collyria against specks in the cornea of the eye.
See also above article 342 (qalimiyā).

383) TINKĀR   Borax

MAIMONIDES:

One also says dinkār. It is the "chrysocolla" (lihām ad-dahab
and lizaq ad-dahab)and the "salt of goldsmiths" (milh as-sāga). Its
Greek name is khrysokolle.

MEYERHOF:

Dioscorides V, 89; Serapion 505; Ibn al-Beithar 431; Tuhfa 401;
'Abd ar-Razzaq 469,516 and 882; Ducros 53

The name tinkār is the Arabic form of the Persian tangār (Vullers I,
469). It is a borax or tetraborate of impure potassium. In industry, one
uses its property of dissolving metallic oxides for the solder of the
metals, from whence its Greek name chrysocolle and its above-mentioned
Arabic translations. In medicine, one uses borax as a detergent, dessi-
cative and antiseptic.

384) TŪDARĪ   Sisymbrium and others

MAIMONIDES:

One also calls it tūdarang; its Greek name is erysimon. It is a
seed which resembles that of the cress (hurf) (fol. 101). There are
two species, a red one and a white one. The red one is the one called
an-nugila in Spanish, the white one is as-sūb.

MEYERHOF:

Theophrastus VIII,1-7; Dioscorides II, 158; Serapion 270; Ibn
al-Beithar 436; 'Abd ar-Razzaq 96; Issa 170,6; Loew I, 527; Ducros 54.

Tudarī is a Persian name. The Arabic name which is derived there-from is vocalized tūdariǧ in most treatises. The plant is the hedge-mustard ("songster's herb", Sisymbrium officinale SCOP., Cruciferaceae), and related species, particularly Sisymbrium polyceratium L. (Hooper and Field (p.171) have noted that the seeds sold in the Persian bazaars under the name of towdri are derived from different Cruciferaceae, above all Lepidium Iberis L., and Matthiola incana R.Br). However, here we are deal-ing with other Cruciferaceae, because the Sisymbriums have yellow flowers. (Maimonides, in one of his medical works, mentions a tūdari asfar!) For the Spanish name nuǧila equivalent to the Latin nucella ("hazel-nut") (Simonet 401), one should think of Cakile maritima SCOP. which has rose flowers and fruits resembling hazel-nuts, but which has another name in Arabic (see above number 325). Ghafiqi (Ms. fol. 61b) still quotes the Spanish name ǧandala for tūdarī; it is perhaps sandalo de agua meaning aquatic mint (Botica. p.751). As to the other name which has no diacritical points, the ʿUmda says that it is written as-sūb (communication from Dr. Renaud). The druggists of Cairo sell the seeds of Sisymbrium officinale under the name of tūdarī iswid ("black tudari"), as a vulnerary, etc. (Ducros). Kohen (p. 126) states having learned from his father that tūdari was a species of cress whose seeds resembled those of the poppy. 'Abd ar-Razzaq gives the synonym asmār.

385) TŪBĀL AN-NUHĀS   Copper scales

MAIMONIDES:

These are scales which become detached (from the metal) when one beats it (with a hammer).

MEYERHOF:

[Dioscorides V,78; Ibn al-Beithar 438; Tuhfa 402.]

The name tūbāl is Persian (as well as tūpāl, Vullers I, 476). It is the equivalent of the Greek lepis ("scale"). The scales of copper were used in medicine in detergent collyria against leukomas and corneal specks.

386) TARANGUBĪN   Manna

MAIMONIDES:

It is that which is called manna (mann) and one also calls it rizq ("provision").

MEYERHOF:

[Serapion 360 and 497; Ibn al-Beithar 408; Tuhfa 269; 'Abd ar-Razzaq 580 and 876; Ducros 223.]

Tarangubīn is the Arabic form of the Persian name tarangubīn ("honey of dew", Vullers I, 440) which designates the sugary exudates observed on certain desert plants. This name corresponds to the mān in the Bible and of Semitic languages in general. It is, however, probable that Biblical manna is not that which in the Middle Ages was called and which today is still called "manna", but rather the edible lichen (Sphoerothallia or Lecanora esculenta), of which we spoke earlier (see numbers 69, ǧawz-ǧundum and 86, dādī).

The ancient Arabic physicians understood manna as a dew which fell from heaven upon plants and which, desiccated, became a type of thick honey. Much has been written about manna, and I refer the reader to the commentary of Renaud-Colin in the Tuhfa. A very complete study was published by the late pharmacist and botanist Alfred Kaiser who himself traveled through the Sinai peninsula in his research on the real manna (A. Kaiser,

Der hautige Stand des Mannafrage, Arbon, Switzerland 1924). According to him, the tree which above all produces manna in the Sinai is a tamarisk (Tamarix nilotica EHRENB. var. Mannifera). The best secretion escapes spontaneously or perhaps as a result of the bite of a gall-insect (Coccus manniparus EHRENB.) and becomes hard during the night. The Bedouins and the monks of the celebrated monastery of St. Catherine gather these concretions and use them as a substitute for sugar. Kaiser, in the Sinai, also observed two other manniferous plants, a wormwood (Artemisia Herba alba ASSO) and a species of Holoxylon (Chenopodiaceae). But these three species do not provide the manna that one finds in the drug bazaars in the Orient. These, as the Persian name tarangubīn indicates, come from Persia, above all from diverse species of Astragalus (Leguminous plants milk-vetch) and Atraphaxis (Polygonaceae). The manna produced by Atraphaxis spinosa L. appears to be the best; the Persians call it šīr-hušk. The manna of milk-vetch is less white and less good. Both are for sale in the bazaars of Cairo under the name mann farsī (Persian manna).

One must still mention the manna produced by two other leguminous plants of the desert, by Alhagi Camelorum FISCH. (Southern Russia, Persia, Afghanistan, Baluchistan) and by Alhagi Maurorum TOURN. (Persia, North Africa). One also finds it as a drug in commerce. The Arabs call the plant al-hāǵ or ʿaqūl. See above article 166. Its manna, according to Ducros, is employed as a vermifuge and laxative, whereas the manna of Atraphaxis is considered as a pectoral.

CHAPTER HĀ'

387) HIYAR ŠANBAR   Cassia-tree

MAIMONIDES:

It is the Indian cucumber (al-qittā' al-hindī) and the Indian

Carob (al-harrūb al-hindī).

MEYERHOF:

[Serapion 169; Ibn al-Beithar 836; Tuhfa 419; 'Abd ar-Razzaq 169;
Issa 42,12; Loew II, 408; Ducros 101.]

Hiyār is the Arabic word which signifies cucumber. Šanbar is the
Arabic form of the Persian name čanbar which designates something round.
Hiyār šanbar and the two Arabic names designate a well-known drug, the
brown-blackish, long and cylindrical pod of the cassia tree (Cassia
Fistula L., Leguminous plants - Cesalpiniae) which is divided by parti-
tions into compartments, and filled by a pulp which is sweetish and lightly
purgative. It is exported from Egyptian Sudan and   India and is sold
in the bazaars of Cairo. In Europe, one sometimes finds it in drug stores
under the incorrect name of "manna".

388) HIYĀR   Cucumber, gherkin

MAIMONIDES:

It is al-qatad and ǧulmātā.

MEYERHOF:

[Theophrastus VII,1-13; Dioscorides II, 135; Serapion 58; Ibn al-Beithar
935; 'Abd ar-Razzaq 741; Issa 62,10; Loew I, 530-535; Ibn 'Awwam II, 223-225.]

Hiyār is the Arabic name of a cucumber smaller than qittā' (see number
343). It is Cucumis sativus L. (Cucurbitaceae), known since the most

remote antiquity, and originating, perhaps, in   Oriental India. The
name qatad(corrupted in our text) is Arabic. Ġulmātā is a Syriac name
(ğalmātā in Freytag I, 298 and Vullers I, 525) which is, however, lacking
in the Syriac (botanic) dictionaries. In medicine, the seeds of the
cucumber are recommended by ancient practicioners as a remedy against inflammation of the liver, of the spleen and of the intestines. Compare also
our articles number 5,54,98,292 and 332 as well as the study of Arabic
Cucurbitaceae by Clément-Mullet (Études sur les noms arabes de diverses
familles de végétaux in the Journal Asiatique, 6th series, vol. 15, pp 90-122,
1870).

389) HANDARŪS   Spelt

MAIMONIDES:

    One also says kandarūs. It is the "Roman barley" (aš-ša'ir ar-rūmī).
It is called isqalya in Spanish and al-'alas in Arabic.

MEYERHOF:

    Dioscorides II, 89 and 96; Serapion 225; Ibn al-Beithar 825 and 1580;
Tuhfa 314; 'Abd ar-Razzaq 340; Issa 183,18; Loew I, 772-776; Ibn 'Awwam II,
46ff.

    Handarūs is the Arabic transcription of khondros of the Greeks. This
name designates grains of wheat or spelt, coarsely ground or crushed, a
type of groats (wheat flower), as well as wheat flower itself. To the
Arabs, it specifically designates spelt and is thus, as 'alas, the translation from the Greek zea,which is the name of Triticum Spelta L. The
Hispanic name is always written isqalya or isqàliya. Leclerc erroneously
corrected it to espelta. One should read isqāliya(Simonet 189), name which
is derived from the Latin scandula and preserved in modern Castilian in

the forms escanda and escana. Ghafiqi (Ms. fol. 177a) has the following
statement: "Zaa (zea). It is al-ᶜalas and in Spanish it is called al-
isqaliya. It is, known seed which resembles wheat and from which one
makes bread. Those who claim that it it as-sult ("stripped barley")
are in error." See our number 270. See also the commentary of Renaud-Colin
in chapter 314 of the Tuhfa. The large spelt was cultivated in Egypt, together
with the grain, since prehistoric times. Its medical use is limited to the
preparation of nourishing soups.

390) **HITMĪ**   Marsh-mallow

MAIMONIDES:

We have explained that it is a wild mallow (hubbāzī barrī). It is
the one called "rose of prostitutes" (ward az-zawān) in the Maghrib and
in Spanish mālba baška (malvavisco). It is also called bantar fīra
(venter frio).

MEYERHOF:

[Theophrastus IX, 15-18; Dioscorides III, 146; Serapion 124; Ibn al-
Beithar 808; Tuhfa 413; 'Abd ar-Razzaq 914; Issa 11,6; Loew II, 230-243;
Ducros 99; Ibn 'Awwam II, 286-288.]

Hitmī is the Arabic equivalent of althaia of the Greeks and designates
the marsh-mallow (Althaea officinalis L., Malvaceae) which is included
in most European pharmacopoeias. It is not a wild marsh-mallow, but the
one cultivated everywhere. The flowers gathered a little before their
opening are dried and sold in the drug bazaars of Cairo under the name
hatmī. Just as in Europe, they serve as a pectoral and bechic. The
Spanish name is still to this day malvavisco (Simonet 328). The other
name was explained to me by M. Renaud according to the manuscript of the
ᶜUmda; one should read bantar frio and it is the Spanish venter frio

meaning "cold abdomen"! But the ʿUmda applies this name to the helleborus which, in Spanish, had the name malvilla or "little mallow" (Renaud).

391) HUSĀ AT-TAʿLAB   Orchis

MAIMONIDES:

It is the plant which is called "fratricide" (qātil ahīhi) and in Spanish aštabaka. It is ġarmūġ and triphyllon as well as satyrion; its name is also orkhis kynos.*

MEYERHOF:

Theophrastus IX,18; Dioscorides III,126-128; Serapion 196; Ghafiqi 140 and 141; Ibn al-Beithar 801-802; Tuhfa 80, 419 and 420; 'Abd ar-Razzaq 916; Issa 129, 8-11; Loew II, 296-298; Ducros 124.

Husā at-taʿlab ("fox's testicle") is the Arabic equivalent of the Greek kynos orkhis meaning "dog's testicle" (Dioscorides III,126). It designates the tubercles of different species of Orchis that are sold in the drug bazaars of the Orient (Orchis Morio L., Orchis hircina L., Orchis papilionacea L., etc.) These tubercles are false-bulbs (axillary buds of subterranean leaves) which renew themselves alternately. Consequently, one is always inflated and juicy, the other limp and withered. This explains the Arabic names qātil ahīhi ("which kills its brother") and al-hāiy wa'l-maïyit ("the living and the dear"). In Europe as well as the Orient, one extracts from these tubercles, the analeptic starch called salep (from the Arabic sahlab). The merchandise sold in France and in England comes from Smyrna; that sold in Egypt, from Syria and from Persia. In the Orient, fresh tubercles pass as aphrodisiacs. I cannot explain aštabaka and ġarmūġ. The first name is undoubtedly Spanish and may be a mutilation

---

* The name is mutilated in the text, the reading is uncertain: perhaps kyrios orkhis; Dioscorides III,127?

of estepilla ("cistus") or estiptica; the second is a Persian form or perhaps a mutilation of ǧawz al-marǧ, synonym of ʿinab at-taʾlab (black night
shade) in 'Abd ar-Razzaq (number 651).

392) <u>HARNŪB</u>   Carob

MAIMONIDES:

   It is that which the people call al-harrūb and in Berber tāslīgwa.

MEYERHOF:

   [Theophrastus I, 11-13 and IV,2,4; Dioscorides I,114; Serapion 114;
Ibn al-Beithar 762; Tuhfa 423; 'Abd ar-Razzaq 920; Issa 45,23; Loew II,
383-407; Ducros 95; Ibn 'Awwam I,227 ff.]

   Harnūb and harrūb are Arabic names borrowed from Hebrew (harrūb)
and from Aramaic (harrūbā). They designate the carob-tree (Ceratonia
Siliqua L., Leguminous plants) and its well-known fruit the carob. This
tree, originating in Palestine (Hehn 340-342), was known to the Greeks
under the names kerônia (Theophrastus) and keration (Dioscorides). It is
widely distributed in all the Mediterranean regions. The Berber name
tāslīgwa is correctly written in our manuscript, according to Dr. Renaud,
and is surely borrowed from the Latin siliqua. One sells the fruits and
the browned and flattened pods in all the bazaars of the Orient. Their
pulp is laxative and bechic.

393) <u>HILĀF</u>   Willow

MAIMONIDES:

   It is as-safsāf and as-sindār and al-ġarab and as-sawhar and as-sāliǧ.

MEYERHOF:

   [Theophrastus III, 13,7; Dioscorides I, 104; Serapion 86; Ibn al-Beithar 816;

Tuḥfa 412 and 438; 'Abd ar-Razzaq 637, 680 and 912; Issa 160, 5,6,8,13;
Loew III, 322-338; Ibn 'Awwam I, 375-377.

In Egypt, the name hilāf designated the Egyptian willow (Salix aegyptiaca
L.) which was already described by Forskal in the 18th centrury, but appears
to have vanished since his time. It still exists in Syria. Safsāf is the
name of Salix Safsāf that one finds along canals, above all in the Nile delta
(Ramis 60ff). Garab is the name of Salix babylonica L., that one also finds
in Egypt. This name, derived from a Semitic root (Arābah of the Bible), first
designated the poplar tree of Mesopotamia (Populus Euphratica OL.), and later
it designated water willows. Sindār is probably a faulty spelling for sabidar,
Arabic form of the Persian sapīd-dār ("white tree"- which designated both the
white willow (Salix alba L.) and the white poplar (Populus alba L., Salicaceae)
(Vullers II, 216). Sawhar is an Arabic name meaning willow as stated in Qamus
(Freytag II, 290), but lacking in the majority of dictionaries (of botany).
Sāliġ is the Arabic-Spanish transcription of the Latin salix (Simonet 579),
in modern Castilian salice. The bark of the young branches of the different
species of Salix contains a tonic and febrifugal principle: Salicin. A very
profound study of Salix aegyptiaca with a complete bibliography recently
appeared in Sweden (B. Floderus. Salix aegyptiaca L., Eine historisch-tax-
onomische Studie, in Arkiv för Botanik, K. Svenska Vetenskapsakademien, vol.
25a, number 11). According to this publication, the land of origin of this
tree is Persia, where it has the name bīd-musk (meaning "musked willow").

394) HĪRĪ   Wall-flower, gilly flower

MAIMONIDES:

One also calls it hīrī asfar.[*]

---

[*] The word asfar is lacking in the manuscript and was supplied by Meyerhof.

It is (fol. 101$^{\vee}$) that which the Egyptians
call al-mant̄ur. There is a wild species; it is the latter that one calls al-
huzāma ("lavender") and also al-bābūna ("camomile").

MEYERHOF:

[Theophrastus VII, 13,9; Dioscorides III,123; Serapion 315; Ibn al-
Beithar 837 and 2181; Tuhfa 422; 'Abd ar-Razzaq 926; Issa 46,20; Loew I, 490;
Ibn 'Awwam II, 256-260.]

Hīrī is the Persian name of the gillyflower, and hīrī asfar or, in
Egypt, mant̄ur asfar is the name of the wall-flower (Cheiranthus Cheiri L.
Cruciferaceae). It is the equivalent of one of the species of leukoion of
Dioscorides. The wild species might be another Cheiranthus just as it might
also be an Erysemum which greatly resembles it. The wallflower is appre-
ciated in medicine as an antispasmodic and diuretic remedy.

395) HUNTĀ   Asphodel

MAIMONIDES:

One also says ǧuntā. It is al-birwāq and it is that which the Berbers
call tiklas (?). Its name in Greek is asphodelos. The root of this plant
resembles a small carrot. It is these roots which are employed (in medicine),
and when they are dried and ground there results a sticky flour: this is al-iǰrās.

MEYERHOF:

[Theophrastus VII, 9-13; Dioscorides II, 169; Serapion 80 and 123; Ibn al-
Beithar 88 and 826; Tuhfa 83 and 421; 'Abd ar-Razzaq 188 and 915; Issa 24,10;
Loew II, 152-156.]

Huntā ("hermaphrodite") and birwāq are Arabic names of the asphodel
(Asphodelus ramosus L., Liliaceae). There are other species of asphodel in
the Near-East. The reading of the Berber name is more than doubtful: Ibn al-

Beithar has tīqliš, Renaud blalūz, etc. (bolbos or loz meaning "almond"?).
In Trabut (p. 37) we find the names tiglich and belwāz for Asphodelus micro-
carpus or cerasiferus. The synonym išrās is contested by Ibn al-Beithar (88),
but appears to be correctly explained by Maimonides. Loew discovered that
the Hebraic word ʿīrīt, like the Syriac ʿirōnā, signifies asphodel, and
simultaneously a sticky substance, in Arabic ġirā' ("paste"). The root of
asphodel simultaneously served as a magical remedy against the evil eye and
as an emolient.

396) HIRWA'   Ricin, Castor-oil plant

MAIMONIDES:

It is tārtaqa (tartago) and it is also called kiki and in Spanish riǧinu
(ricino). The Chinest castor-oil plant (al-hirwaʿ as-sinī) is ad-dand.

MEYERHOF:

Theophrastus I, 10,1; Dioscorides IV, 161; Serapion 317; Ibn al-Beithar
771; Tuhfa 7,56,81,415; 'Abd ar-Razzaq 89,331 and 414; Issa 156,17; Loew I,
608-611.

Hirwa' is the Arabic name of the castoi-oil plant (Ricinus communis L.,
Euphorbiaceae), in Greek kroton, in Latin ricinus. These two names designate
the capricorn-beetle (coleopter) and were applied to the seeds of the castor-
oil plant which resemble small spotted scarabs. Kiki is a name which is
derived from the Egyptian k',k', and also from the Hebrew qiqāyōn, because
the plant and its seed were well-known in ancient Egypt (Keimer I, 120).
Nevertheless, Egyptologists still doubt that k',k', is identical with ricin.
Tartago is the Spanish name of another Euphorbiaceae, Euphorbia Lathyris
(see above māhūdāna number 178) (Simonet 396); dand refers to croton
(see above number 97). The seeds and oil of ricin are still in usage everywhere.

397) <u>HAWH</u>   Peach

<u>MAIMONIDES</u>:

It is the "Persian apple" (<u>at-tuffah al-fārisī</u>) and the "Persian
fruit" (<u>at-tawra al-fārisiyya</u>). The Syrians call it <u>ad-durrāqin</u> and one
of its species is known by the name of <u>az-zahrī</u> ("flowery"); we have mentioned it in chapter <u>fā'</u>

<u>MEYERHOF</u>:

[Dioscorides I, 115; Serapion 417; Ibn al-Beithar 830; Issa 149,5;
Loew III,159; Ibn 'Awwam I, 315.]

We have above encountered (see number 314) a species of peach called
"flowery" (<u>firsik</u> or <u>hawh zahrī</u>) cultivated in Spain. Here Maimonides speaks
of the peach in general. The name "Persian apple" is the translation of
<u>Persikon mêlon</u> of Dioscorides, and the other Arabic name has nearly the
same meaning. The land of origin of the peach is perhaps China   It was
introduced from Persia into the Roman Empire during the first century (Hehn
320 ff). The Latin name was <u>duracina</u>,which one transcribed into Greek
<u>dôrakinon.</u> (This name is preserved in modern Greek in the form <u>rhodakinon</u>).
From the latter name is derived the Arabic-Syrian name <u>durrāqin</u> which remains
in usage by the Syrians until the present day (Post I,449; see also Simonet 180).

In medicine, the peach was employed as a refresher during fevers, and
the leaves of the peach tree were used for rubbings.

398) <u>HŪLANGĀN</u>   Galingale

<u>MAIMONIDES</u>:

It is <u>kisrūdārā</u> in Persian, and it is <u>al-hawsarā</u>.

<u>MEYERHOF</u>:

[Serapion 417; Ibn al-Beithar 829; <u>Tuhfa</u> 411; 'Abd ar-Razzaq 906 and 918;
Issa 10,13; Loew III,497; Ducros 100; Dymock III,437-443.]

Hūlangán or hawlingán are names derived from the Persian hawalingán, name of the rhizome of galingale. There are several types: a large one, a light one and a small one. The latter is sold in the bazaars of Cairo, and it is derived from Alpinia officinarum HANCE. (Zingiberaceae), whereas Alpinia Galanga WILLD. ("the large galingale") originates from Java and is cultivated in the Oriental Indies. Hance, who in 1868 found a wild Alpinia in China, thinks that the name hūlangán is derived from the Chinese kao-lian-kian; but Laufer (545 ff) contests this etymology and derives the name from the Sanskrit kulanga, name which passed into Persian in the form hawalingan. The correct form of the second name means "wood of king Chosroes ("royal wood"). The third name seems mutilated: it should read either husraw-dārū (Persian for "wood of Chosroes") or husrawán (Dozy I, 371; "royal, magnificant"). The rhizome of galingale, sold in Cairo in cylindrical pieces as thick as a finger, has an aromatic odor and tart taste (Ducros). It is sold as an aphrodisiac and it is mixed into certain electuaries (manzūl), which sometimes contain narcotics.

399) HARBAQ   Hellebore

MAIMONIDES:

Its Greek name is artīqis (narthêx?) There are two species: one white and one black. The name of the white one in Spanish is malbīla (malvilla); another of its species is called halbīnak (?)

MEYERHOF:

Theophrastus IX, 8-17; Dioscorides 148-149; Serapion 121; Ibn al-Beithar 772-773; Tuhfa 425; 'Abd ar-Razzaq 910; Issa 92, 18 and 19; Loew III, 119 ff; Ducros 94.

The Arabic name harbaq is derived from the Syriac hūrbaknā or hūrbekānā

(Loew) which nevertheless seems to be borrowed from another language. It designates the hellebore (Helleborus albus and niger L., Ranunculaceae), well-known drug, which should not be confused with veratrum or white hellebore (Veratrum album L., Colchicaceae). The small roots of the black hellebore are still sold in the bazaars of Cairo under the name harbaq iswid. They are used as a drastic purgative, vermifuge and sternutatory. The Greek name artīqis is perhaps a mutilation of narthêx or the species Antikyrikos mentioned by Dioscorides (IV, 149), whose name passed into the Syriac translation. In Simonet (410), we find the name artīqiš or urtīqaš as a Spanish term which designates nettles (in modern Castilían ortigas). The Spanish name malvilla is found in Simonet (328) and has the meaning "small mallow". The name halbīnak (or other analagous name since there are no diacritical points) is probably an approximation of the Greek helleboros or the Syriac hūrbaknā.

400) HARDAL   Mustard

MAIMONIDES:

The white one is called isfandār, and the wild one (fol. 102^z) al-harša. It is said that the name of the whole plant is al-haršā' and that of its seed al-hardal.

MEYERHOF:

Theophrastus VII,1-5; Dioscorides II, 154; Serapion 101; Ibn al-Beithar 767; Tuhfa 417; 'Abd ar-Razzaq 909; Issa 169; 17 and 21; Loew I, 516-527; Ibn 'Awwam II, 252 ff.

Hardal is an Arabic name, related to other Semitic names (Assyrian hardinnu, uncertain; Hebrew-Mishnaic hardal; Syriac hardêlā). It designates mustard in general, known to the ancient Egyptians, called by the Greeks nâpy

(Theophrastus) and sinapi (or sinêpi, Dioscorides). It is the white or
black mustard (Sinapis or Brassica alba L., Brassica nigra KOCH. or
Brassica sinapioides) and the wild mustard (Sinapis arvensis L.), all
cruciferaceae. The latter is called al-harsá ("the harsh one") in Arabic.
Isfandār is a faulty spelling for isfandān, Arabic form of the Persian is-
pandān meaning "mustard seed" (Vullers I, 91). The seed of black mustard is
utilized in medicine as a rubefacient and irritant, and in cooking as a condiment, but in the Orient much less than in the West. See above numbers 218
(labsān) and 322 (sināb).

401) HAŠHĀŠ   Poppy

MAIMONIDES:

The white one is the one which is called an-nuʿmān al-abyad; the
wild one is tārahīra (?) and the "frothy poppy" (al-hashāš az-zabadi) is
the one which is called peplos in Greek.

MEYERHOF:

Theophrastus IX, 8-20; Dioscorides IV, 64-66 and 167; Serapion 502;
Ibn al-Beithar 794-797; Tuhfa 414; 'Abd ar-Razzaq 905; Issa 134,6-8; Loew
II, 364-370; Ducros 98; Ibn 'Awwam II, 128-131.

The Arabic name hashāš is onomatopoeitic and designates something
which produces a clicking or similar sound. This is the case with heads of
dried poppy shaken by the wind in the fields. Hashāš is today in Arabic the
generic name for all poppies. Poppy was well-known to the ancient Egyptians
but was introduced rather late into near Asia. It was frequently confused with the anemone (nuʿmān).Nuʿmān abyad here is probably the somni-
ferant poppy (Papaver somniferum L.) and its varieties. It is this one
which has been cultivated for thousands of years and whose latex, extracted
by incision of the green fruits, collected, agglomerated and desiccated,

constitutes opium. Its cultivation in Egypt is prohibited since half
a century, but one still sells the heads of poppy (rās el-hušhāš) in
the bazaars, and one uses them to make children sleep by giving them a
beverage produced by the infusion of these heads. It is an unfortunate
practice which is widespread in all the Orient. The name tārahīrā seems
to be to be Berber (tadjira in Trabut number 184). Hašhāš zabadī is the
translation from the Greek mekôn aphrôdes and designates a type of silenus.

402) HARRĀTĪN   Earthworms

MAIMONIDES:

    These are worms which are found in moist earth when one digs into
it. Their name in Spanish is at-tartāniya and one also calls them
"strings of the earth" (ʿurūq al-ard) and "grease of the earth" (šahmat
al-ard). However, the Maghribians apply the name šahmat al-ard to a
small quadriped animal with streaked paws of the species of the gecko
(sāmm abras).

MEYERHOF:

    Dioscorides II, 67; Serapion 112; Ibn al-Beithar 789 and 1314; Tuhfa
416; Damiri II,123ff; 'Abd ar-Razzaq 908.

    Harrātīn (common plural) designates something which is fashioned round.
These are earthworms (Lumbricus terrestris L.) which played a certain role
in popular medicine in all lands. In Europe, one used them as compresses
against contusions; in the Orient, ground with oil, against all sorts of in-
flammations and against luxations and fractures. The Arabic names are
translations of the Greek name gês entera meaning "viscera of the earth".
The Spanish name is no longer in use; Simonet (538) derives it from the
Latin teredines meaning "worms". Kohen (p. 130 line 4) has at-tartiyar,

undoubyedly a copyist's error for <u>at-taritan</u>. The small striped
"gecko" is without doubt the speckled salamander (<u>Salamandra maculosa</u>
LAUR.), because Damiri mentions that <u>sahmat al-ard</u> is also the name of
a small animal which is not burned by fire, a superstition which is attached to the salamander since antiquity. In 'Abd ar-Razzaq (679) the
synonymous terms <u>šahmat al-ard</u> and '<u>urūq al-ard</u> designate mushrooms.

CHAPTER GAIN

403) GĀFIT — Eupatory, elecampane and diverse plants

MAIMONIDES:

It is that which the Arabs call at-tubbāq. It is al-ʿarār and al-ǧātǧāt
and in Spanish maškāniya (moscato), that which is al-labarda (olivarda).
Its name in Berber is tarrahla. There are four species of gāfit, and one
also calls it yerba balqaʿira (pulguera), which signifies "herb of fleas"
(Šaǧarat al-barāǧīt).

MEYERHOF:

[Dioscorides IV, 41; Serapion 91; Ibn al-Beithar 1618 and 1448; Tuhfa
434; Issa 7,11; 98,18 and 150,20-25; Loew III,188 ff, I 421-424 and 1446;
Ducros 171; Dymock I, 582 ff and II, 508 ff.]

Gāfit is the Arabic equivalent of Eupatorios of Dioscorides which
has been identified with agrimony (Agrimonia Eupatoria L., Rosaceae).
Ibn al-Beithar (1618) argues against the identification of this plant with
tubbāq or (in Berber) tirhilā, which would be the equivalent of konyza of
the Greeks (Fleabane. Inula conyzoides D.C., Compositae). See above number
375 (šahmānaǧ). Ibn al-Beithar also states that the physicians of Iraq,
of Syria and of Egypt employed a different plant "having an extreme bitter-
ness, with blue flowers, etc." and strongly purgative. In that,he is
correct, because in the bazaars of Cairo, the druggists to this day sell,
under the name gāfit hindi ("Indian gafit"), a dried plant which Ducros
erroneously identifies with agrimony. It is a Gentianacea and we learn in
Dymock (II, 508) that it is Gentiana dahurica FISCH. (synonym Gentiana
decumbens L.), plant from Turkestan which is sold in the Persian and Indian
bazaars under the name gāfis or gul-i-gāfis. The Persian physicians

erroneously identified it with <u>Teupatorios</u> of Dioscorides. The flowers
are long and blue, and the taste is very bitter, as indicated by Ibn al-
Beithar. It is this plant which is sold in the bazaars of Cairo, as a
detergent and astringent. One employs it in a decoction for internal
and external usage.

As to the other names given by Maimonides, ʿarār and g̱atg̱āt, these
designate Compositae, above all the species of <u>Pulicaria</u> (in Spanish
<u>pulguera</u>)(Simonet 466). The Arabicized Hispanic name maškāniya is identi-
fied by Simonet (380) as muškātu or muškīnu equal to the Castillian
<u>moscato</u> or <u>mosquino</u> meaning "herb of flies". The other name is mutilated
both in our manuscript as well as in all the manuscripts of Ibn al-Beithar:
<u>labārda</u>, <u>barmanda</u>, <u>ramida</u>, etc. One should here read <u>ulibārda</u> meaning
<u>olivarda</u> from the low Latin <u>olivaria</u> (Simonet 405), and in Ibn al-Beithar
<u>ramido</u> (Simonet 481) or <u>ramita</u> (Laguna 399).

404) <u>G̱ĀR</u>   Laurel

<u>MAIMONIDES</u>:

It is <u>ar-rand</u> as well as <u>al-irmid</u> and in Persian <u>ad-dahmast</u>. Its
seed is called <u>al-gar</u> and <u>habb ad-dahmas</u>; its name in Spanish is <u>arbaqa</u>
(lorbaco).

<u>MEYERHOF</u>:

Theophrastus III,3; IV,16 etc.; Dioscorides I, 78; Serapion 192;
Ibn al-Beithar 1619; <u>Tuhfa</u> 437; 'Abd ar-Razzaq 243,355 and 785; Issa
105,20; Loew II, 119-123; Ibn 'Awwam I, 226 ff.

G̱ār is the Arabic name of the laurel (<u>Laurus nobilis</u> L.) and the
equivalent of the Greek daphnê. The land of origin of this plant, which
played such a major role in the religious rites of the Greeks and the

Romans, is probably in Asia Minor from where it spread out toward the West and the East (Hehn 171-175). The names rand and dahmast are Persian (Vullers I, 943 and II,54). ʿIrmid is an Arabic name which designates duckweed or a species of jujube (Zizyphus Spina Christi), but never the laurel. There is here an error either on the part of the author or on the part of the copyist. The Spanish name was mutilated in the text (arbāqa); it should read lurbāqa meaning lorbaco or orbaco derived from the Latin lauri bacca (Simonet 316).

The use of laurel in medicine has nearly ceased. The fruits and the seeds of the laurel were used as a stomachic and as an ingredient in certain collyria in ophthalmopathies.

The Biblical-Hebrew name which probably designated the laurel is ʾoren, in Hebrew-Mishnaic ʾorānim (Loew),in Syriac ʿārā; these three names are related to the Arabic ġār.

405) GUBAĪRĀ   Sorb tree and others

MAIMONIDES:

It is the name of the fruit of the tree which is called al-muštahā, and the name of the herb called bulāyu (poleo).

MEYERHOF:

[Theophrastus II,2; III,15; Dioscorides I,120; Ibn al-Beithar 1627; Tuhfa 436; Issa 151,18; Loew II,245-249; Ibn ʿAwwam I, 302 ff.]

Al-ġubaïrā' is an Arabic name which has the sense of "the small gray one" and designates numerous trees and their fruits. Issa cites no less than nine. We will only mention the best-known one, the service-tree (Pirus Sorbus GAERTN.) that we have already encountered in number 330 (qarāsiyā).

The Arabic word <u>al-mustahā</u> has the sense of "the appetizing one"
and also designates the sorb tree (Dozy I,797 and Simonet 381 ff), but
in addition the common medlar-tree and the azarole-tree. See the commentaries of Renaud-Colin and of Dozy. Finally, the name <u>ġubairā'</u> still
designates the pennyroyal (<u>Mentha Pulegium</u> L., see above number 309,
<u>fawdana</u>), as Maimonides indicates by the Spanish name <u>poleo</u>.

The fruit of the sorb tree was used against intestinal afflictions
because of its constipating effect.

End of the Book

Praise be to G'd as it is fitting!

INDEX SECTION
(for Hebrew, Greek and Copte indices, see Meyerhof's edition).

The numbers in all the indices refer to the drug or
remedy numbers and not to the page numbers.

- 296 -

INDEX OF LATIN NAMES

Abies pectinata, 341.

— webbiana, 38.

Acacia, 12, 278.

— arabica, 12, 278.

— Farnesiana, 324.

— Senegal, 278.

— Seyal, 278.

— tortilis, 278.

acetosella, 350.

Achillea fragrantissima, 337.

Aconitum Anthora, 81.

Acorus Calamus, 125, 329

acriones, 325

Adiantum Capillus Veneris, 182.

Aeluropus littoralis, 251

— repens, 251.

Aframomum Melegueta, 82

Agrimonia Eupatoria, 403

Agropyrum repens, 251

Ajuga Chamaepitys, 190

Albersia Blitum, 53, (var. obe-
    racea).

Alkanna tinctoria, 376

Alhagi camelorum, 386

— manniferum, 166

— Maurorum, 166, 386.

Allium Ampeloprasum, 198.

— ascalonicum, 198.

— Porrum, 198.

— rotundum, 198.

— Victoriale, 282.

Aloe Perryi, 318.

— succotrina, 318

— vera, 318

Aloexylum Agallochum, 113.

Althaea officinalis, 390.

Alyssum saxatile, 370

Amaracus Dictamnus, 242

amarum, 114

Ambrosia maritima, 3.

Ammi Visnaga, 94.

Ammoperdix Heyl, 169.

Anacyclus Pyrethrum, 299.

— valentinus, 49.

Anagallis arvenis, 16.

— coerulea, 16.

Anagyris foetida, 180.

Anamirla paniculata, 178.

Anarrhinum orientale, 17.

Anchusa italica, 211.

— tinctoria, 376.

Andropogon Martini, 329.

INDEX OF LATIN NAMES (cont'd)

- 298 -

INDEX OF LATIN NAMES (cont'd)

Baliospermum montanum, 97.

Balsamodendron africanum, 230.

— Mukul, 230.

belladonna, 179.

Berberis vulgaris, 17, 241.

Beta vulgaris, 361.

Bdellium aegyptiacum, 230.

bitumen judaicum, 138.

Brassica Erucastrum, 74.

— oleracea, 184.

bolus armeniaca, 172.

Borrago officinalis, 211.

Boswellia Carteri, 188.

Brassica alba, 400.

— Napus, 273.

Brassica nigra, 400.

— sinapioides, 400.

Bryonia alba, 312.

— dioica, 313.

Caccabis Chukar, 169.

Cachris, 364.

Caesalphinia-Bonduc, 355.

Caesalphinia Bonducella, 67, 311, 355.

Cakile maritima, 325, 384.

Calamintha Acinos, 47.

— officinalis, 47.

calcarium, 366.

Calendula arvensis, 55.

— officinalis, 55.

Calotropis (procera), 178

calx, 260.

Calycotome, 88.

Cameleo vulgaris, 165.

Cannabis sativa, 58, 348.

Capparis spinosa, 197.

Capsicum Tournefort, 113.

Cardamine pratensis, 195, 334.

Carduncellus pinnatus, 362.

Carnabadium, 195

Carthamus, 44.

— tinctorius, 300.

Carum Carvi, 195.

— copticum, 167, 193, 250.

Carum nigrum, 193

— Petroselinum, 196.

Cassia Absus, 167.

— acutifolia, 267.

— augustifolia, 267.

— fistula, 387.

— obovata, 267.

— Tora, 324.

Castanea vesca, 335.

— vulgaris, 335.

Castor fiber, 79.

Cedrus Deodara, 22.

Celtis australis, 309.

INDEX OF LATIN NAMES (cont'd)

INDEX OF LATIN NAMES (cont'd)

INDEX OF LATIN NAMES (cont'd)

INDEX OF LATIN NAMES (cont'd)

INDEX OF LATIN NAMES (cont'd)

INDEX OF LATIN NAMES (cont'd)

INDEX OF LATIN NAMES (cont'd)

INDEX OF LATIN NAMES (cont'd)

INDEX OF LATIN NAMES (cont'd)

INDEX OF LATIN NAMES (cont'd)

INDEX OF IBERIC NAMES
(Hispanic, Castilian, Catalanian, Portuguese, etc.)

abobriella, 115.

abobrilla, 312.

absus, 271.

acebuche, 130.

acederilla, 150, 350.

aceite, 131.

aceituna, 120.

acerola, 132.

acetosilla, 350.

achethiella, 350.

aciana, 333.

acíbar, 318.

aconito saludable, 81.

aguazul, 24.

ajedrea, 319.

albahaca, 48.

albaricoque, 233.

albayalde, 29.

albedarrumbe, 40.

albihar, 49.

alcachofa, 154.

alcaparra, 197.

alcarceña, 80, 185.

alfalfa, 346.

alholva, 153.

aljonjoli, 268.

almartaga, 239.

alpiste, 143.

altabaquillo, 207.

alubia, 210.

antora, 81.

archaquil, 182.

archo-bellitho, 179.

asarabácara, 21.

asaro, 21.

aulaga, 88.

azarcon, 28.

azebre, 318.

azevre, 318.

azogue, 139.

azufaifa, 291.

barella espinosa, 24.

barrena, 372.

bastlísco, 77.

bedarangi, 40.

belesa, 367.

bellota, 42.

bertonica, 189.

blito, 53.

bobrella, 21.

bobrinella, 312.

buebra (redonda), 133.

butticella, 207.

calabazuela, 133.

calamento, 255.

calza, 260.

cambronera, 344.

INDEX OF IBERIC NAMES (cont'd)

INDEX OF IBERIC NAMES (cont'd)

INDEX OF IBERIC NAMES (cont'd)

INDEX OF IBERIC NAMES (cont'd)

INDEX OF ACCADIAN AND SYRIAN NAMES

allūnu, 42.

ašlu, 9.

āsu, 10.

buṭnu, 66.

dulbu, 93.

giparu, 204.

ḫallūru, 80.

ḫardinnu, 400.

ḫaṣbu, 60.

ḫaššu, 240.

karāšu, 198.

kir-ra, 138.

kamtu, 192.

kamūnu, 193.

ḳupru, 168.

kurkanu (?), 205.

kusibirru, 183.

ladunu, 208.

laptu, 273.

lubanu, 188.

murāru, 240.

ñānḫū, 259.

nina, 259.

qaqullu, 116.

qaraš, 198.

qiššū, 343.

šamašammu, 268.

šamrañu, 351.

šibittu, 363.

šimru, 351.

siltu, 270.

šūšu, 271.

INDEX OF ARABIC NAMES

INDEX OF ARABIC NAMES (cont'd)

318 -

INDEX OF ARABIC NAMES (cont'd)

— Harmas, 276.

asad al-ard, 237.

asaf, 197.
asal, 90, 372
'asal al-lubnā; 228.

— al-qina, 339.

— Dāwūd, 36.

— tamr, 103.

— zaitūn, 36.

ašāǧ, 124.

ašaq, 124.

asārūn, 21.

ašbalt, 138.

ašbant, 138.

ašbaṭānna, 125.

ašbaṭila, 125.

asfārāǧ, 111.

asfiyūs, 52.

'asfur, 300.

'asīr ad-dubb, 328.

— al-munk (al-mahk), 271.

ašiyābardīn, 294.

ašiyāf barf, 294.

ašku-bardīn, 294.

asmār, 384.

asqūdūriyūn, 282.

asrīs, 367.

aštabaka, 391.

astafilīna, 73.

asṭarak, 228.

astiyālla, 350.

astūhūdus, XI.

'ašūr, 333.

'āšūrā, 125.

atariyūn, 282.

'atfa, 202.

atl, 9.

'atm, 130.

atmūd, 27.
atmat, 311, 351
atmūt, 311.

atrār, 17.

'atsān, 92.

atwān, 17.

atwār, 17.

'awsāǧ, 294.

'awsiǧ, 148, 294, 315.

'awt, 275.

azāǧ, 179.

azfār aṭ-ṭīb, 15.

azzāz, 222.

bābalūn, 292.

bābūna, 39, 394.

bābūnaǧ, 20, 39.

(bābūnig), 20.

INDEX OF ARABIC NAMES (cont'd)

bābūnak, 39.

bābūnag, 39.

badanğ, 67.

bāḏarūğ, 48.

baḏaward, 44, 253.

baḏīlubā, 325.

bādranbūya, 40.

bādrangūya, 40.

bādzahr, 316.

ba ēterān, 337.

bāftirag (?), 237.

bahārina (?), 73.

bahār, 49.

bahas̆, 205.

bahman, 50.

bahram, 300.

bahramān, 300.

bahrāmağ, 64.

bahrāmiğ, 64.

bahūr ʿarabi, 188.

balābis, 198.

balāḏur, 62.

balantāyin, 213.

balīra, 190, 209.

balīs̆a, 367.

balīz, 172.

ball, 57.

ballūṭ al-arḍ, 189.

balmānda, 58.

baltamīn, 285.

bān, 112.

banafsağ, LXII

banğ, 58.

baniyūla, 115.

banṭafilūn, LXV, 263.

bantarfīra, 390.

banūla, 190.

baqdūnis, 196.

bāqilā, 41.

bāqillā, 41.

baql, 285.

Baqla hamqāʾ, 59.

  — bārida, 207.

  — ḏahabiyya, 331.

  — ḥurāsāniyya, 150

  — murra, 114.

  — yahūdiyya, 190, 229.

  — yamāniyya, 53.

baqlat al-anḏār, 184.

  — al-anṣār, 184.

  — ar-Rūm, 331.

baqq, 91.

baqs, 9.

bāranğ, 257.

INDEX OF ARABIC NAMES (cont'd)

INDEX OF ARABIC NAMES (cont'd)

INDEX OF ARABIC NAMES (cont'd)

INDEX OF ARABIC NAMES (cont'd)

INDEX OF ARABIC NAMES (cont'd)

farbiyūn (furbiyūn), 25

farfaǧ, 59.

farfaǧīn, 59.

farfaḥ, 59.

farfaḥīn, 59.

farfīz, 59.

farfūs, 107.

farīqa, 153.

farsaḫ, 314.

fašaǧ, 332.

fašaršīn, 313.

fašīrā, 312.

fašrā, 312.

fašrasīn, 313.

fasrīqūn, 134.

fasfasa, 346.

fasūḫ, 124.

fawāniyā', 304.

fawdanaǧ, 242.

— nahrī, 309.

fawfal, 311.

fawtanaǧ, 309.

fāzahr, 316.

fāzahraǧ, 316.

fāzūl, 210.

fiḍḍiyya, 303.

fīl, 315.

filzahra, 315.

fīlzahraǧ, 148, 315, 316.

filfilmūya, 310.

firsik, 314, 397.

fisfisa, 346.

flēya, 309.

flēyyu, 309.

flīsun, 309.

frašinu, 212.

fū, 305.

fūḍanaǧ, 242.

fūḍanaǧāi, 242.

fuǧl barrī, 217.

fula'ifula, 308.

fulful as-Saqāliba, 308, 319.

fulful as-Sūdān, 161.

fuqqāḥ al-arḍ, 39.

fuqqāḥ es-sūringān, 276.

fūl, 41.

full, 57, note.

fula'ifala, 113, 259.

fulaifila, 113.

furfīr, 59.

fuššala, 174.

fuṭr, 192.

gabbār, 234.

gābār, 147.

gadī, 135.

INDEX OF ARABIC NAMES (cont'd)

ǧaʿda (ǧuʿda), 72.

ǧadwār, 81.

   — andalusī, 81.

ġāfit, 403.

   — hindī, 403.

ġāfiṭ, 403.

ǧaft al-ballūṭ, 42, 83.

ġaïm, 5.

ǧalidūniya, 241.

ġāliǧun, 309.

ġāliubsīs (?), 364.

ġalla qrisṭa, 190.

gamām, 5.

ǧamhūrī, 84.

ǧamlāǧ, 370.

ǧamlāǧ, 370.

ǧamlīǧ, 370.

ǧamlōǧ, 370.

ǧamlūǧ, 370.

ǧamr al-arḍ, 69.

ǧānat qabṭa, 190.

ġanǧabānsa, 275.

ǧantiyānā, 77.

ǧantūria, 333.

ġār, 404.

ġarab, 393.

ǧarāsiya, 371.

ǧar-bawwā, 71, 116.

ǧarǧantīya, 209.

ǧarǧar, 379.

ǧarǧaritiyya, 55.

ǧargīr, 74.

ǧarmūǧ, 391.

ǧarmūz, 53.

ġarqud, 294.

ǧass, 78.

ġāsūl, 24, 345.

ġasūniš, 20.

ǧatǧāṭ, 403.

ġatta, 124.

ǧāwašīr, 76.

ǧāwars, 70.

   — hindī, 70.

ǧawlaq, 88.

ǧawz Bawwā, 71, 82.

   — ǧandum, 69.

   — ǧīnā, 8.

   — ǧundum, 69, 86.

   — kundum, 69.

   — aṭ-ṭīb, 71.

ǧawz al-Hind, 82, 257.

   — maʿkul, 82.

   — al-marǧ, 201

   — hindī, 101.

— mātā, 82.

— mātil, 82.

— al-qayy', 82.

— ar-ru'yān, 367.

— as-sarw, 82.

— aš-širk, 82.

— as-Sūdān, 82.

— aṭ-ṭarfā, 200.

ǧazar, 73

— afrangi, 94.

— barri, 94, 360.

ǧazmāzik, 200.

ǧazmāziǧ, 200.

gedūr faqqūs el-homār, 292.

gelawīn, 114.

gerdeq, 294.

gernūnes, 196, 340.

ǧibs al-farrānīn, 78.

ǧibs (zaǧāǧī), 78.

ǧibsīn, 78.

ǧidr al-banafsig, 34.

ǧidwār, 81.

ǧilbān, 80.

gilbān, 80.

ǧillawz, 42.

ǧinšīla, 358.

gīr, 260.

ǧir al-farrānīn, 221.

ǧirā', 395.

— al-baqar, 321.

ǧirǧir, 41, 74.

girǧīr al-kalb, 163n.

ǧirǧir al-mā', 340.

gōzet eṭ-ṭib, 71.

ǧu'aida, 72.

ġubairā', 72.

ġubairat al-ayyil, 309, 405.

ǧubn an-naḥl, 68.

ǧufarrā, 204.

ǧul, 106, 121.

— 121.

ǧulanǧubīn, 84.

ǧulbān, 80.

ǧullabān, 80.

ǧulubbān, 80.

ǧulǧabin, 85.

ǧulǧulān, 268.

— ḥabaši, 268.

— maṣrī, 268.

ǧulhum, 294.

ǧulmāṭā, 388.

ġumlūl, 344.

ǧummār, 68.

INDEX OF ARABIC NAMES (cont'd)

ǧundbādastar, 79.

ǧundabādustur, 79.

ǧuntā, 395.

habad, 158.

ḥabaq; plur. aḥbāq, 47, 48.

 — al-baqar, 39.

 — bustānī, 256.

 — al-fīl, 236.

 — kirmānī, 360.

 — al-mā᾽, 309.

 — nabaṭī, 48.

 — nahrī, 309.

 — qaranfulī, 47.

 — ar-rā῾ī, 337.

 — a῾-šuyūh, 235.

 — at-timsāḥ, 309.

ḥabaq tūrunǧī, 40.

ḥabāqā, 147.

ḥabaṭ, 342.

ḥabb al-aǧab, 159.

 — al-῾azīz, 161.

 — al-ārāk, 220.

 — al-῾arūs, 194.

 — al-balasān, 324.

 — al-bān, 378.

 — ad-dahmas, 404.

 — al-faqd, 308.

 — al-hāl, 116.

 — al-mulūk, 97, 330, 371.

 — an-nīl, 159.

 — an-nīla, 126.

 — an-nisā᾽, 14.

 — al-qulb, 326.

 — ar-rās, 155.

 — aṣ-ṣabīb, 155.

 — ar-rašād, 163.

 — as-samna, 348.

 — as-si᾽bān, 155.

 — at-tīl, 348.

 — az-zalam, 161.

ḥabba ġāliya, 378.

 — ḥaḍrā᾽, 66, 156.

 — ḥulwa, 19.

 — sawdā᾽, 167, 365.

 — sōda, 193.

ḥabbat al-baraka, 365.

 — al-ḥabīd, 158.

ḥabl al-masākīn, 207.

hadaba, 120.

ḥadaǧ, 158.

ḥaḍamān, 217.

ḥadībiyya, 55.

ḥadid al-ḥarqūs, 357.

ḥaḍrā᾽, 237.

ḥafā᾽, 46.

INDEX OF ARABIC NAMES (cont'd)

INDEX OF ARABIC NAMES (cont'd)

INDEX OF ARABIC NAMES (cont'd)

INDEX OF ARABIC NAMES (cont'd)

INDEX OF ARABIC NAMES (cont'd)

INDEX OF ARABIC NAMES (cont'd)

INDEX OF ARABIC NAMES (cont'd)

INDEX OF ARABIC NAMES (cont'd)

INDEX OF ARABIC NAMES (cont'd)

INDEX OF ARABIC NAMES (cont'd)

INDEX OF ARABIC NAMES (cont'd)

INDEX OF ARABIC NAMES (cont'd)

INDEX OF ARABIC NAMES (cont'd)

INDEX OF ARABIC NAMES (cont'd)

INDEX OF ARABIC NAMES (cont'd)

INDEX OF ARABIC NAMES (cont'd)

- 344 -

INDEX OF ARABIC NAMES (cont'd)

INDEX OF ARABIC NAMES (cont'd)

INDEX OF ARABIC NAMES (cont'd)

INDEX OF ARABIC NAMES (cont'd)

INDEX OF ARABIC NAMES (cont'd)

INDEX OF ARABIC NAMES (cont'd)

INDEX OF ARABIC NAMES (cont'd)

INDEX OF ARABIC NAMES (cont'd)

INDEX OF ARABIC NAMES (cont'd)

INDEX OF ARABIC NAMES (cont'd)

INDEX OF BERBER NAMES

INDEX OF BERBER NAMES (cont'd)

tistīwĭn, 65.

uhkāl, 60.

INDEX OF SANSCRIT NAMES & INDIAN DIALECTS

INDEX OF SANSCRIT NAMES & INDIAN DIALECTS (cont'd)

INDEX OF PERSIAN NAMES

INDEX OF PERSIAN NAMES (cont'd)

INDEX OF PERSIAN NAMES (cont'd)

jīva, 139.

kabābā, 194.

kabast, 158.

kāh-rubā, 199.

kākanğ, 201.

kākuna, 201.

kalkalānağ, 101.

kangar, 154.

kapak, 169.
kašna, 185
kasnā, 185.

kasnak, 185.

kašt bar kašt, 202.

kazmāzak, 9.

kil-dārŭ, 266.

kisrā-dāru, 398.

kunğur, 362.

kunkur, 362.

kupurrā, 204.

kūšad, 77, 273.

māhī, 224.

māhūb-dāna, 97.

maibahuša, 265.
mai-puhta, 84
mai-sūsan, 247.

mahk, 271.

māmiran, 205.

mar-čuba, 111.

marg-i-mūš, 377.

marmāhūr, 40, 235.

marmāhūz, 235.

marzanğuš, 236.

matk, 271.

mawīzak, 155.

māzariyūn, 237.

merdum-giyāh, 216.

mūm, 234, 244.

mūmiyā'ī, 234.

mūrd afšurağ, 245.

murdār-sang, 239.

mušk-tiramšir, 242.

nahšal, 73.

nānahwāh, 259.

nār-mušk, 250.

nargi, 254.

nārgil, 287.

nargis, 254.

našāsta, 261.

nīlūpar, 252.

nisrīn, 253.

palanğ-mišk, 47.

panğ-angušt, 308.

pānīd, 289.

parr-i-Siyāwušān, 182.

INDEX OF PERSIAN NAMES (cont'd)

INDEX OF PERSIAN NAMES (cont'd)

INDEX OF CHINESE NAMES

www.ingramcontent.com/pod-product-compliance
Lightning Source LLC
Chambersburg PA
CBHW081339190326
41458CB00018B/6050